Breast Cancer Management
– Early and Late

Contributors:

Thomas H. Ackland
Charles B. Anderson
Michael Baum
Diana Brinkley
Florence C. H. Chu
Robert W. Crichlow
George Crile, Jr.
G. A. Dalton
Hugh L. Davis, Jr.
William L. Donegan
Arthur J. Donovan
Thomas B. Ferguson
Bernard Fisher
C. S. B. Galasko
John S. Lyon
John A. McCredie
James P. Neifeld
P. E. Robin
Guy F. Robbins
Charles L. Roper
G. Keith Stillwell
Basil A. Stoll
Paul Strickland
Douglass C. Tormey
Robert G. Twycross

Breast Cancer Management –Early and Late

Edited by

Basil A. Stoll

Honorary Consultant Physician to the Radiotherapy and Oncology Departments, St. Thomas' Hospital and Royal Free Hospital, London.

1977

A WILLIAM HEINEMANN MEDICAL BOOKS PUBLICATION
Distributed by
YEAR BOOK MEDICAL PUBLISHERS, INC.,
35 E. WACKER DR., CHICAGO

First published 1977

ISBN 0-8151-8272-4

Library of Congress Catalog Card Number: 77-72660

Distributed in Continental North, South and Central America, Puerto Rico, Hawaii and the Philippines by

Year Book Medical Publishers, Inc.,

by arrangement with

William Heinemann Medical Books, Ltd

Printed in Great Britain

Contents

Editor

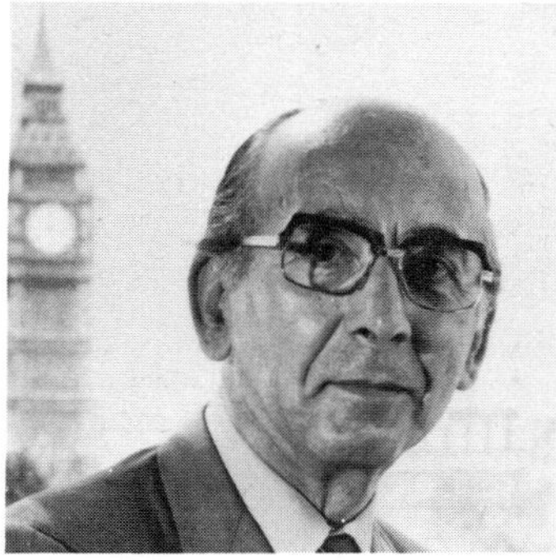

Basil A. Stoll, F.R.C.R.
Honorary Consultant Physician to Radiotherapy and Oncology Departments at St. Thomas' Hospital and Royal Free Hospital, London, U.K.

Principal Authors

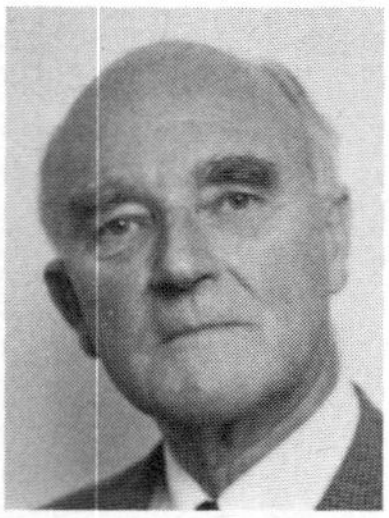

Thomas H. Ackland, M.D., M.S., F.R.C.S., F.R.A.C.S., F.A.C.S.
Consultant Surgeon, Royal Melbourne Hospital, Melbourne, Victoria, Australia.

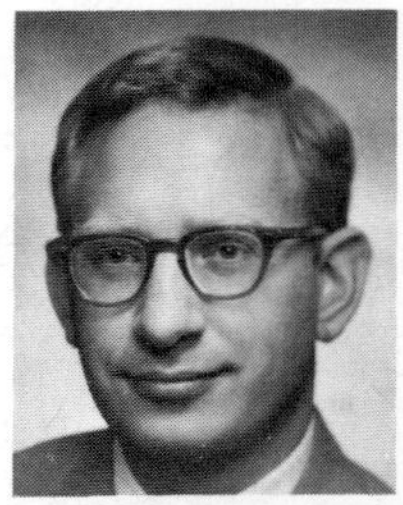

Charles B. Anderson, M.D., F.A.C.S.
Associate Professor of Surgery, Washington University School of Medicine: Chief Transplantation Surgery, Barnes Hospital, St. Louis, Missouri, U.S.A.

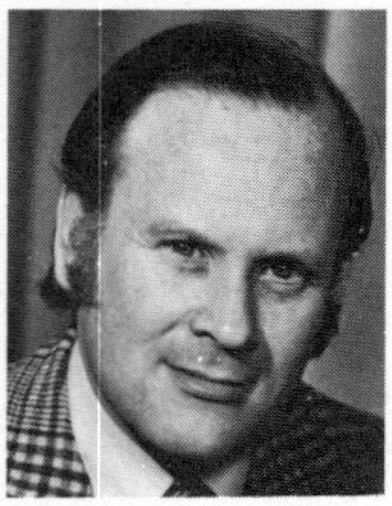

Michael Baum, Ch.M., F.R.C.S.
Senior Lecturer, Department of Surgery, Welsh National School of Medicine; Honorary Consultant Surgeon, University Hospital of Wales, Cardiff, U.K.

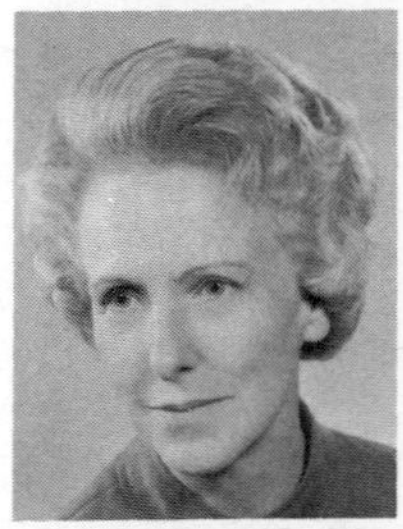

Diana Brinkley, M.B., D.M.R.T.
Consultant in Radiotherapy and Oncology, King's College Hospital, London, U.K.

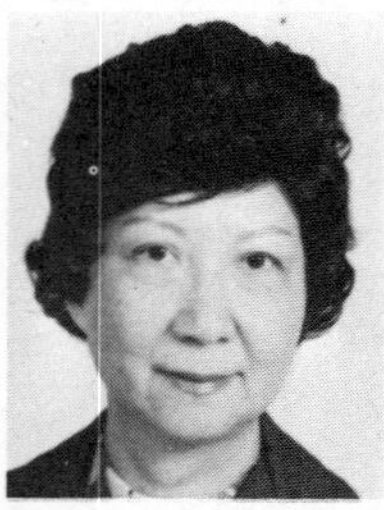

Florence Chu, M.D., F.A.C.R.
Acting Chairman Radiation Therapy Department, Memorial Hospital, Clinical Professor of Radiology, Cornell University Medical College, New York, U.S.A.

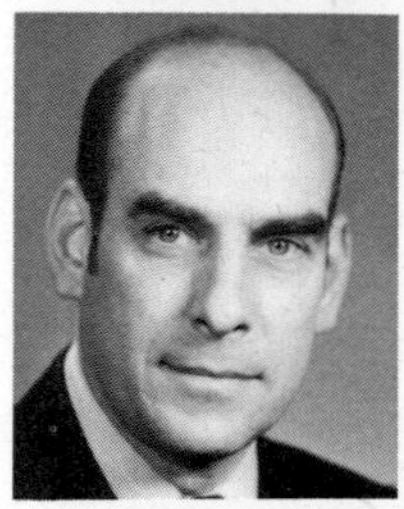

Robert W. Crichlow, M.D.
Associate Professor of Surgery, Dartmouth Medical School: Staff Surgeon Mary Hitchcock Memorial Hospital, Hanover, New Hampshire, U.S.A.

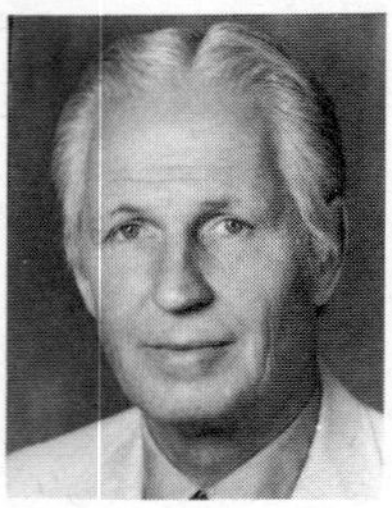

George Crile, Jr., M.D., F.A.C.S.
Emeritus Consultant, Department of General Surgery, Cleveland Clinic, Cleveland, Ohio, U.S.A.

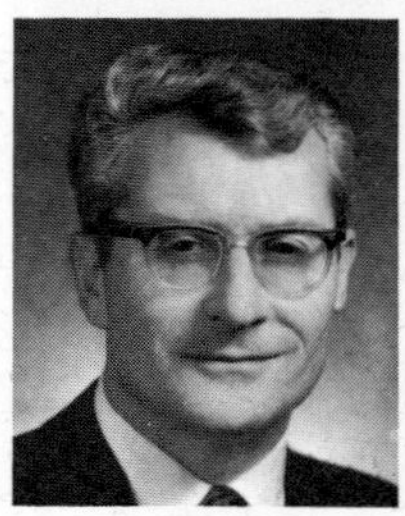

Hugh L. Davis, Jr., M.D.
Associate Professor of Human Oncology and Medicine University of Wisconsin: Special Assistant to Associate Director, Division of Cancer Treatment, N.C.I. Bethesda, U.S.A.

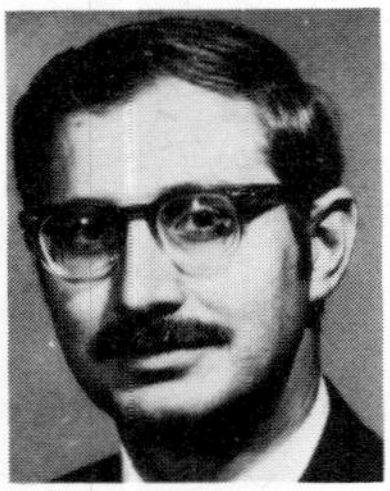

William L. Donegan, M.D.,
Professor of Surgery, Medical College of Wisconsin:
A.C.S. Professor of Clinical Oncology, Milwaukee Division,
Milwaukee, Wisconsin, U.S.A.

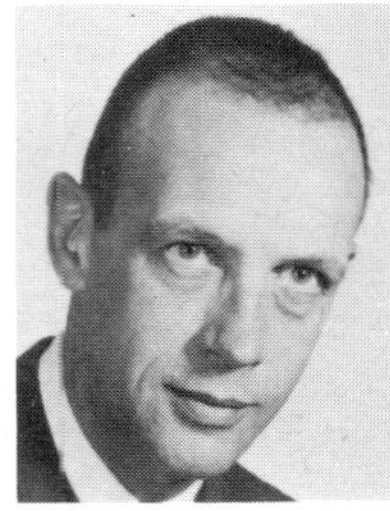

Arthur J. Donovan, M.D.
Professor and Chairman, Department of Surgery, University
of South Alabama College of Medicine, Mobile, Alabama,
U.S.A.

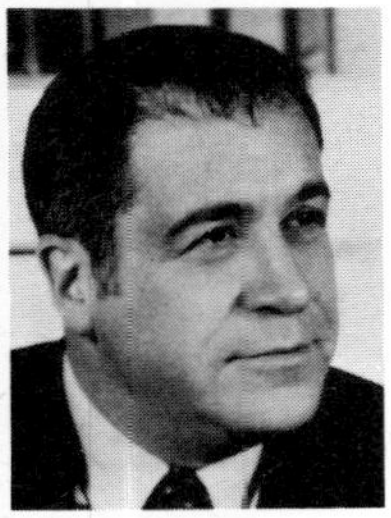

Bernard Fisher, M.D., F.A.C.S.
Professor of Surgery and Director of Oncology, University of
Pittsburgh School of Medicine, Pittsburgh, Pa., U.S.A.

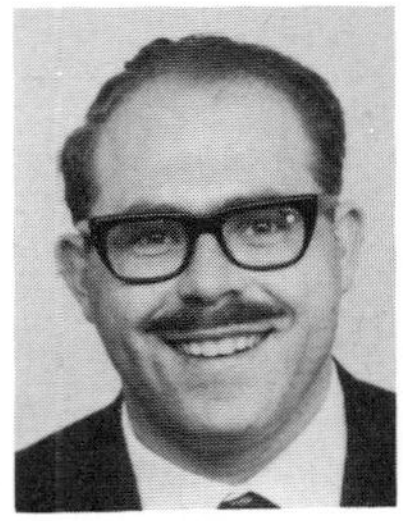

C.S.B. Galasko, Ch.M., F.R.C.S. (Eng.), F.R.C.S. (Edin.)
Professor of Orthopaedic Surgery, University of Manchester,
Lancashire, U.K.

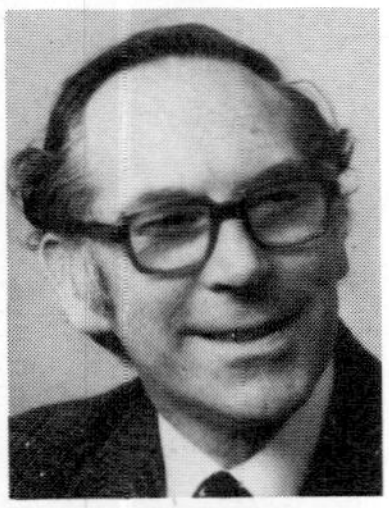

John S. Lyon, M.R.C.P., M.R.C. Psych.
Consultant Psychiatrist, Basingstoke District General
Hospital, Basingstoke, Hampshire, U.K.

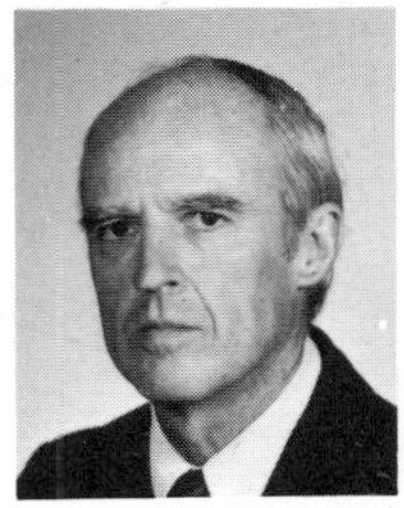

John A. McCredie, F.R.C.S. (E. & Edin.) F.R.C.S.(C.),
F.A.C.S.
Associate Professor of Surgery and of Therapeutic Radiology,
University of Western Ontario; Research Associate, Ontario
Cancer Treatment and Research Foundation, London,
Canada.

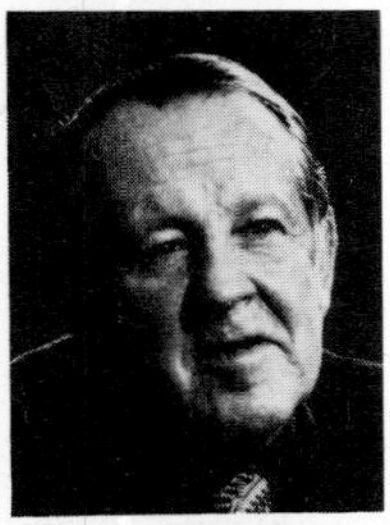

Guy F. Robbins, M.D.
Senior Attending Breast Service, Department of Surgery;
Director of Cancer Control and Rehabilitation, Memorial
Sloan-Kettering Cancer Center, New York, U.S.A.

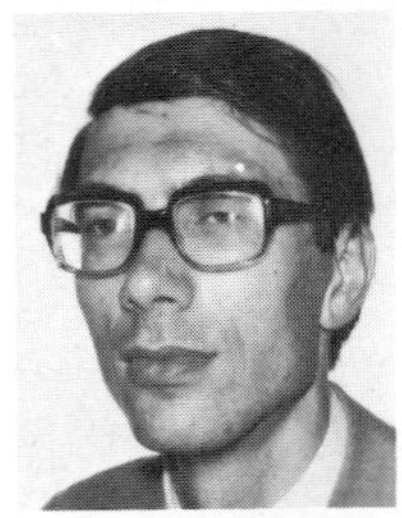

P. E. Robin, M.D., F.R.C.S.
Consultant Otolaryngologist, Dudley Road Hospital,
Birmingham, U.K.

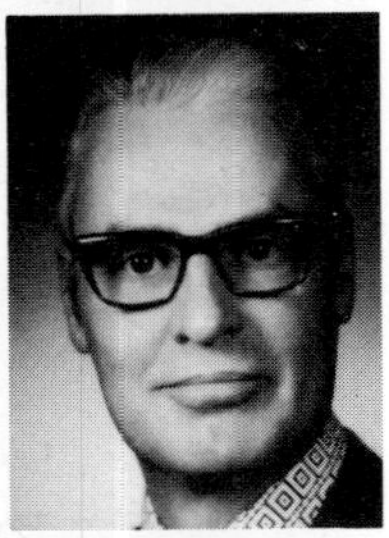

G. Keith Stillwell, M.D., Ph.D.
Professor and Chairman, Department of Physical Medicine
and Rehabilitation, Mayo Medical School and Mayo Clinic,
Rochester, Minnesota, U.S.A.

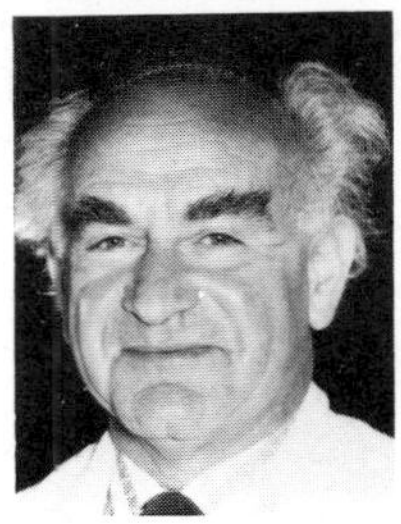

Paul Strickland, F.R.C.P., F.R.C.R.
Consultant Radiotherapist, Mount Vernon Hospital,
Northwood, Middlesex, U.K.

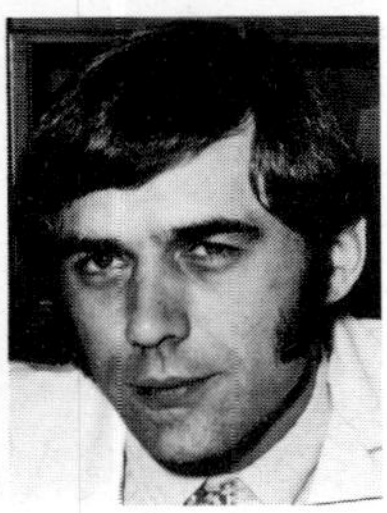

Douglass C. Tormey, M.D., Ph.D.
Associate Professor, Department of Human Oncology and
Medicine, University of Wisconsin, Madison, Wisconsin,
U.S.A.

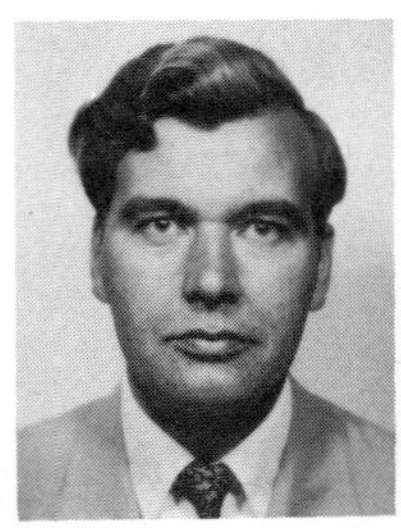

Robert G. Twycross, M.A., B.M., M.R.C.P.
Consultant Physician, Sir Michael Sobell House, Churchill
Hospital, Oxford, U.K.

Preface

In recent years, considerable doubts have been expressed as to the effectiveness of traditional surgical techniques aiming at the cure of early breast cancer. At the same time, the value of adjuvant radiotherapy relative to its damaging effects, has come into doubt. Much of the questioning is based on increasing evidence that only a minority of women found to have "early" breast cancer will have a normal expectation of life. Increasing emphasis is therefore being placed on the possible use of systemic therapy at an earlier stage of the disease, and the avoidance of useless and possibly harmful treatment directed at the primary site of disease.

The recent literature on the topic is vast and controversial and it may be timely to assess in one volume where we stand currently in the management of both early and late breast cancer and its special aspects. Leading specialists from both sides of the Atlantic have been asked to review current thinking in their particular field of breast cancer and to provide a scientific justification for the methods they practise in its management.

A remarkable consensus of opinion is found among the authors on major principles; differences are based mainly on our inability to judge accurately the degree of spread of the tumour and the defence reactions of the host. A new concept is emerging that policies need to be adapted to each individual because breast cancer is not only heterogeneous histopathologically but also biologically and immunologically. For such an approach, it is obvious that the management of breast cancer must be multidisciplinary.

The book is planned in three sections—management of "early" disease, palliation of advanced disease and management of special problems arising in the course of the disease. Many reviews of cancer treatment tend to highlight recent scientific or technical developments. In this book the aim has been to apply our advancing knowledge to better the quality of life of the patient with breast cancer. Length of survival is merely one measure of the efficacy of treatment. If the majority of patients cannot be cured, the quality of their survival becomes all-important.

Basil A. Stoll

London, 1977

SECTION 1

Treatment Aiming at Cure

Chapter

1

MICHAEL BAUM

The Curability of Breast Cancer

"It is now, as it was then, as it may ever be,
Conceptions from the past blind us to facts
which almost slap us in the face."
W. S. Halsted (1908)

It has to be accepted that there is a degree of uncertainty concerning the curability of breast cancer. Rather than simply shelve this question as being irrelevant to the day-to-day treatment of the disease, it may be more fruitful to consider what lessons can be learnt from this very uncertainty as to the biological nature of the disease.

Accepting at the outset that 20-30% of patients diagnosed as early breast cancer will have a normal expectation of life after local therapy, and that only about a quarter of these are the ones with axillary node involvement detected in the mastectomy specimen, it is surely complacent to continue our current practice in an uncritical way, subjecting at least 70% of women showing primary disease to a futile mutilating procedure.

Discussion of the problem will therefore be divided under the following sub-headings:

- Does "early" diagnosis improve the cure rate?
- Survival after treatment of "curable" breast cancer.
- The natural history of untreated breast cancer.
- The metastatic potential of breast cancer.
- Alternative concept concerning the nature of breast cancer as a first step towards improving the cure rate of the disease.

DOES "EARLY" DIAGNOSIS IMPROVE THE CURE RATE?

Macdonald (1951) coined the phrase "biological predeterminism" to explain the behaviour of solid tumours in man. In a closely argued classical paper he attempted to ridicule the conventional approach to cancer therapy. He postulated that if a period of localized tumour growth is associated with either subjective or objective evidence of its presence, treatment should be able to produce a 100% cure. Therefore, providing that patients are educated to recognize these signs and symptoms, and on recognition proceed to get medical advice without delay, cure rates should continue to improve, eventually to the 100% level.

However, in spite of a health education programme in the U.S.A. directed at the early diagnosis of cancer, and launched 20 years before Macdonald wrote his paper, the age adjusted death rates for cancer were increasing rather than decreasing. Furthermore, he presented data which suggested that "delay" on the part of the patient did not affect the stage at presentation of the tumour; the results of treatment for breast cancer were little different if the patient delayed for 1 month or 12 months.

He concluded therefore that the outcome of treatment is predetermined by the biological nature of the disease:

> This preoccupation with therapeutic seizure of time by its neoplastic forelock rests on the assumption that the cancer is treated more efficiently during the nebulous period when it is yet limited to its site of origin. . . . The wide range of biological potential exhibited by human cancer is determined early in the preclinical phase of the disease—apparently early cancer by historical and dimensional criteria may be biologically late.

Park and Lees (1951), writing in the same year as Macdonald, expressed a similar point of view. Starting with the null hypothesis that cancer is incurable until it is proved curable, they postulated that proof is impossible because the natural history of breast cancer is not known. They suggested that there was no "available time margin" between the time that the tumour reached diagnosable proportions and its dissemination.

This view was supported by evidence which failed to relate improved survival to shorter patient delay. Again their conclusion was that the outcome is predetermined by variations in the growth rate, infiltrative power and metastatic potential of the breast cancer, in addition to its chronological age. But host factors, such as age and general health, may also be important.

McKinnon (1954) took the argument one step forward. He postulated that there might be two types of breast cancer; a metastasising variety which would be incurable and a non-metastasising variety which would be curable. The former would present as Stages II, III and IV disease whilst the latter would present as Stage I disease.

The same theme was taken up again by Devitt in 1965. By this time the subject of cancer immunology was developing and the host defence factor could be inserted into the equation of biological predeterminism. Surely if the lymph node, which must be the most hostile environment for a cancer cell, becomes the focus of an established metastasis, then the biological war between tumour and host is already lost. Or as Devitt succinctly put it: "Metastases to axillary nodes are an expression of a poor prognosis rather than a determinant".

More recently Devitt (1976) has reviewed the evidence that "early" cancers are slow growing tumours and "late" cancers are aggressive tumours. He notes that the interval between treatment and recurrence, and that between recurrence and death are longer for those cancers which are diagnosed "early" than for those diagnosed "late". He concludes that the timing of initial treatment appears to have little influence on the growth behaviour of breast cancer as reflected in survival rates.

However, this conclusion cannot go unchallenged and it would be invidious to ignore the recently reported Screening Program of the New York Health Insurance Plan (Strax et al., 1967). This study included 62,000 women of 40-64 years of age, 31,000 of whom were randomly selected and offered screening by clinical examination and mammography on four occasions at annual intervals. The published results indicate that in the screened population breast cancer was detected at an earlier stage and that deaths within 7 years of enrolment were reduced by approximately one-third among the women over the age of 50 years.

This would seem powerful evidence for the traditional concept of an arithmetic spatial progression related to duration of the disease. Unfortunately, however, the treatment standards in the two populations were not controlled and the histology of the lesions detected are not reported. It is therefore vitally important that this experiment is confirmed before the clamour for a National Screening Programme pressurizes the government into diverting enormous sums of money from other areas where it might be more effectively directed towards the reduction of mortality from breast cancer.

SURVIVAL AFTER TREATMENT OF "CURABLE" BREAST CANCER

When reporting the results of therapy for breast cancer, whether from a retrospective analysis or from a prospective trial, it is conventional to use the 10 year survival as marking some kind of end-point. For example, in McKay and Sellars (1965) series of nearly 10,000 patients, there was a 10 year crude survival of 51.1% for Stage I disease (T1-2, No, Mo) and of 23.8% for Stage II disease (T1-2, NI, Mo). However, a significant proportion of women with breast cancer are already in their 6th decade or older at diagnosis and will inevitably be dying from incidental disease over this 10 year period.

As a concession to this factor, adjustments are

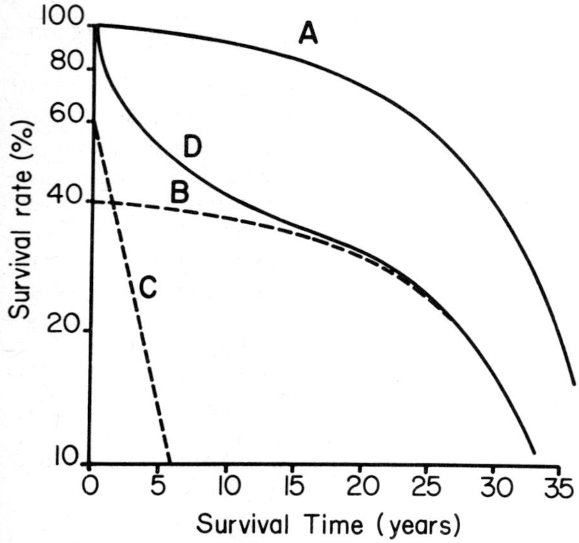

Figure 1. Definition of the cured group after treatment for cancer: Curve A, survival characteristics of age matched control population. Curve B, cancer treated group dying off at same rate as controls. Curve C, cancer treated group who are not cured. Curve D, composite survival (B and C) of all cancer treated group. (After Haybittle, 1964.)

usually made according to actuarial life tables, to give a corrected survival rate. Using such an adjustment, the overall 10 year survival rate of 30.4% in McKay and Sellars series becomes 37.5%. Again, Cutler (1968) reporting on a collected series of 1,760 cases quotes 10 year crude survival rates after a more detailed breakdown based on clinical and pathological criteria of patients subjected to "curative" treatment. These results vary from 86% for T1 primaries without cutaneous or lymph node involvement to 11% for T3 primary tumours with ulceration of the overlying skin and pathological involvement of the axillary nodes. The same two groups of patients have a corresponding annual mortality rate after treatment of 0.02 and 0.20.

Unfortunately, 10 year survival rates for breast cancer, whether crude or corrected, give no real indication of the size of the cured group within the population, because of the uncertainty as to the natural history of the disease as described later in this chapter. It is common to see recurrence of breast cancer at intervals of 15 to 20 years after apparently successful treatment of the original primary. This fact makes the problem of defining a cured group for breast cancer extremely difficult. Assuming that the population under consideration continues to die at a steady rate from breast cancer (*vide infra*), the death rate from other pathology accelerates to such an extent as to mask almost completely the cancer-associated deaths.

Bearing this in mind, the most satisfactory method of defining the cured group is probably that adopted by Haybittle (1964) as illustrated in Figure 1. Curve A describes the survival characteristics of an age matched control population. Curve D describes the survival of patients treated for cancer. The shape of Curve D can be attributed to two subpopulations, one a cured group dying off at the same rate as the control population (B), and the second an uncured group with an accelerated death rate (C). The point at which curve D parallels curve A can be taken to mean that an excess risk of death no longer exists for the treated group, and so in practical terms they can be considered cured. Extrapolation of curve D from the point of parallelism to the origin gives an index of the population of patients in the originally treated group who were in fact cured.

Applying these criteria for cure, Brinkley and Haybittle (1968) have analysed the long term results in 704 patients treated in the Cambridge area between 1947 and 1950. This group of patients probably represented the total pool of cases treated by surgery and radiotherapy in that period. In their original analysis, Brinkley and Haybittle described a 15 year crude survival of 16.6% (age corrected to 24.3%), with a third of the 10 year survivors failing to live for 15 years. Furthermore, 6% of the 15 year survivors had recurrent disease present. At the 15 year mark, parallelism had not yet occurred but they predicted that such would be the state of affairs at 18 years with a cured group representing 20% of the original total. It is worth commenting at this point, that 24% of their "cured" group had histological evidence of nodal involvement at the time of primary therapy.

More recently Brinkley and Haybittle (1975) have published a further report on this series, when all patients had been followed up for at least 22 years. The survival curves up to 25 years for the treated and the control populations are shown in Figure 2. It can be seen that parallelism between the expected and the observed curves seems to be occurring after 21 years, providing a "cured" percentage for the whole group of 18.5%, and a "cured" percentage for those presenting with "early" breast cancer of about 30%.

However, it is of particular importance to note that although the death rates between 20 and 25 years for the treated and control groups were identical, eight out of 23 deaths after 20 years in the treated series were from cancer of the breast, which is 16 times the number that would be expected in the normal population. Since the total death rates are similar, it implies that a woman who lives for 20 years with metastatic breast cancer "on her person" is less

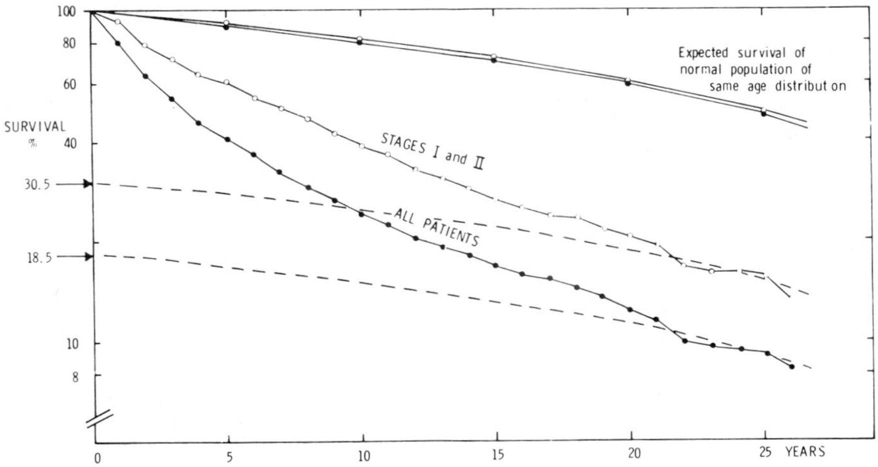

Figure 2. The 25 year survival of patients treated for breast cancer, compared with age matched control population. From Brinkley and Haybittle (1975). Reprinted by permission of Editor *Lancet.*

likely to die of *other* causes. This fact alone would support the biological concept of cancer control by host factors.

A similar state of affairs was noted by Bloom et al. (1970), who reported an abnormally high survival rate for women treated for medullary carcinoma of the breast. He suggested that this type of cancer might represent an immunogenic tumour growing within a woman who was highly immunocompetent and, as such, resistant to disease that would normally carry off less immunocompetent individuals. An alternative explanation might be that women followed up for breast cancer have an overall better standard of medical supervision, and incidental disease might be diagnosed and treated at an earlier stage. So, to use Brinkley and Haybittle's own words: "To define 'cure' in terms of the general population mortality may have its limitations".

What constitutes a cure?

There have been several other series with prolonged follow-up of cases for 15 to 30 years after primary therapy. The extremes of opinion that emerge are surprising, varying from extreme optimism to extreme pessimism bordering on nihilism.

At the most optimistic extreme we have the report of Adair and his colleagues (1974) from the Memorial Hospital, New York. They report a 30 year follow-up of a cohort of 1,458 cases treated by radical mastectomy between 1940 and 1943. Over this long period only 6.8% of patients were lost to follow-up, 826 died of carcinoma of the breast, 349 died of other causes and 184 are still alive. A third of the group alive at 30 years had histological evidence of nodal involvement in their mastectomy specimen. Only 4% of all deaths from the original cancer occurred between 20 and 30 years after mastectomy. They considered that 300 of the original series were "practical cures" after 20 years, having achieved a normal life span. The actuarial 30 year survival rate was 38%.

Campos (1972) also paints a reasonably optimistic picture from his analysis of 391 cases treated by radical mastectomy at the University of Michigan between 1940 and 1955. He concluded that 99% of the cancer mortality had occurred at the 15th anniversary, providing an actuarial survival rate of 74.2% for node-negative cases and 20.9% for node-positive cases at that point in time. However, he is careful not to define his cured population, as his analysis demonstrates that death from carcinoma of the breast proceeds as an orderly phenomenon manifested by an exponential function. As such, the chance of dying from cancer does not diminish with time and the number of patients dying during equal periods is a fixed proportion of those who were alive at the beginning of the period.

An identical conclusion was reached by Mueller and Jeffries (1975) from a study of the death rate of an unselected group of 1,500 women with carcinoma of the breast. Within the first 3 years after diagnosis there was an accelerated death rate but thereafter for the 15 years of the study, the actuarial survival curve was expressed by a single exponential function suggesting a constant rate of dying with a 50% mortality at 5.9 years. The figures indicated that any woman developing breast cancer had a greater than

80% chance of dying of that disease and the younger she was at diagnosis the greater the chance of an eventual cancer-related death. Expressed in an alternative way the percentage of women dying each year was a fixed proportion (8%) of those at risk, with the exception of the higher risk in the first 3 years.

A note of moderate pessimism is sounded by Myers (1973) on behalf of the end-results group of the National Cancer Institute. He reviews data collected from 100 hospitals throughout the U.S.A. relating to 63,000 cases of breast cancer treated between 1940 and 1969. He notes that there has been no improvement in the survival rate after treatment for the last 20 years. He also points out that the survival rate of the treated group relative to an age-matched population continues to show a downward slope up to 25 years, even for those women treated for localized disease. Myers interprets these data as suggesting a failure to cure the disease and concludes as follows: "Apparently, reduction of the excess risk of dying of breast cancer even for localized disease, awaits some new therapeutic method".

At the extreme of pessimism we have the report by Bond (1968) of the long term follow up of 6,775 cases of "early" breast cancer treated in the United Birmingham Hospitals. For each of the 25 years after treatment he calculated the ratio of cancer deaths to death from other causes. Plotting these data on semilogarithmic paper produced a straight line, and the 15% of women surviving 25 years still carried a 1 in 5 risk of dying of breast cancer when their average age was 80. He interpreted this information to mean that in all cases the cancer had disseminated before diagnosis and was therefore incurable with the methods then available.

This interpretation was, however, challenged by Haybittle (1968) following an alternative analysis of the same data. He demonstrated that the death rate from cancer in the Birmingham series was not constant (which would suggest incurability), but decreased exponentially with time. Using his extrapolated actuarial mathematical model, Haybittle calculated that well over a quarter of the patients in the Birmingham series could be considered cured, a figure close to that achieved in the Cambridge series (Brinkley and Haybittle, 1975).

From the foregoing it can be seen that there is no unanimity as to what constitutes a cure for breast cancer. For practical purposes we may consider that 20-30% of women treated for apparently localized cancer of the breast will have a normal expectation of life. The doubt still remains as to whether all patients having been diagnosed as suffering from the disease would ultimately die of the cancer if they lived long enough! Furthermore, the impact of treatment has to remain an open question. How many of these long term survivors would have lived out their natural life span without any treatment? As will later be shown, there does not exist an adequate control population of untreated "early" breast cancer in the literature to make such a comparison.

THE NATURAL HISTORY OF UNTREATED BREAST CANCER

In spite of the supposed improvements in the diagnosis and treatment of breast cancer, and in the face of an increased public awareness of the significance of lumps in the breast, the mortality rates for breast cancer in England and Wales demonstrate a disturbing upwards trend (see Table 1).

There are four possible explanations for this trend. Firstly, a greater proportion of the female population may be developing the disease. This would be in keeping with observations relating breast cancer incidence to an increase in the proportion of the older age groups in the population, although it would be difficult to argue that this alone accounted for the increase in the decade 1963-73 for England and Wales. Secondly, death registration for breast cancer may be more complete than in the past. This again is unlikely as regional cancer registries have been fully operational for the period covered by Table 1.

Table 1 Crude mortality rates per 100,000 population (England and Wales) for breast cancer

Years	*1952-7*	*1961-3*	*1969*	*1970*	*1971*	*1972*	*1973*
Reference	*Campbell (1968)*	*Campbell (1968)*	*Registrar General's Statistical Review*				
All ages	36.5	38.9	43	43	45	44	45
25-44	–	–	13	14	14	14	14
45-64	–	–	77	78	78	78	79
65-74	–	–	111	109	118	115	122
75+	–	–	161	158	171	169	170

A third possible explanation is that treatment may have become less effective. This is unlikely, as no reported prospective trial for the primary disease had demonstrated a meaningful superiority of one therapeutic modality against another (Fisher, 1973). Finally, and to my mind the most likely explanation, the biological nature of the disease may be changing towards a more aggressive form. For this and other reasons it is essential to take a critical look at our knowledge of the natural history of breast cancer which, after all, is the only reliable index of its biological nature.

In 1880, Gross published a treatise on breast cancer which provides a clear insight into the status of the disease in the immediate pre-Halsted era. He describes a series of 616 cases, 70% of whom had skin infiltration on presentation and in 25% of whom the skin was ulcerated; 64% had extensive involvement of axillary nodes and 27% had obvious supraclavicular nodal involvement. As a result of the attitude of that time that the risks of surgery outweighed the meagre benefits offered by such treatment, he considered it ethical to follow the natural course of 97 cases who received nothing other than "constitutional support".

From this study he described how skin infiltration appeared on average 14 months after a tumour is first detected, ulceration occurred on average six months after that, and fixation to the chest wall after a further two months. Invasion of the other breast was seen if the patient lived on average 32 months after the lump first appeared. The average time for the appearance of enlarged axillary nodes was 15 months in those few cases presenting with what today would be staged as T1-2, N0, M0 disease; 25% of these untreated cases exhibited obvious distant metastases within 1 year and 25% after 3 years while 5% of this series died 5 years or more after presentation.

Since then, a number of additonal series of untreated breast cancer have been reported. For example, Greenwood (1926) described a 6 year follow-up of 651 cases of untreated breast cancer with only 60 of the group remaining alive at the end of this period. Daland (1927) reported a series of 100 patients who were considered either inoperable or unfit for surgery, or who refused the offer of an operation. The average duration of life in this group was 40.5 months, being 42.8 months for those considered operable and 29 months for those considered inoperable. Similar reports appeared subsequently (Wade, 1946; Shimkin, 1951).

The study that has attracted the most attention in recent years is that of Bloom (1968). His data came from the records of 250 women dying of breast cancer in the Middlesex Hospital cancer ward between 1905-33. Of this group 95% died of breast cancer and 97% presented with Stage III or Stage IV disease. The survival rates from alleged onset of symptoms were 18% at 5 years, 3.6% at 10 years and 0.8% at 15 years. The mean survival for his series was 2.7 years which compares well with that of 1,728 untreated cases he was able to collate from other sources, which had a mean survival of a little over 3 years. The reasons for withholding treatment in Bloom's series are important to note and were as follows: old age or infirmity 35%, disease considered too advanced 30%, early death 15.4%, and treatment refused 19.6%.

There are several criticisms that can be levelled against the studies I have so far quoted, which invalidate their use as a baseline against which to judge the "curative" effect of conventional therapy. Firstly, as with all retrospective uncontrolled series there must be an element of selection. Why was treatment withheld? It is quite obvious that in the majority of cases, with the exception of those refusing treatment, they were a group with an exceptionally poor prognosis to begin with. Secondly, they all represent women seeking medical attention at a time in the early years of this century, when many women were content to co-exist with a breast lump until they died of old age or were knocked down by a Hansom cab!

Is the biology of breast cancer changing?

Most important of all, these studies may not be relevant to today's problem because it is likely that the biological nature of the disease has changed over the last 50 years. Bloom attempts to refute this suggestion by describing 86 cases observed between 1902-33 from whom pathological material suitable for the grading of malignancy was similar to that found today. Histological grading, although giving some index of prognosis, can in no way be considered the sole indicator of the biological propensity of an individual cancer. In the light of recent developments in our knowledge, host factors must be considered to carry equal weight.

In this respect, it is relevant to note a recent paper by Fisher and Taylor (1973). They analysed the grade of malignancy and the histological evidence of host response in a large contemporary series of breast cancers, and compared their findings with a review of the histology of a similar series collected a decade before. In general they found an increase in the less favourable grades of malignancy and a fall in the number of cases demonstrating a lymphocyte stromal response or sinus histiocytosis of the regional nodes.

It is therefore possible that the early series of untreated cancers may underestimate the lethal nature of today's disease, and this is in accordance with my interpretation of the mortality statistics quoted at the start of this section.

It would, of course, be inconceivable to suggest that we add a control group of untreated women when a new prospective trial for the treatment of early breast cancer is launched. However, the closest approximation to such a group comes from the report of Mackay and Sellars (1965). They published a statistical review of all cases of breast cancer seen at the Ontario Cancer clinics between 1938 and 1956. The 9,742 cases analysed accounted for about 40% of all new cases of breast cancer arising in the province of Ontario during this period. Among this group were 145 well documented cases who received no treatment of any kind. Although 100 of these cases were untreated because of late stage of disease or poor general condition, the rest were unwilling or unable to attend for treatment. As in previous series, they tended to be older, to have delayed longer before presentation and to have presented with more advanced disease.

A careful note was made in this series of the date the patient first became aware of the lump, and as a result, it was possible, with a fair degree of accuracy, to calculate survival rates from the date of clinical presentation of the disease. Unfortunately, the follow-up data are available for only a 5-year period but at least this group represents a relatively contemporary population, a proportion of whom would be considered eligible for inclusion in today's clinical trials for early breast cancer. The 5-year survival from first recorded symptoms for the whole untreated group was 35.2%, with a median interval between first symptom and death of 47 months. A most surprising figure. however, is the 68.8% 5-year survival after the first symptom in those untreated patients presenting with localized disease. Such a figure does not compare unfavourably with many treated series, although this could well be an artifact resulting from selection and the small number in the sample.

This brings us to the question raised earlier. Is carcinoma of the breast inevitably a fatal condition or could there be a group of women living in blissful ignorance of their cancer and eventually dying of other causes? This question is virtually impossible to answer with any degree of confidence, but the suggestion that such a state of affairs might exist comes from postmortem studies and anecdotal evidence based on case reports.

Sandison (1962) reported a large autopsy study of the human breast in an unselected consecutive series of 800 female postmortems, carried out at the Western Infirmary, Glasgow, over a 5-year period. He reported a 0.77% incidence of occult breast cancer in women dying of disease other than mammary carcinoma. The majority of these cases occurred in the 8th decade and he points to the analogy of occult carcinoma of the prostate in postmortem series. In addition there were three cases with overt but untreated breast cancer in the total series. But, as Sandison (1975) points out, most routine postmortems pay scant attention to the breast and to collect the type of information required would demand an enormous planned effort.

Anecdotal evidence that breast cancer is not inevitably fatal if untreated, is by its very nature suspect. The author has personal experience of four well documented cases of women who refused treatment for their breast cancer for 7, 10, 13 and 16 years respectively. Three of these are still alive and well with the cancer in situ, and one recently died of carcinoma of the stomach with the still localized breast primary weighing 2 Kg. However, the best documented case in the literature is reported by Steckler and Martin (1973). They described a 38-year-old woman with histologically proved cancer who refused mastectomy and was then followed for 20 years before she consented to surgery! We will never know how many of the cases we see in our everyday practice carry such a favourable natural history.

THE METASTATIC POTENTIAL OF BREAST CANCER

Arguments concerning the curability of breast cancer may become obscure in that a lump removed from a patient who thereafter lives a normal span of years can be claimed not to have been a cancer in the first place. However, in spite of this danger, it is still reasonable to question the absoluteness of a diagnosis of cancer based on the histological examination of a biopsy specimen. All pathologists readily admit that there are grey areas in the field of the histopathology of tumours.

Difficult sections are often circulated for a consensus opinion. The dividing lines between epithelial hyperplasia, intraduct carcinoma and early invasive ductal carcinoma are not clear-cut. Furthermore, sclerosing adenosis is notoriously difficult to diagnose, and Urban and Adair (1949) reported that 90% of such cases were being classified as carcinoma up until 1949.

Although it is unlikely that any mistakes would be made among the sub-group with axillary metastases found at the time of mastectomy, there must inevitably be some doubts as to the true diagnosis in the long term survivors after mastectomy. Nonetheless, it would help in the development of the subsequent argument, if it were conceded that all apparently cured women have had a truly invasive carcinoma of the breast.

The factors that determine at which point in time a localized cancer will disseminate cells into its lymphatic drainage or into the general circulation are not fully understood. Nor for that matter is there a clear understanding of the factors that decide whether a shed malignant cell will successfully establish a metastasis. It is more than likely that both events represent a complex equation involving the rate of replication of the cancer cell, the invasive aggressiveness of the cancer, the anatomical access to lymph or vascular channels, the chronological age of the tumour, the defence mechanisms of the patient and factors within the "soil" of the target sites.

It is reasonable to assume that, all other things being equal, the greater the number of times the original transformed cell has replicated itself, the greater the opportunity for dissemination. If the growth rate of a tumour is assumed to be constant (expressed by its doubling time), and the size of the tumour at diagnosis is measured, a rough estimate can be made of the number of doublings that have occurred in the pre-clinical phase of its growth. If the number of doublings between inception of the growth and clinical presentation are small then the chances of spread before treatment are small. However, if the clinical phase of tumour growth merely represents the last chapter of a prolonged silent but sinister story of cellular proliferation, then, if that tumour has any metastatic potential, spread will have occurred before diagnosis is possible and the disease must be considered incurable by conventional local therapy.

Several authors have attempted to estimate doubling times of breast cancer based on a variety of clinical and radiological measurements. Collins et al. (1956) estimated growth rates from serial chest X-rays of patients with pulmonary metastases. Philipe and Le Gal (1968) utilized cutaneous nodules to determine growth rate, whilst Kusama et al. (1972) calculated the doubling time by observing the growth patterns of the primary lesion. All authors are agreed that there is a wide scatter in the growth rates of breast cancers, with doubling times varying between a few days and several months.

One of the most interesting and perhaps most meaningful studies of this nature was reported by Gershon-Cohen et al. (1963). They reviewed serial mammograms of the lesion taken prior to biopsy in 18 patients with breast cancer. They discovered that the doubling time of the tumours varied between 23 and 209 days. For convenience the tumours were divided up into three groups, fast growing with a doubling time of less than 75 days, slow growing with a doubling time of more than 150 days and an intermediate group with doubling times betwen 75 and 150 days. On the premise that a clinically detectable tumour of 1.0 cm has undergone 30 doublings if the original cell was $10\,\mu$ in diameter, they estimated that fast growing tumours originated about 2 years before clinical presentation whilst slow growing tumours would originate up to 17 years before becoming clinically diagnosable.

They therefore suggested that therapy is, on average, instituted only during the final third of the life cycle of breast cancer. Yet in their experience a difference of 1.5 cm in the diameter of a tumour, representing only three or four doublings, increases the metastatic rate from 30% to 60%. Thus, although most tumours would appear to have had ample opportunity to disseminate before clinical presentation, it still might be conceivable that some tumours need to attain a certain clinical size before colonizing, and should be curable by entirely local measures.

Using similar reasoning, Bond (1968) reached a less optimistic conclusion. In 9,341 cases he plotted the size of the tumour at presentation against the alleged duration from first detection by the patient. This plot appeared to yield two lines, which he interpreted as suggesting either one type of tumour with changing growth rate, or two types of tumour of different growth rates. If the latter explanation was correct, this would suggest the existence of fast growing tumours with a 90-day doubling time, and slow growing tumours with a 450-day doubling time. The former would originate an estimated 8 years before detection whilst the latter might arise 42 years before detection.

Extrapolating the data in the other direction, to the time of appearance of bone and pulmonary metastases of a given diameter, Bond suggested that a primary tumour only 10 cells in diameter was originally responsible for the successful establishment of a proportion of these secondary growths. Furthermore, a primary tumour of only 1 mm in diameter containing 10^6 cells is capable of metastasising and causing death in 20% of patients within 8 years.

However, these and similar arguments must be considered doubtful because they are based on three unproven assumptions. Firstly, the assumption that

the growth rate of the primary and its metastases are constant throughout the life cycle of the tumour; secondly, that once established, the primary or its secondaries develop full growth rate immediately without any latent period; thirdly, the assumption that all tumour masses consist of malignant cells which are packed together in a homogeneous sphere and are all subdividing in concert.

The evidence supporting the variability of growth rate and the dormancy of malignant tumours has recently been reviewed by Devitt (1976). Quoting his own studies and referring to the work of Brennan (1966), Smithers (1968) and Skipper (1971), he concludes that both primary and secondary tumours have a finite maximal volume and their growth rate plateaus with time. Therefore, judging the doubling time of a metastasis on the basis of an increase from 2 to 4 cm diameter gives ludicrously prolonged estimates of the tumour's duration. As, for example, the case quoted by Smithers (1968) of a patient with lung metastases from breast cancer whose primary would have arisen long before birth if judged on the criteria of the doubling time of her metastases.

Evidence of dormancy in the malignant cell has been described in the classical experiments of Fisher and Fisher (1959). Although the exponential growth characteristics of a rapidly proliferating cancer may give the impression of a sudden metastatic shower, it is equally likely that the showers of secondary deposits often seen after a long recurrence-free interval, are provided by dormant cells which were kept in check by host factors, until some event disturbed the delicate tumour host balance.

Finally, it is obvious that whereas a 1 mm tumour *may* theoretically contain 10^6 active tumour cells and *nothing* else, a 1 cm tumour certainly will consist of other elements such as a necrotic tissue, vascular spaces and connective tissue. Furthermore, of those malignant cells present, only a fraction will be proliferating and a significant proportion will be dying off. This involves consideration of cellular kinetics which is outside the scope of this chapter but can be referred to in publications such as Tubiana (1971). Nevertheless, it should be emphasized that the growth rate of a tumour depends on the proportion of proliferating cells to all cells present (expressed as the growth fraction and estimated as 40% for breast cancer, according to Tubiana), and also on the mean cell cycle time. Both of these may alter as the tumour itself influences its surrounding environment.

The arguments of Gershon-Cohen and Bond are therefore doubtful, but they are important in having stimulated us to think about the preclinical phase of tumour development which surely must predetermine the outcome of treatment.

ALTERNATIVE CONCEPT CONCERNING THE NATURE OF BREAST CANCER AS A FIRST STEP TOWARDS IMPROVING THE CURE RATE OF THE DISEASE

The vast majority of breast cancer cases met with in everyday practice in this country must be considered incurable by whatever criterion is chosen. The failure to improve survival rates in breast cancer over the last 20 years is due in large part to the clinicians who have rigidly maintained what must now be considered obsolete concepts concerning the nature of the disease. If the current generation of clinicians are to make a significant impact on mortality rates, they must as a first step reject the simplistic mechanistic view of the disease which has led to more and more aggressive local therapy, with greater morbidity but no apparent gain.

As a first step we should accept the idea that breast cancer is a systemic disease until proved otherwise. The assumption that dissemination has not occurred until it is proven, must be dropped. Secondly, it has to be accepted that breast cancer is not a single homogenous entity but behaves as if it were in fact, a multitude of diseases.

Slack et al. (1969) produced a mathematical model from the results of the National Surgical Adjuvant Breast Project which suggested that there were at least two types of breast cancer. One-fifth of all cases appeared to be fast growing tumours with a short delay in reporting symptoms, and carrying 3 to 8 times the average risk of nodal involvement and 2 to 6 times the average risk of occult metastases; the other four-fifths comprised slow growing tumours. I feel that even this is an oversimplification related to the limitations of this type of mathematical analysis.

I would like to propose theoretical groupings of breast cancer types based on the data described in this chapter. These are shown in Table 2 together with the implications regarding therapy for each type. Other similar theoretical classifications are possible.

We can individualize treatment only if we can identify the type of breast cancer on presentation. At present, the best we can do is to recognize the exceptionally poor prognostic significance of positive nodal histology or positive scans, and to introduce systemic therapy for these patients at an early stage. With greater refinement in prognostic indicators and with the use of more effective non-toxic anticancer agents, the appalling mortality rate for breast cancer will finally be controlled. Available resources might

Table 2 Theoretical groupings of breast cancer

Type		*Biological nature*	*Therapeutic implications*
I		Non-metastasising (rare)	
	A	Single focus	Curable by "lumpectomy"
	B	Multifocal	Curable by simple mastectomy
II		Metastasises to regional lymph nodes with only late vascular spread (rare)	Curable by radical mastectomy or simple mastectomy plus regional radiotherapy. Node dissection or irradiation could be performed electively rather than prophylactically
III		Metastasises via blood stream	
	A	Disseminates before either radiographically or clinically detectable. Nodal involvement acts as index of unfavourable tumour host/balance (probably the most common type)	Incurable by local therapy alone. Demands adjuvant systemic therapy
	B	Disseminates in period between becoming radiologically apparent but before clinically obvious (rare)	Curable by local therapy alone if detected at mass screening by mammography
	C	Disseminates at any period after it becomes clinically detectable (rare)	Curable by local therapy alone if detected by patient herself or at mass screening by clinical examination, before it has metastasised

better be turned in this direction rather than to the establishment of a National Screening Programme which can only benefit that small group of patients whose cancer metastasises as its grows from radiological to clinical proportions. This is a relatively short period in the life cycle of any breast cancer.

Acknowledgements

I wish to sincerely thank Dr. John Haybittle for his helpful advice and for supplying important source material. I also wish to acknowledge the invaluable secretarial assistance of Miss Sheila Herbert.

REFERENCES

Adair, F., Berg, J., Joubert, L. and Robbins, G. F. (1974). Long term follow up of breast cancer patients: The 30 year report. *Cancer 33*, 1145.

Bloom, H. J. G. (1968). Survival of women with untreated breast cancer—Past and present. In *Prognostic Factors in Breast Cancer* (Eds A. P. M. Forrest and P. B. Kunkler). Edinburgh: E. & S. Livingstone Limited.

Bloom, H. J. G., Richardson, W. W. and Field, J. R. (1970). Host resistance and survival in carcinoma of the breast—study of 104 cases of medullary carcinoma in a series of 1,411 cases of breast cancer followed for 20 years. *British Medical Journal 3*, 181.

Bond, W. H. (1968). The influence of various treatments on survival rates in cancer of the breast. In *Treatment of Carcinoma of the Breast*, Excerpta Medica Foundation, p. 1.

Brennan, M. J. (1966). Indices of response to breast cancer therapy. In *Clinical Evaluation in Breast Cancer*, p. 141 (Eds J. L. Hayward and R. D. Bulbrook). London: Academic Press.

Brinkley, D. and Haybittle, J. L. (1968). A 15 year follow up study of patients treated for carcinoma of the breast. *British Journal of Radiology 41*, 215.

Brinkley, D. and Haybittle, J. L. (1975). The curability of breast cancer. *Lancet 2*, 95.

Campbell, H. (1968). Breast Cancer in Wales. In *Prognostic Factors in Breast Cancer*, p. 50 (Eds A. P. M. Forrest and P. B. Kunkler). Edinburgh: E. & S. Livingstone Limited.

Campos, J. L. (1972). Observations on the mortality from carcinoma of the breast. *British Journal of Radiology 45*, 31.

Collins, V. P., Loeffler, R. K. and Tivey, H. (1956). Observations on growth rates of human tumours. *American Journal of Roentgenology 76*, 988.

Cutler, S. J. (1968). The prognosis of treated breast cancer. In *Prognostic Factors in Breast Cancer*, p. 20 (Eds A. P. M. Forrest and P. B. Kunkler). Edinburgh: E. & S. Livingstone Limited.

Devitt, J. E. (1965). The significance of regional lymph node metastases in breast carcinoma. *Canadian Medical Association Journal 93*, 289.

Devitt, J. E. (1976). Clinical prediction of growth behaviour. In *Risk Factors in Breast Cancer*, p. 110 (Ed. B. A. Stoll). London: Heinemann Medical.

Daland, E. M. (1927). Untreated carcinoma of the breast. *Surgery, Gynecology and Obstetrics 44*, 264.

Fisher, B. (1973). Co-operative clinical trials in primary breast cancer. A critical appraisal. *Cancer 31*, 1271.

Fisher, B. and Fisher, E. R. (1959). Experimental evidence in support of the dormant tumour cell. *Science 130*, 918.

Fisher, E. R. and Taylor, M. (1973). Changing pattern of some pathologic parameters of mammary carcinoma. *Cancer 32*, 1380.

Gershon-Cohen, J., Berger, S. M. and Klickstein, H. S. (1963). Roentgenography of breast cancer moderating concept of "biologic predeterminism". *Cancer 16*, 961.

Greenwood, M. (1926). A report on the natural duration of cancer; reports on public health and medical subjects, No. 33. London: H.M.S.O.

Gross, S. W. (1880). *A practical treatise of tumours of the mammary gland.* New York: D. Appelton & Co.

Halsted, W. S. (1908). The training of the surgeon. In *Surgical papers by William Stewart Halsted*, Vol. 2. Baltimore: The Johns Hopkins Press, 1924.

Haybittle, J. L. (1964). The cured group in series of patients treated for cancer. *Anglo-German Medical Review 2*, 422.

Haybittle, J. L. (1968). The cured group in a series of treated breast cancer patients. *British Journal of Radiology 41*, 639.

Kusama, S., Spratt, J. S., Donegan, W. L., Watson, F. R. and Cunningham, C. (1972). The gross rates of growth of human mammary carcinoma. *Cancer 30*, 594.

Macdonald, I. (1951). Biological predeterminism in human cancer. *Surgery, Gynecology and Obstetrics 92*, 443.

MacKay, E. N. and Sellers, A. H. (1965). Breast cancer at the Ontario Cancer Clinics, 1938-1956. A statistical review. Medical Statistics Branch, Ontario Department of Health.

McKinnon, N. E. (1954). Control of cancer mortality. *Lancet 1*, 251.

Mueller, C. B. and Jeffries, W. (1975). Cancer of the breast: Its outcome as measured by the rate of dying and causes of death. *Annals of Surgery 182*, 334.

Myers, M. H. (1973). In *Breast Cancer: A challenging problem*, p. 87 (Eds M. L. Griem, E. V. Jensen, J. E. Ultmann and R. W. Wissler). London: Heinemann Medical.

Park, W. S. and Lees, J. C. (1951). The absolute curability of cancer of the breast. *Surgery, Gynecology and Obstetrics 93*, 129.

Philippe, F. and Legal, Y. (1968). Growth of 78 recurrent mammary cancers. *Cancer 21*, 461.

Registrar General's Statistical Review of England and Wales (1973). Part I (A) Medical. London: H.M.S.O.

Sandison, A. T. (1975). Personal communication.

Sandison, A. T. (1962). An autopsy study of the human breast. N.C.I. Monograph No. 8. U.S. Department of Health Education and Welfare.

Shimkin, M. D. (1951). Duration of life in untreated cancer. *Cancer 4*, 1.

Skipper, H. E. (1971). Kinetics of mammary tumour cell growth and implications for therapy. *Cancer 28*, 1479.

Slack, N. H., Blumenson, L. E. and Bross, I. D. J. (1969). Therapeutic implications from a mathematical model characterizing the course of breast cancer. *Cancer 24*, 960.

Smithers, D. W. (1968). Clinical assessment of growth rate in human tumours. *Clinical Radiology 19*, 113.

Steckler, R. M. and Martin, R. G. (1973). Prolonged survival in untreated breast cancer. *The American Journal of Surgery 126*, 111.

Strax, P., Venet, L., Shapiro, S. and Gross, S. (1967). Mammography and clinical examination in mass screening for cancer of the breast. *Cancer 20*, 2184.

Tubiana, M. (1971). The kinetics of tumour cell proliferation and radiotherapy. *British Journal of Radiology 44*, 325.

Urban, J. A. and Adair, F. E. (1949). Sclerosing adenosis. *Cancer 2*, 625.

Wade, P. (1946). The natural history of untreated carcinoma of the breast. *British Journal of Radiology 19*, 272.

Chapter

2

C. S. B. GALASKO

Screening for the Potentially Curable Patient

The detection of metastatic involvement is a prerequisite in the management of the patient who presents with an apparently "early" mammary carcinoma. This patient requires basic investigation to determine the extent of the disease before starting treatment. If she has a tumour localized to the breast, then some form of radical local therapy is indicated. If, however, the tumour has disseminated, adjuvant therapy either in the form of chemotherapy, hormonal therapy or radiotherapy may be indicated in addition to local treatment.

The minimal initial screening should consist of a careful examination of the breasts and regional lymph nodes and a full general examination. An X-ray of the chest is essential. Basic blood tests should include a blood count, sedimentation rate and a biochemical profile which will include some simple liver function tests and an estimation of the alkaline phosphatase level. Mammography of both breasts is desirable and, where facilities exist, skeletal scintigraphy should be carried out. Where skeletal scintigraphy is not available, routine radiographic skeletal surveys may be helpful.

When a patient has even minor symptoms or signs suggestive of metastatic involvement of any particular organ, this needs to be investigated specifically. Liver function tests, hepatic scintigraphy and ultrasound examination may be necessary if hepatic metastases are suspected. Cerebral scintigraphy and computerized transaxial tomography (EMI brain scan) are used if cerebral metastases are suspected.

LYMPH NODE METASTASES

The commonest site of dissemination of cancer is to the regional lymph nodes, which must be examined carefully at the time of initial presentation. Their operability by the TNM system includes either no regional lymph node involvement (N0) or early involvement (N1); the disease is advanced if the axillary nodes are fixed (N2) or the supraclavicular lymph nodes are involved (N3).

Unfortunately, clinical examination of the lymph nodes is relatively inaccurate. Attempts have been made to improve the accuracy by lymphangiography

and lymph node scintigraphy but the results have been disappointing (Kett et al., 1972). Some surgeons, therefore, consider it essential to biopsy the ipsilateral axillary nodes and even the internal mammary nodes at the time of mastectomy.

The prognosis is closely related to the number and level of axillary nodes involved. Thus, Haagensen (1956) reported a 79% 5 year survival in patients with negative axillary nodes, 66% where there were only one or two nodal metastases, 37% where three to seven lymph nodes were involved and 15% if more than seven nodes were affected. Urban (1960) reported an 83% 5-year survival in patients with negative nodes, 65% in those with low axillary nodal involvement, 45% where the mid-axillary nodes were involved and 28% in patients with high axillary nodal involvement.

However, Huvos and his colleagues (1971) found that the prognosis was related to the size as well as to the extent of axillary nodal involvement. Where the metastases were less than 2 mm in diameter (micrometastases), the survival rates were much better than where the metastases were 2 mm or larger (macrometastases). Overall they reported an 82% 8-year survival rate in patients with no axillary nodal involvement, 71% where only the lowest nodes were involved and 55% where the axillary lymph nodes were involved at all levels.

Where only the lowest nodes were involved, the survival rate was 94% for patients with micrometastases and 62% for those with macrometastases. Where all levels were involved, the survival rate for patients with micrometastases was 59%, whereas it fell to 29% where there were macrometastases. Johnstone (1972) reported an 83% 5-year survival in patients where there was no axillary nodal involvement, 60% where the axillary lymph nodes were involved and 29% where the apical or internal mammary nodes were infiltrated.

DISTANT DISSEMINATION

The main factor in determining the patient's prognosis is the presence or absence of distant dissemination and the skeleton is the commonest site of distant metastases from mammary carcinoma (Coley, 1949; Geschickter and Copeland, 1949; Abrams et al., 1950; Willis, 1952; Ackerman and del Regato, 1954; Haagensen, 1956; Cole, 1964). Garland (1954) reviewed 60 patients with distant metastases from mammary carcinoma and found that the first manifestations occurred in the skeleton in 30%, in the chest wall, lymph nodes or mediastinum in 28%, lungs in 20%, liver in 9%, brain in 3% and in miscellaneous sites in 10% of patients. Fisher and his colleagues (1968) found that 26% of their patients developed skeletal metastases whereas 19% developed pulmonary, 15% lymphatic, 9% gastrointestinal and 1% cerebral metastases. It seems reasonable, therefore, that the skeleton and lung fields should be carefully examined for metastases in all cases when a patient first presents with mammary carcinoma.

Skeletal metastases

Although the skeleton is the commonest site of distant metastatic involvement, conventional methods of detecting skeletal metastases are not very sensitive. Galasko (1972) investigated 86 patients with advanced mammary carcinoma, all of whom had skeletal metastases evident on X-ray. Only 65% of the patients complained of pain, tenderness was elicited in 16% and the serum alkaline phosphatase level was raised in 66%. The serum calcium, urinary calcium, inorganic phosphorus and lactic dehydrogenase were of even less diagnostic assistance.

Cuschieri (1973) found that the urinary hydroxyproline was persistently elevated in many patients who subsequently developed skeletal metastases and suggested that its measurement may be a sensitive index of the presence of occult skeletal metastases. The measurement of the hydroxyproline–creatinine ratio is even more sensitive (Guzzo et al., 1969), the urinary hydroxyproline being elevated in only 50% of patients known to have skeletal metastases, whereas the urinary hydroxyproline/creatinine ratio was increased in 83% of these patients.

Roberts and his colleagues (1975) found an abnormal hydroxyproline/creatinine ratio in 11 of 14 patients with mammary cancer, whose skeletal scintigram was positive although their X-rays were normal. However, they also reported a high false negative rate in patients with established metastatic disease. The urinary hydroxyproline/creatinine ratio is probably more accurate than the serum alkaline phosphatase level but there is still a high rate of false negatives in patients with radiologically established skeletal metastases.

Radiographic examination is also inaccurate. Edelstyn and his colleagues (1967) found that at least 50% of the bone, in the beam axis of the X-ray, must be destroyed before the lesion will be seen radiologically.

During the past few years scintigraphy has been shown to be more accurate and sensitive than conventional methods for the early detection of skeletal metastases (Table 1). Galasko (1972) investi-

Table 1 Detection of skeletal metastases: comparison between radiography and scintigraphy

Authors	*No. of investigations*	*Scintigram more accurate*	*X-ray more accurate*	*No difference*
Charkes and Sklaroff (1965)	156	34	5	117
Simpson and Orange (1965)	62	34	3	25
Briggs (1967)	83	29	1	53
French and McCready (1967)	57	12	4	41
Harmer et al. (1969)	159	49	6	104
Milner et al. (1971)	100	17	9	74
Galasko (1972)	50	36	0	14
Gnekow et al. (1972)	359	32	11	316
Robinson and Constable (1973)	42	5	0	37
Shearer et al. (1974)	314	32	18	264

gated by scintigraphy a group of 50 patients with advanced mammary carcinoma. In 25 of them (50%) bone metastases were evident on the X-rays which were taken when the patient first attended. Yet 42 patients (84%) had lesions evident on their Fluorine-18 scintigram taken with a gamma camera within a few days of the radiographic skeletal survey. (Jaffe (1958) found that approximately 85% of mammary carcinoma patients had skeletal metastases at autopsy examination.) In 36 (72%) of Galasko's patients additional lesions were seen on the scintigram, yet in 17 of these patients the radiographic skeletal survey was entirely normal. These additional lesions, which were found only on the scintigram, have since been confirmed either on subsequent X-rays or at autopsy.

A more crucial question is the accuracy of skeletal scintigraphy for the early detection of skeletal metastases in patients with apparently "early" mammary carcinoma and in whom there is no other evidence of dissemination of their disease. To answer this, I investigated a group of 50 women with apparently "early" mammary carcinoma and each patient had a careful clinical examination, a radiographic skeletal survey and an X-ray of her chest. In a previous study (Galasko, 1972) we had found that of 138 consecutive patients who were thought to have an operable mammary carcinoma, one patient had hepatomegaly (which on biopsy contained tumour cells), one patient had asymptomatic pulmonary metastases shown on her chest X-ray and four patients had skeletal metastases evident on their skeletal radiographs.

In this second study the primary tumour was operable (i.e. T1, T2) except in two patients with large breasts where it was T3 by size. There was no fixity of the primary tumour and the lymph nodes were either N0 or N1. There was no clinical evidence of dissemination of the disease and the liver function tests, radiographic skeletal survey and chest X-rays were entirely normal. Each patient also had a skeletal scintigram using ^{18}Fluorine and the gamma camera and in 12 (24%) patients, lesions were found on the scintigram. The women with positive scintigrams were treated in an identical manner to those with normal scintigrams, namely, by mastectomy and post-operative radiotherapy.

The patients have been followed up for 5 years and the scintigraphic findings have been confirmed in all the patients with a positive scintigram. The time taken for the confirmation of these lesions, either on subsequent X-rays or at autopsy, is shown in Table 2. Ten (83%) of the patients with a positive scintigram have died from their mammary carcinoma during the 5-year period (Table 3). During the same period, only 10 (26%) of the patients with a negative scintigram have developed evidence of either local recurrence or dissemination of their disease and eight (21%) have died from their mammary carcinoma. Three patients with a negative scintigram have died from intercurrent disease and at autopsy there was no evidence of residual tumour.

At 5 years, two (17%) of the patients with a positive scintigram were alive but both had dis-

Table 2 Patients with apparently "early" mammary cancer: the time taken for radiological or autopsy confirmation of the skeletal scintigraphic finding

Time taken	*% of patients*
3 months	33
6 months	42
12 months	50
18 months	50
2 years	83
3 years	83
4 years	92
5 years	100

Table 3 The 5 year follow-up in 50 patients subjected to skeletal scintigraphy at the time of presenting with apparently "early" mammary carcinoma

	Scintigram		
	+ ve	*– ve*	*Total*
No. of patients	*12*	*38*	*50*
Developed advanced disease	12 (100%)	10 (26%)	22 (44%)
Died from cancer	10 (83%)	8 (21%)	18 (36%)
Died from other causes	0	3 (8%)	3 (6%)
Alive 5 years	2 (17%)	27 (71%)	29 (58%)
Alive with metastatic disease	2 (17%)	2 (5%)	4 (8%)
Alive with no evidence recurrence	0	25 (66%)	25 (50%)

seminated carcinoma. This compares with 71% of the patients with a negative scintigram who were alive at 5 years but two (5%) of whom had developed advanced disease. Thus, at 5 years, none of the patients with a positive scintigram were alive and apparently free from tumour, compared with 66% of the patients with a negative scintigram. Similar detection rates for "occult" metastases have been reported by Citrin et al. (1975) and Blair (1975).

The results of this study confirmed that skeletal scintigraphy is more accurate than conventional methods for the staging of mammary carcinoma. The results also indicated that occult skeletal metastases, which are found by a skeletal scintigram in a patient who has no other evidence of disseminated disease, are highly significant and indicate the patient's prognosis. The presence of such lesions suggests that the patient has a very poor prognosis and that probably some form of adjuvant therapy is required in addition to local surgery or radiotherapy.

Pulmonary metastases

The lung is the next most common site of distant metastases from mammary carcinoma. Asymptomatic lesions can occasionally be found on routine radiographs. Lung tomography has been shown to detect occult metastases, particularly those from osteosarcoma, at a much earlier stage than routine radiographs. However, there is insufficient information as to its value in the routine screening of patients with apparently "early" mammary carcinoma.

Pulmonary scintigraphy is probably no more accurate in detecting these lesions. Ali and his colleagues (1971) investigated 21 patients with nodular pulmonary metastases. They frequently found ventilatory defects in the vicinity of single metastases, and in patients with multiple metastases defects in the pulmonary blood flow and ventilation were commonly observed in the vicinity of the tumour masses. However, they they found that scintigraphy was no more accurate than conventional radiology in detecting these lesions.

Standard X-rays of the chest should be obtained in all patients with mammary carcinoma before undertaking surgery, as asymptomatic pulmonary metastases may be found occasionally in patients with apparently "early" mammary carcinoma (Galasko, 1972). Lung tomography and pulmonary scintigraphy are probably not indicated as routine screening procedures although where pulmonary metastases are suspected and routine radiographs are normal, pulmonary tomography and scintigraphy may be of value.

Hepatic metastases

The early diagnosis of hepatic metastases is extremely difficult. By the time the patient develops hepatomegaly and particularly umbilicated nodules, the metastases are usually very large. Nevertheless, the abdomen should be examined when the patient first presents and occasionally an enlarged liver may be the only suggestion of dissemination of the disease in a patient with an otherwise apparently "early" carcinoma. One such patient was found in 138 consecutive patients with mammary carcinoma who were thought to have an operable tumour (Galasko, 1972).

The value of routine biochemical liver function tests in the assessment of patients with apparently "early" mammary carcinoma has not been adequately defined. Occasionally these tests are reported abnormal, suggesting metastatic involvement, when there is no clinical evidence of hepatic involvement. On the other hand, the liver function tests were reported normal in my 50 patients with apparently "early" mammary carcinoma, although 22 (44%) developed disseminated carcinoma (including hepatic involvement in many) within 5 years (Table 3).

Table 4 The detection of hepatic metastases by scintigraphy in patients with clinical suspicion of hepatic involvement. Lesions subsequently confirmed at autopsy, laparotomy or by biopsy

Author	*No. of patients*	*Scintigram correct*
Nagler et al. (1963)	548	461 (83%)
McAfee et al. (1965)	112	101 (90%)
Ariel et al. (1969)	196	169 (85%)
Ferrier et al. (1969)	155	131 (84%)
Poulose et al. (1969)	54	45 (83%)
Bieler et al. (1972)	100	90 (90%)
Castagna et al. (1972)	109	81 (74%)
Lunia et al. (1975)	581	449 (77%)

Hepatic scintigraphy is probably more accurate for the early detection of hepatic metastases (Table 4). Nevertheless, the metastasis must be large before it can be detected on the hepatic scintigram. Thus, Friedell and his colleagues (1957) and Wagner and his colleagues (1961) found that the minimum size lesion that could be seen on the hepatic scintigram was 2 to 2.5 cm in diameter where the tissue was 10 cm thick. Where the tissue was only 5 cm thick, a lesion 1.5 cm in diameter could be seen. It has been suggested by others that a lesion must be at least 4.5 cm in diameter if it lies in the centre of the right lobe, or 1.8 cm in diameter if it is peripheral, before it will be visualized on the scintigram (Vidrih and Higgins, 1971).

Ozarda and his colleagues (1962) found at autopsy that in 41% of patients with hepatic involvement, the largest hepatic metastases were less than 2 cm in diameter. It is surprising therefore that so many authors have reported an 80% or higher detection rate by scintigraphy for hepatic metastases (Table 4). This may be because the patients examined had already developed symptoms suggestive of hepatic involvement, and these results therefore give no indication of the value of hepatic scintigraphy for screening patients with occult disease.

Castagna and his colleagues (1972) investigated 109 patients in whom the liver was subsequently examined, either at laparotomy or autopsy. They found that the scintigram was correct in 81 (74.3%) patients; there were 12 (11%) false positives and 16 (14.7%) false negatives. Of the 53 patients with proven hepatic metastases, 41 (78%) had lesions demonstrable on the scintigrams. Ferrier and his colleagues (1969) found that hepatic scintigraphy was more accurate than biochemical liver function tests or blind needle biopsy for the detection of hepatic metastases.

Jasinski and his colleagues (1969) found a 20% incidence of hepatic metastases on routine hepatic scintigrams, in patients with mammary carcinoma admitted for radiotherapy. Nathan (1972) studied 88 patients with mammary carcinoma and in 59 the scintigram was normal although nine of these patients developed evidence of hepatic metastases within a few months. The scintigram was abnormal in 14 and suspicious in 15 patients. In a follow-up of several months, 17 (58%) of these patients developed hepatic metastases but, it is possible that with a longer follow up, metastases would have become apparent in some of the other 12 patients.

During the past few years ultrasonography of the liver has been developed (McCarthy et al., 1967, 1970) and is able to differentiate between cysts and solid tumours (Taylor et al., 1974). It is not widely used but with further technological improvements, may become useful for screening the liver for metastases. Another more exciting development is the EMI whole body scanner. This is still in its prototype form but if it proves as successful as the EMI brain scanner it may become the method of choice for detecting hepatic and pulmonary metastases.

In summary, the value of routine biochemical liver function tests and hepatic scintigraphy in patients with an apparently "early" mammary carcinoma is still questionable, but a careful abdominal examination should be part of the routine clinical examination of every patient presenting with mammary carcinoma. A full battery of liver function tests is not necessary for routine screening purposes, and the few tests which form part of the modern biochemical profile are probably all that is required. There does not seem to be sufficient indication, at the moment, for routine scintigraphy or ultrasonography.

If, on the other hand, the physician suspects that a particular patient may have developed hepatic metastases, then more detailed liver function tests, hepatic scintigrams and even ultrasound examination of the liver may help to confirm the diagnosis.

Table 5 Results obtained by cerebral scintigraphy in patients with symptoms suggestive of cerebral metastases. The lesions were subsequently confirmed at surgery or autopsy

Author	*No. of patients*	*Scintigram +ve*
Burrows (1972)	179	166 (89%)
Jansen et al. (1973)	34	32 (94%)
Klopper et al. (1973)	41	38 (93%)
Brooks et al. (1974)	47	36 (77%)

Cerebral metastases

Cerebral metastases from mammary carcinoma occur relatively infrequently compared with skeletal, pulmonary or hepatic metastases. There does not seem to be any indication for routine screening for cerebral metastases in a patient with apparently "early" carcinoma. However, where a patient develops symptoms or signs suggestive of cerebral metastases, then further investigation is essential.

Until recently, cerebral scintigraphy was probably the method of choice for the diagnosis of cerebral metastases. It is relatively simple, non-invasive, sensitive and highly accurate (Table 5). Multiple areas of increased uptake are usually seen on the scintigram but a solitary metastasis cannot be differentiated from a primary brain tumour nor from a variety of benign lesions which concentrate the radiopharmaceutical. The overall diagnostic accuracy is approximately 90% (Table 5).

During the past few years the computerized transverse axial scanner (EMI) has been developed (Ambrose, 1973; Paxton and Ambrose, 1974). This is an accurate radiological method of investigating cerebral metastases, but a major drawback is the high cost of the instrumentation. Centres which have been fortunate enough to obtain an EMI scanner report that there has been a marked reduction in the number of cerebral scintigrams which they now carry out. Paxton and Ambrose (1974) reviewed 650 patients, 232 of whom were thought to have a cerebral neoplasm. The EMI scan was positive in 34 of the 35 patients with supratentorial metastases, and in 6 of the 11 patients with infratentorial cerebral metastases.

There is no information as to the value of routine cerebral scintigraphy or EMI scanning in patients with apparently "early" mammary carcinoma, nor at the moment is there any indication for cerebral screening in such cases. These investigations probably should be reserved for the patient suspected of having developed cerebral metastases.

Metastases at other sites

Metastases from mammary carcinoma have been diagnosed in practically every region of the body. As stated at the outset, a careful general physical examination should be part of the routine examination of every patient presenting with mammary carcinoma but special screening of the less common sites of metastatic involvement is not indicated unless she shows symptoms or signs suggesting their involvement.

TUMOUR LOCALIZING AGENTS

Organ scintigraphy or radiology can detect metastases only in that specific organ. What is required in screening for mammary carcinoma is a simple method of detecting cancer at all sites, irrespective of whether the tumour is primary or secondary, or whether it involves the skeleton or the soft tissues. Over the past few years many attempts have been made to find tumour localizing agents.

The two most successful to date have been radioactive tagged bleomycin and ^{67}Ga. Overall they have a high percentage accuracy for the detection of tumours which are obvious on clinical or radiological examination but the detection rate of occult lesions has been disappointing. Lavender et al. (1971) using ^{67}Ga, detected 6 of 15 primary mammary carcinomata, and Higasi and his colleagues (1972) also using ^{67}Ga, detected 8 of 16 mammary carcinomata. Merrick and his colleagues (1975) using ^{111}In tagged bleomycin, detected 5 out of 6 mammary carcinomata.

The detection rate of skeletal metastases has been high although very few cases have been reported (Hisada et al., 1974). Higasi and his colleagues (1972) detected pulmonary metastases in 5 of 10 patients whereas Kinoshita and his colleagues (1974) using ^{67}Ga, detected pulmonary metastases in all 18 patients they studied.

The detection rate for hepatic metastases has been very disappointing. Suzuki and his colleagues (1971) using ^{67}Ga, found hepatic metastases in only 1 of 15 patients, and Grove and his colleagues (1974) using a variety of isotopes, detected metastases in 4 of 6 patients.

HUMORAL TUMOUR MARKERS

Another approach has been to look for a humoral tumour marker in patients with malignant disease. To be of value it must be tumour specific, present in the serum, decrease with successful treatment of the tumour and increase again should the tumour recur. This factor should also be readily measurable. One of the more promising methods has been to look for macromolecules associated with foetal tissue growth.

Carcinoembryonic antigen (CEA) was described by Gold and Freedman in 1965. Unfortunately, it is not tumour specific and it has been found in approximately 52% of patients with carcinoma of the breast, 73% of cancers of the colon and rectum, 92% of cancers of the pancreas, 67% of cancers of the liver and 60% of miscellaneous gastro-intestinal carcinomata. It is also found in 4% of patients with benign mammary tumours and 7% of patients with fibroadenosis, 9% of patients with polyps of the colon and rectum, 21% of patients with inflammatory disease of the colon, 42% of cirrhotics and 53% of patients with acute pancreatitis (Dykes and King, 1972; Laurence and Neville, 1972; Laurence et al., 1972; MacSween et al., 1972).

Its most important use may be in the detection of recurrence. A raised CEA level usually returns to normal if the tumour has been totally extirpated and the first sign of recurrence may be the reappearance of CEA in increasing titres. This has been found helpful in patients with carcinoma of the colon and rectum but is said to be of little value in patients with mammary carcinoma (Laurence et al., 1972).

Another foetal humoral factor is alpha foeto-protein. This is more tumour specific and although it is present in a variety of tumours, its level is not raised in patients with inflammatory disease. However, it is of very little value either in detection, assessment of the extent of the disease or assessment of recurrence in mammary carcinoma (Laurence and Neville, 1972). A variety of other foetal antigens and enzymes are being studied, but so far none appear to be of value in screening for metastases in patients with early mammary carcinoma.

CONCLUSION

There seems at present to be very little role for tumour localizing radio-pharmaceuticals or measurement of humoral tumour markers in the screening of patients with mammary carcinoma, except as a research investigation. It may be possible, however, in the future, to use one of these techniques not only for the early detection of mammary carcinoma, but also for the assessment of the extent and site of dissemination and for the early diagnosis of recurrence. The ideal method should not be organ specific but allow one to detect tumour at all sites, primary and secondary.

At the moment, the skeletal scintigram would appear to be the most sensitive method of staging mammary carcinoma and assessing the prognosis. Careful histological examination of the axillary lymph nodes and the hydroxyproline/creatinine ratio may also give a useful indication as to the prognosis.

Medicine is going through an era of rapid technological advances, and during the past few years, scintigraphy, ultrasonography and more recently the EMI scanners, have been developed. It is probable that during the next decade, new and highly sophisticated equipment will be developed, which will increase the accuracy and sensitivity of current techniques for diagnosing distant metastases, thus accurately assessing the extent of mammary carcinoma.

REFERENCES

Abrams, H. L., Spiro, R. and Goldstein, N. (1950). Metastases in carcinoma: analysis of 1,000 autopsied cases. *Cancer 3,* 74.

Ackerman, L. V. and del Regato, J. A. (1954). *Cancer, Diagnosis, Treatment and Prognosis.* 2nd edit., C. V. Mosby, St. Louis.

Ali, M. K., Howe, C. D. and Miller, J. M. (1971). Regional pulmonary function in metastatic carcinoma to the lung studied with Xenon-133. *Cancer 27,* 460.

Ambrose, J. (1973). Computerized transverse axial scanning (tomography): Part 2. Clinical application. *British Journal of Radiology 46,* 1023.

Ariel, I. M., Molander, D. and Galey, D. (1969). Hepatic gamma scanning. An aid in determining treatment policies for cancer involving the liver. *American Journal of Surgery 118,* 5.

Bieler, E. U., Meyer, B. J. and Jansen, C. R. (1972). Examination of the liver using radio-active Rose Bengal. *South African Medical Journal 46,* 1772.

Blair, J. S. G. (1975). Does early detection of bone

metastases by scanning improve prognosis in breast cancer? *Clinical Oncology 1,* 185.

Briggs, R. C. (1967). Detection of osseous metastases. Evaluation of bone scanning with ^{85}Sr. *Cancer 20,* 392.

Brooks, W. H., Mortrara, R. H. and Preston, D. (1974). The clinical limitations of brain scanning in metastatic disease. *Journal of Nuclear Medicine 15,* 620.

Burrows, E. H. (1972). False-negative results in brain scanning. *British Medical Journal 1,* 473.

Castagna, J., Benfield, J. R., Yamada, H. and Johnson, D. E. (1972). The reliability of liver scans and function tests in detecting metastases. *Surgery, Gynecology and Obstetrics 134,* 463.

Charkes, N. D. and Sklaroff, D. M. (1965). In *Progress in Clinical Cancer,* p. 235 (Ed. I. Ariel). New York: Grune and Stratten Inc.

Citrin, D. L., Bessant, R. G., Greig, W. R., McKeller, N. J., Furnival, C. and Blumgart, L. H. (1975). The application of ^{99m}Tc phosphate bone scan to the study of breast cancer. *British Journal of Surgery 62,* 201.

Cole, M. P. (1964). The place of radiotherapy in the management of early breast cancer. A report of two clinical trials. *British Journal of Surgery 51,* 216.

Coley, B. L. (1949). *Neoplasms of Bone and Related Conditions.* New York: Hoeber.

Cuschieri, A. (1973). Urinary hydroxyproline excretion in early and advanced breast cancer—a sequential study. *British Journal of Surgery 60,* 800.

Dykes, P. W. and King, J. (1972). Progress report. Carcinoembryonic antigen (CEA). *Gut 13,* 1000.

Edelstyn, G. A., Gillespie, P. J. and Grebbell, F. S. (1967). The radiological demonstration of osseous metastases. *Clinical Radiology 18,* 158.

Ferrier, F. L., Hatcher, C. R. Jr., Achord, J. L. and Abbott, O. S. (1969). The value of liver scanning for detection of metastatic cancer. *American Surgeon 35,* 112.

Fisher, B., Ravdin, R. G., Ausman, R. K., Slack, N. H., Moore, G. E. and Noer, R. J. (1968). Surgical adjuvant chemotherapy in cancer of the breast; results of a decade of co-operative investigations. *Annals of Surgery 168,* 337.

French, R. J. and McCready, V. R. (1967). The use of ^{18}F for bone scanning. *British Journal of Radiology 40,* 655.

Friedell, H. L., MacIntyre, W. J. and Rejali, A. M. (1957). A method for the visualization of the configuration and structure of the liver. Part A. Preliminary clinical investigations. *American Journal of Roentgenology 77,* 455.

Galasko, C. S. B. (1972). Skeletal metastases and mammary cancer. *Annals of the Royal College of Surgeons of England 50,* 3.

Garland, L. H. (1954). The rationale and results of simple mastectomy plus radiotherapy in primary cancer of the breast. *American Journal of Roentgenology 72,* 923,

Geschickter, C. F. and Copeland, M. M. (1949). *Tumours of Bone.* Philadelphia: Lippincott.

Gnekow, W. C., DeNardo, G. L., Poole, G. J. and Kriss, J. P. (1972). Review of a 5-year experience with the radiostrontium bone scintiscan. *California Medicine 117,* 1.

Gold, P. and Freedman, S. O. (1965). Specific carcinoembryonic antigens of the human digestive system. *Journal of Experimental Medicine 122,* 467.

Grove, R. B., Reba, R. C., Eckelman, W. C. and Goodyear, M. (1974). Clinical evaluation of radiolabeled bleomycin (bleo) for tumor detection. *Journal of Nuclear Medicine 15,* 386.

Guzzo, C. E., Pachas, W. N., Pinals, R. S. and Krant, M. J. (1969). Urinary hydroxyproline excretion in patients with cancer. *Cancer 24,* 382.

Haagensen, C. D. (1956). *Diseases of the Breast,* p. 629. Philadelphia: W. B. Saunders Co.

Harmer, C. L., Burns, J. E., Sams, A. and Spittle, N. (1969). The value of Fluorine-18 for scanning bone tumours. *Clinical Radiology 20,* 204.

Higasi, T., Nakayama, Y., Murata, A., Nakamura, K., Sugiyama, M., Kawaguchi, T. and Suzuki, S. (1972). Clinical evaluation of ^{67}Ga-citrate scanning. *Journal of Nuclear Medicine 13,* 196.

Hisada, K., Tonami, N., Hiraki, T. and Ando, A. (1974). Tumor scanning with ^{169}Yb-citrate. *Journal of Nuclear Medicine 15,* 210.

Huvos, A. G., Hutter, R. V. R. and Berg, J. W. (1971). Significance of axillary macrometastases amd micrometastases in mammary cancer. *Annals of Surgery 173,* 44.

Jaffe, H. L. (1958). *Tumors and Tumorous Conditions of the Bones and Joints.* Philadelphia: Lee & Febiger.

Jansen, C. R., Meyer, B. J., Bieler, E. U. and Du Toit, D. (1973). Brain scintigraphy in the diagnosis of intracranial lesions: Comparative scanning with ^{169}Ytterbium diethylene triamine penta acetic acid and ^{203}mercury chlormerodrin. *South African Medical Journal 47,* 232.

Jasinski, W. K., Malinowska, J. and Mackiewicz, H. (1969). In *Medical Radioisotope Scintigraphy,* Vol. II, p. 507. Vienna: International Atomic Energy Agency.

Johnstone, F. R. C. (1972). Results of treatment of carcinoma of the breast based on pathological staging. *Surgery, Gynecology and Obstetrics 134,* 211.

Kett, K., Lukács, L. and Varga, G. (1972). Diagnostic value of lymphography of the arm in the preoperative diagnosis of early metastases in breast cancer. *American Journal of Surgery 123,* 712.

Kinoshita, F., Ushio, T., Maekawa, A., Ariwa, R. and Kubo, A. (1974). Scintiscanning of pulmonary diseases with ^{67}Ga-citrate. *Journal of Nuclear Medicine 15,* 227.

Klopper, J. F., Rossouw, D. S. van Heerden, P. D. R., Malan, C. and Potgieter, J. (1973). Brain scanning with ^{99m}Tc-pertechnate. A comparative study in 2,000 cases. *South African Medical Journal 47,* 1792.

Laurence, D. J. R. and Neville, A. M. (1972). Foetal antigens and their role in the diagnosis and clinical management of human neoplasms. A review. *British Journal of Cancer 26,* 335.

Laurence, D. J. R., Stevens, A. U., Bettelheim, R., Darcy, D., Leese, C., Turberville, C., Alexander, P., Johns, E. W. and Neville, A. M. (1972). Role of plasma carcinoembryonic antigen in diagnosis of gastrointestinal, mammary and bronchial carcinoma. *British Medical Journal 3,* 605.

Lavender, J. P., Lowe, June, Barker, J. R., Burn, J. I. and Chaudhri, M. A. (1971). Gallium^{67} citrate scanning in neoplastic and inflammatory lesions. *British Journal of Radiology 44,* 361.

Lunia, S., Parthasarathy, K. L., Bakshi, S. and Bender, M. A. (1975). An evaluation of ^{99m}Tc-Sulfur colloid liver scintiscans and their usefulness in metastatic workup. A review of 1,424 studies. *Journal of Nuclear Medicine 16,* 62.

McAfee, J. G., Ause, R. G. and Wagner, H. N. Jr. (1965). Diagnostic value of scintillation scanning of the liver. *Archives of Internal Medicine 116,* 95.

McCarthy, C. F., Read, A. E. A., Ross, F. G. M. and Wells, P. N. T. (1967). Ultrasonic scanning of the liver. *Quarterly Journal of Medicine 36,* 517.

McCarthy, C. F., Rhys Davies, E., Wells, P. N. T., Ross, F. G. M., Follett, D. H., Muir, K. M. and Read, A. E. (1970). A comparison of ultrasonic and isotope scanning in the diagnosis of liver disease. *British Journal of Radiology 43,* 100.

MacSween, J. M., Warner, N. L., Bankhurst, A. D. and MacKay, I. R. (1972). Carcinoembryonic antigen in whole serum. *British Journal of Cancer 26,* 356.

Merrick, M. V., Lavender, J. P., Poole, G. W., Stradling, P., Thakur, M. L. and Walter, L. H. (1975). ^{111}In-labelled bleomycin; clinical experience as a diagnostic agent in tumours of the thorax and abdomen. *British Journal of Radiology 48,* 279.

Milner, T. H., Maynard, C. D. and Cowan, R. J. (1971). Evaluation of ^{85}Sr. bone scans and roentgenograms in 100 patients. *Archives of Surgery 103,* 371.

Nagler, W., Bender, M. A. and Blau, M. (1963). Radioisotope photoscanning of the liver. *Gastroenterology 44,* 36.

Nathan, B. E. (1972). Unpublished data.

Ozarda, A. and Pickren, J. (1962). The topographic distribution of liver metastases: its relation to surgical and isotope diagnosis. *Journal of Nuclear Medicine 3,* 149.

Paxton, R. and Ambrose, J. (1974). The EMI scanner. A brief review of the first 650 patients. *British Journal of Radiology 47,* 530.

Poulose, K. P., Reba, R. C., DeLand, F. H. and Wagner, H. N. Jr. (1969). Role of liver scanning in the preoperative evaluation of patients with cancer. *British Medical Journal 4,* 585.

Roberts, J. G., Williams, M., Henk, J. M., Bligh, A. S. and Baum, M. (1975). The hypronosticon test in breast cancer. *Clinical Oncology 1,* 33.

Robinson, M. R. G. and Constable, A. R. (1973). Strontium-87m and the Gamma camera in the study of bone metastases from carcinoma of the prostate. *British Journal of Urology 45,* 173.

Shearer, R. J., Constable, A. R., Girling, M., Hendry, W. F., and Fergusson, J. D. (1974). Radioisotopic bone scintigraphy with the Gamma camera in the investigation of prostatic cancer. *British Medical Journal 2,* 362.

Simpson, W. J. and Orange, R. P. (1965). Total body scanning with ^{85}Sr in the diagnosis of metastatic bone disease. *Canadian Medical Association Journal 93,* 1237.

Suzuki, T., Honjo, I., Hamamoto, K., Kousaka, T. and Torizuka, K. (1971). Positive scintiphotography of cancer of of the liver with ^{67}Ga citrate. *American Journal of Roentgenology 113,* 92.

Taylor, K. J. W., Carpenter, D. A. and McCready, V. R. (1974). Ultrasound and scintigraphy in the differential diagnosis of obstructive jaundice. *Journal of Clinical Ultrasound 2,* 105.

Urban, J. A. (1960). Treatment of early cancer of the breast. *Postgraduate Medicine 27,* 389.

Vidrih, V. E. and Higgins, H. P. (1971). Accuracy of liver scintiphotography using a plastic and water phantom. *Canadian Journal of Surgery 14,* 273.

Wagner, H. N. Jr., McAfee, J. G. and Mozley, J. M. (1961). Diagnosis of liver disease by radioisotope scanning. *Archives of Internal Medicine 107,* 324.

Willis, R. A. (1952). *The Spread of Tumours in the Human Body,* 2nd edit. London: Churchill.

Chapter

3 GUY F. ROBBINS

The Case for Radical Surgery

There is a choice of treatment for every woman with potentially curable breast cancer and it must be based on the fullest extent of clinical and pathological data available in her case. The objectives of good treatment are local control of the disease and good quality and length of survival, and comparison of results should be based upon treatment regimens with "quality control" of their surgery, pathology and radiation therapy (Robbins, 1974). In our opinion, the standardization of staging and of the other criteria used in reporting end-results would aid considerably in dispelling the confusion that exists, among the medical profession and public alike, on the best way to treat women with potentially curable breast carcinoma.

CHOICE OF PROCEDURE

There are five operations which are performed in the primary treatment of women with potentially curable breast carcinoma (Table 1). The choice, in our opinion, depends upon the clinical and pathological findings demonstrated prior to definitive treatment. But fundamentally, we must accept the fact that neither multicentric involvement of the breast, nor the histologic status of ipsilateral axillary and internal mammary lymph nodes, can be effectively determined prior to study of the surgical specimens by a pathologist.

Partial mastectomy is performed if the patient's medical status is such that she cannot tolerate more extensive surgery. The probable existence of multicentric areas of breast carcinoma and metastatic involvement of lymph nodes is recognized but disregarded in these circumstances. Radiation therapy to the breast and axilla is administered once the wound has healed.

A modified radical mastectomy involves total mastectomy including the pectoral fascia, but preserving the pectoralis major and usually the pectoralis minor. In addition, the axillary nodes and fat and the nodes between the pectoral muscles are removed. It is used when treating non invasive breast carcinoma, or for invasive carcinoma provided that the dominant mass is less than 1 cm in diameter and situated in the

outer half of the breast (Wallace and Champion, 1972; Wanebo et al., 1974). Women over 65 years of age, and those whose general condition makes them borderline operable, should be subjected to a modified radical mastectomy in the presence of invasive carcinoma (Berg and Robbins, 1961; Schottenfeld and Robbins, 1971). Post-operative radiation therapy is frequently used as adjunct therapy in these cases (Table 2).

The majority of women with invasive carcinoma of the breast are, however, subjected to the so-called classical radical mastectomy. The removal of the breast, pectoral muscles and axillary fat and lymph nodes by block dissection meets the objectives of dealing with multicentric deposits of cancer in the breast and with axillary lymph nodes which may or may not be involved. In addition, the nodes beneath the pectoral muscles, which at times do contain metastatic disease, are excised. Studies have shown that there are lymphatics coursing through the muscles which may contain metastatic tumour, and large deep-seated dominant masses spread in this manner all too frequently.

Urban's data documenting the incidence of internal mammary nodal involvement when the dominant mass is located centrally or in the inner half of the breast are impressive (Robbins and Urban, 1972), and his policy of performing an extended radical mastectomy has been adopted by our staff (Urban and Baker, 1952; Urban, 1964; Urban and Marjani, 1971). However, the addition of en bloc dissection of the internal mammary nodes (with small segments of the overlying ribs and adjacent pleura) to the classical radical mastectomy is a formidable procedure, and not recommended unless the surgeon is part of a specialized team. The morbidity and mortality rates at our institution are minimal. If an extended radical mastectomy is not performed for central or inner quadrant invasive lesions we believe that adjunct radiation therapy should be used.

The fifth operation mentioned for patients with breast carcinoma—total mastectomy—has few indications when treating women with potentially curable breast carcinoma. In order to perform an adequate total mastectomy, the tail of the breast, which extends into the adjacent axilla, must be removed and in so doing, inevitably a few nodes will be removed at the same time. We are not aware that morbidity or mortality risks are increased by removing *all* nodes of the lower axilla.

Since positive axillary nodes are found in 17% of cases where the dominant mass is less than 1 cm in diameter (Table 3), we believe that there is real cause to continue our policy of never performing less than a modified radical mastectomy in treating breast carcinoma, unless there are medical contraindications (Robbins, 1974). Our specific criteria of inoperability for cure have not changed since established by Dr. Frank Adair nearly 40 years ago. These are inflammatory carcinoma, positive supraclavicular nodes, a

Table 1 Types of mastectomy practised in the treatment of breast carcinoma

Partial (tylectomy)	Usually the removal of one quadrant of breast
Total	Total breast removal, including the tail of the breast
Modified radical	Removal of total breast, fascia of pectoral muscles, pectoralis minor muscle (sometimes preserved), fat and nodes between muscles and axillary fat and nodes
Radical	Removal of total breast, pectoralis muscles, fat and nodes of axilla
Extended radical	Same as in a radical mastectomy plus en bloc removal of internal mammary nodes

Table 2 Indications for specific surgical procedures in patients with breast carcinoma

Partial mastectomy (tylectomy)	Very poor medical risk patient
Total mastectomy	Poor medical risk patient
Modified radical mastectomy	Fair medical risk patient—especially older women and non-invasive breast cancer including Paget's disease with no mass. Invasive breast cancer in outer half of breast less than 1 cm in diameter
Radical mastectomy	Outer half of breast if lesion is more than 1 cm. Inner half and central lesions if extended radical is contra indicated or considered excessive surgery
Extended radical mastectomy	Central or inner quadrant lesions for invasive carcinoma other than low grade histologically unless medical contra indications exist

swollen ipsilateral arm, distant metastases and poor medical condition.

EVALUATING RESULTS OF PROCEDURES

There is widespread agreement on many of the factors which affect prognosis in breast carcinoma, but unfortunately, "quality control" of the primary treatment (expertise of the surgeon, pathologist and radiation therapist) is rarely considered when comparing survival rates among patients. These quality factors may be just as important in evaluating the use of adjunct chemotherapy or immunotherapy.

In a recent report comparing radical mastectomy and total mastectomy, some of the specimens in the latter group were said to contain as many as 20 nodes while some of the radical mastectomy specimens had only two or three nodes! It is not unusual to have patients referred to our center who supposedly have been subjected to total mastectomy and axillary dissection but who, at the time of secondary procedures, are found to have residual breast tissue and gross quantities of axillary fat and nodes.

The defence of conservative and/or radical surgery must be presented in a standard form and unless this is done, the reported results are not comparable. Rissanen (1969) reports similar ten-year survival figures from partial mastectomy plus radiation therapy as from radical mastectomy. Unfortunately, the two groups of patients were quite different in that there was a preponderance of women with small lesions (less than 2 cm) in the group treated conservatively.

The percentage of patients in each stage of disease must be listed and there must be a specific definition as to the findings included under each stage. Staging should be pathologic–surgical rather than clinical, as there is nearly 33% error in clinical staging of axillary nodes (Robbins and Urban, 1972). The staging system developed by the American Joint Committee for Cancer Staging and End Results is recommended. Series that have an unusually high percentage of Stage 0 and 1 cases are obviously going to report superior survival rates (Mustakallio, 1972).

In evaluating a specific procedure the average number of nodes removed should be given (Urban et al., unpublished). Reports on modified radical, radical or extended radical mastectomy specimens which contain four or five lymph nodes reflect either poor surgical technique or inadequate gross examination of the axillary segment of the specimen. Not only must the total number of nodes be listed, but also the number involved at each of the three levels of the axilla (and in the internal mammary areas when an extended radical procedure was performed). The proportion of microscopic to macroscopic node involvement should be given too. Better survival rates can be expected if there is a relatively lower proportion of cases with more than four nodes or with apical nodes involved, or if there is a relatively higher proportion of microscopic to macroscopic nodal involvement (Huvos et al., 1971).

Ideally, the tumor size as measured in the pathology laboratory should be quoted rather than the size based on clinical judgement, since a considerable discrepancy is often found. A series with an unusually high percentage of small tumors will obviously have better survival figures.

Certain histological types of cancer are less prone to metastasize and carry a good prognosis (Adair et al., 1974), e.g. adenoid cystic, lobular, medullary with lymphoid infiltrate, colloid, papillary and comedo with minimal stromal invasion (Table 4). Series with an above average proportion of these types of cancer will have superior survival rates. Therefore in evaluating any given series, it is important to list the percentage of the different histologic types. For instance, the higher 10 year survival rates in Japanese women may be a reflection

Table 3 Percentage distribution of positive tagged axillary nodes as related to size of lesion (Memorial Hospital, 1940-1943). (Level 1—lower axilla. Level 2—mid axilla. Level 3—apex axilla)

Size (cm)	*No. of patients*	*Positive nodes (%)*	*Level 1 (%)*	*Level 2 (%)*	*Level 3 (%)*	*Percent of all patients*
<1	35	17	11	3	3	3
1-1.9	219	43	17	11	15	18
2-2.9	334	47	18	9	19	28
3-3.9	246	61	18	10	38	21
4-4.9	141	64	14	14	36	12
>5	219	74	12	11	51	18
Total	1,194	54	16	9	29	100

of their unusually high proportion of medullary carcinoma.

An analysis of the cases by nuclear grade, i.e. undifferentiated, moderately differentiated or well differentiated, must be given. Series with a relatively high percentage of well differentiated cancers will have a much better survival rate.

Too often conclusions are drawn as to the efficacy of a procedure based on a series with a relatively small number of cases. Series must contain an adequate number of cases to allow for proper statistical evaluation. Also in evaluating the results of different operations it is important to know where and by whom they were done since survival rates will differ between good and poor techniques regardless of the operation performed. Survival rates are better in centers with highly trained breast surgeons as compared to hospitals where the breast surgery is performed by a surgeon who does only an occasional mastectomy (Table 5).

It is important to note what percentage of cases received adjuvant therapy in addition to surgery. If radiotherapy was used as an adjuvant then the percentage of cases receiving it, and the technique and dosage used must be given. It is uncertain whether either pre- or post-operative radiotherapy increases survival rates but series in which it is used as a routine have a significantly lower percentage of local recurrences (Robbins et al., 1966).

Any use of radiotherapy either alone or in combination with a mastectomy procedure poses the problem of possible complications at a later date. When given to the chest wall after mastectomy, it makes breast reconstruction relatively impossible. As yet, there are no firm conclusions as to the effect on survival rates of adjunct chemotherapy or immunotherapy (see Chapter 6), or of prophylactic castration based on estrogen receptors (see Chapter 8). If they are used this should be so designated in the report.

The cosmetic result of any given procedure is becoming increasingly important in its evaluation. Procedures that preserve the breast in whole or in part must be judged as to whether they cause unsightly scars and breast deformity, or radiation-

Table 4 Per cent relative survival by histologic type (Memorial Hospital, 1940-1943)

Reprinted by permission Editor *Cancer*. (Patients with tumor of unknown size or rare types not tabulated)

Type	*No. of patients*	*Years of survival (%)* 5	10	15	20	25	30
Comedo	66	84	77	74	74	74	74
Lobular	126	57	42	37	34	34	34
Medullary	62	69	68	65	62	58	58
Colloid	37	76	72	62	62	55	55
Papillary	18	89	65	65	65	65	65
Grade I-II duct	245	80	64	56	52	48	45
Grade III-IV duct	696	50	39	33	31	29	29
Grade III-IV duct with plasma cell border	135	64	56	52	49	49	49

Table 5 Per cent survival at 5 years in relation to TNM staging. Memorial Hospital compared with American Joint Committee for Cancer Staging and End Result Reporting*

(Reprinted by permission, Editor *Cancer*)

Stage	*Memorial* No. of patients	5 year survival (%)	*American Joint Committee* No. of patients	5 year survival (%)
I	66	95.6†	385	85
II	176	71.8	1,284	66
III	62	53.0	273	45

* Based upon a review of over 2,500 white patients, under 65 years of age at the time of diagnosis, treated by radical mastectomy between 1940-57. The survival statistics were limited to patients with infiltrating ductal carcinoma and adenocarcinoma, not otherwise specified. The comparison of end results between each group by TNM stage was adjusted for the proportion of cases by each TNM category within each stage.

† $0.02 < P < 0.05$. Stages II and III were not significantly different between each series.

induced texture changes in the skin or in the breast itself. Mastectomy procedures must be evaluated as to whether they avoid the unsightly axillary hollow defect, and as to whether they lend themselves to later breast reconstruction. In this regard, the percentage of cases requiring skin grafting must be listed since it not only detracts from the cosmetic appearance but is also makes breast reconstruction practically impossible.

Arm and shoulder function and the degree of arm edema are important in evaluating the various procedures. Not only must the percentage of patients with significant arm edema be given but it must be based on a uniform rule of measurement (see Chapter 21). In our practice significant arm edema is defined as an increase in the forearm circumference of 3 cm or more as compared to the other side.

Reports of local recurrence rates must include recurrences both in the chest wall, in any remaining breast tissue and in the axilla. The total percentage of local recurrence in patients with potentially curable breast cancer must be subdivided according to the percentage in each stage. Series that report only recurrences in the chest wall and consider those arising in remaining breast tissue or axilla to be new cancers, obviously give a falsely favorable impression.

In comparing surgical techniques, each series must offer an equal chance of curing the patient, and for this reason, full evaluation of the disease extent before treatment is essential. This should include a full medical work-up and a chest radiograph. Preoperative bone scans and/or skeletal surveys are done only on those patients with significant bone pain or those whose tumors are borderline operable, i.e. tumor mass larger than 5 cm with extensive axillary metastases and a moderate amount of skin edema. We found a 19% incidence of bone metastases at 10 years in our 1960 cohort of 304 sequentially treated women who had been designated as potentially curable (Robbins et al., 1972). Many of them first demonstrated bony metastasis more than 5 years after their primary surgery (Figure 1).

The frequency of simultaneous or subsequent breast carcinomas developing in the opposite breast is well documented (Urban, 1969; Robbins et al., 1972). Routine mammography of the opposite breast prior to initial treatment and as an adjunct to long-term follow-up of women with breast carcinoma has become routine in our institution. Urban's data derived from biopsy of the opposite breast have resulted in our acceptance of this procedure as part of the primary treatment for women with noninvasive or invasive breast carcinoma which is considered to be potentially curable.

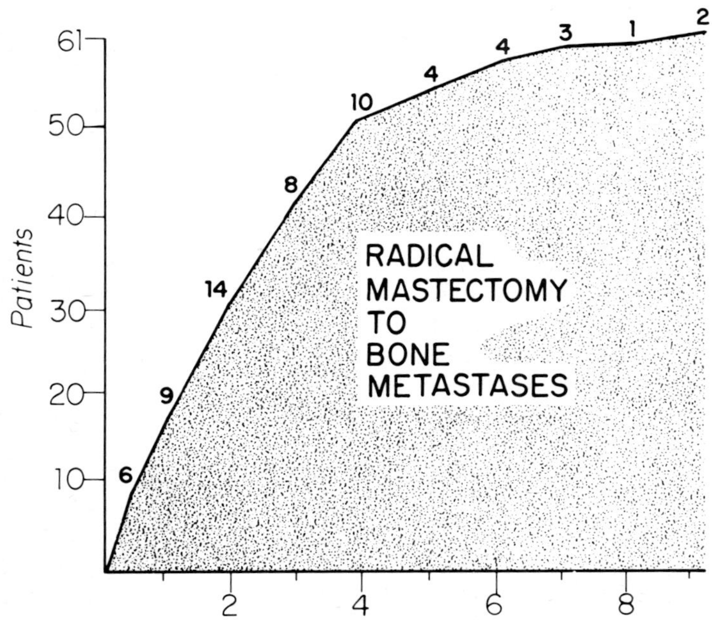

Figure 1. Delay before appearance of bone metastases following radical mastectomy in 304 patients (Memorial Hospital, 1960). (Reprinted by permission, Editor *Cancer.*)

CURRENT SURGICAL PRACTICE

A search of the literature will find support for practically every type of surgical procedure (Crile et al., 1973). However, a recent survey by the New York Metropolitan Breast Cancer Group, an unofficial organization consisting of specialists in different disciplines who have a major interest in treating breast carcinoma, reveals that the vast majority of the surgeons answering the questionnaires have not been stampeded into utilizing less than a total mastectomy plus an axillary dissection. The survey was conducted at several scientific meetings during 1975.

Five hundred surgeons answered the questionnaire. In no way does this document show what is being done by a majority of American surgeons. It does show, however, that those answering believe firstly in the multicentric origin of breast cancer and their inability to recognize its existence prior to treatment. Secondly, they wish to know the histologic status of the axillary nodes, not only in developing an overall basis for prognosticating survival, but also in deciding adjunct therapy, be it post-operative radiation therapy or chemotherapy (Table 6).

The reported surgical procedures varied with the histological type of carcinoma, the location and size of the primary tumor and the status of the axillary nodes (both clinical and histological). Those surgeons who have been in practice for over 20 years tend to perform more radical mastectomies than modified radicals if the nodes are positive. This group also seems to utilize postoperative adjunct therapy (X-ray therapy and chemotherapy) more frequently than the other surgeons.

BASIS OF OUR POLICY

It is our firm opinion that until the presence or absence of multicentric deposits of carcinoma in the breasts and the histologic status of the lymph nodes in the adjacent axilla and internal mammary chain can be demonstrated prior to surgery, one must assume they are involved until proven otherwise. The results of our treatment also form a major basis for our policy.

(1) Presence of multicentric disease

The classic studies of Qualheim and Gall (1957) and Gallager and Martin (1969) have unequivocally demonstrated that carcinoma of the breast is a diffuse process involving the entire breast epithelium. Shah et al. (1973) and Rosen et al. (1975) have recently reported on two groups of women who were treated at Memorial Hospital between 1964 and 1966. In 508 women diagnosed as having potentially curable breast carcinoma, the dominant mass was removed together with a generous portion of grossly normal appearing breast. Usually this amounted to one-fourth of the breast (quadrectomy).

Following subsequent definitive surgery, the mastectomy specimens and their axillary components were subjected to an extensive histologic search for residual area of breast carcinoma. Shah's study demonstrated residual or multicentric carcinoma in 59% of the mastectomy specimens after local excision of the dominant mass plus adjacent grossly normal tissue. If the whole organ study technique of Gallager and Martin had been used, the yield of residual and multicentric mammary carcinoma would have been much higher. The size of the primary lesions was directly related both to the incidence of residual or multicentric carcinoma in the breast and to the presence of axillary node involvement.

Rosen et al. (1975) recently reported a study to determine, by pathologic examination, how often carcinoma might remain in the breast and axilla after partial mastectomy. The operation was simulated in 204 complete mastectomy specimens removed

Table 6 Surgical procedures used for breast cancer patients, as reported by 500 surgeons (see text)

Procedure	*In situ lobular and purely intraductal*	*Low grade invasive carcinoma*	*Infiltrating duct carcinoma* Inner or center	*Outer half*
	(%)	*(%)*	*(%)*	*(%)*
Partial mastectomy and X-ray therapy	2.0	1.75	0.3	0
Subcutaneous mastectomy	6.0	2.25	0	0
Total mastectomy*	50.0	50.0	8.2	4.0
Modified radical*	34.0	34.0	44.0	67.0
Radical mastectomy*	10.0	10.0	44.0	29.0
Extended radical*	0	0	3.5	0

* With or without adjunct therapy.

because of the presence of invasive carcinoma. As far as could be determined on gross examination, the entire primary lesion was included in the quadrant which was excised in the simulated procedure.

Among 100 women with primary lesions less than 2 cm in diameter, 26% had carcinoma in the breast which remained after simulated partial mastectomy and 6% also had axillary node metastases. When the primary lesion was more than 2 cm in diameter, 38% of patients had carcinoma in the residual breast after simulated partial mastectomy, and 29% also had axillary metastases. After simulated partial mastectomy, carcinoma was found in the residual breast in 80% of patients with lesions in the sub-areolar area, in contrast with 25-35% of patients where the primary carcinoma was in one of the four quadrants.

None of the nine patients with medullary or colloid carcinomas smaller than 2 cm had axillary metastases or carcinoma in the breast outside of the primary quadrant. The findings also suggested that a familial history of breast carcinoma, or a large primary lesion may be associated more often with multifocal disease. However, factors such as age at diagnosis, axillary status, and the mammogram report could not be correlated with the presence of carcinoma in the breast tissue after the primary had been removed by a simulated partial mastectomy.

(2) Determination of axillary nodal status

With few exceptions surgeons admit the fallibility of clinical assessment of the malignant status of axillary nodes. Atkins et al. (1972) report a 25% error in determining axillary nodal status in patients with Stage I and II breast carcinoma. Wallace and Champion (1972) also confirm the inadequacy of clinical staging of axillary nodes. Rosen et al. (1975) reported 31% false negatives and 40% false positives for tumors of pathologic size less than 2 cm in diameter, and 48% false negatives and 24% false positives for tumors larger than 2 cm.

The exploration of the axilla at the time of surgery has been suggested as an effective method of determining the histologic status of the nodes. A review of pathology reports at Memorial Hospital revealed that estimates from gross examination by the pathologists dissecting the mastectomy specimens differed from their microscopic findings in 25% of cases. This is not surprising since microscopic nodal involvement may be limited to a 1-2 mm area and on the other hand hyperplastic nodes of 2 cm diameter may show no metastatic involvement.

A few investigators have suggested a beneficial effect on the host resistance from leaving axillary nodes at the time of surgery (Fisher and Fisher, 1972). Hammond and Rolley (1970) have failed to confirm that such a procedure in mice protects the host against tumor growth, and the better long-term survival among women with micrometatases compared to those with macroscopic axillary metastasis (Huvos et al., 1971) substantiates Hammond's observations. It seems unrealistic to expect major tumor destructive capabilities from such a minor portion of a patient's reticulo-endothelial system.

It is essential to know the true status of the axillary lymph nodes before embarking on an adjunct chemotherapy program after primary treatment. Until we can accurately determine the involvement status of lymph nodes without their removal, it seems that the use of the only accurate diagnostic procedure (histological study) must be continued.

One cannot assume that small invasive cancers are not capable of metastasizing to adjacent axillary nodes. The Memorial Hospital (1940-43 series of 1,458 patients reported by Adair et al. (1974) and that reported by Shah et al. (1973) present an almost identical incidence of positive axillary nodes in relation to the size of the dominant area of invasive carcinoma. Among patients with lesions less than 1 cm in diameter (pathologist measurements) 17% had positive nodes (Table 3). The percentage increases with the size of the lesion and 74% of patients with lesions greater than 5 cm were found to have positive nodes. Thus, even in the so-called "early cases", one frequently finds evidence of axillary metastasis.

If therefore, one is to achieve maximum local control, an attempt must be made to thoroughly remove the axillary fat and nodes. Many of these involved nodes have only microscopic involvement and an accurate clinical evaluation of the axillary contents is not possible.

(3) Results of treatment

The 1973 TNM Classification (see Appendix) was utilized by Schottenfeld et al. (1975) in a report on 304 potentially curable patients with invasive breast carcinoma who were treated at Memorial Hospital during 1960. We believe that these data represent the results of selecting a treatment regimen to fit the individual situation (Table 7).

There were 66 patients (22%) classified under Stage I, 176 (58%) under Stage II, and 62 (20%) under Stage III (Table 8). The standard radical operation was employed in most patients, and post-

operative radiation therapy was administered to 89 patients who had either inner quadrant lesions or more than a single positive axillary node. There were 82 patients (27%) in whom the nodal status was misclassified clinically, the ratio of false positives being 26%, and of false negatives, 27%.

The overall 10-year survival was 59.7%. The 10-year end-results diminished significantly in relation to advancing clinical stage of disease, namely 90.9% (±6.9%) for Stage I, 57.1% (±7.3%) for Stage II and 33.9% (±11.8%) for Stage III patients. () indicates 95% confidence limits. Increase in tumor size and more extensive microscopically proven axillary disease were each associated independently with diminishing survival rates at 5 and 10 years. The 10-year survival in patients with pathologically negative axillary nodes was 71.5%, and in patients with pathologically positive axillary nodes, 48.3% (Table 9).

Quality of survival is a major consideration in evaluating a specific treatment regimen for breast carcinoma. The Breast Service at Memorial Hospital has a structured rehabilitation program for post-mastectomy patients (Schottenfeld and Robbins, 1970) and during the past 6 years, this has been expanded by the involvement of long term post-mastectomy patients, social workers, physical therapists, and nurses (Schmid et al., 1974). Both physical and emotional readaptation to society are being evaluated (Winick et al., 1975). Women with personality defects will probably react poorly to breast cancer regardless of what procedure is performed but a program stressing "intelligent concern, not unreasonable fear" has been quite successful.

Shaw (1968) reports on a survey of quality of survival among his personal series of 115 patients undergoing radical mastectomy. He stated that minor symptoms were fairly common but serious disability was rare. Atkins stated that his patients subjected to tylectomy and radiation therapy had problems of

Table 7 Type of treatment and TNM staging of breast cancer

(Reprinted by permission, Editor *Cancer*)

	Stage I		*Stage II*		*Stage III*	
*Procedure**	*No.*	*(%)*	*No.*	*(%)*	*No.*	*(%)*
Total	66	100	176	100	62	100
Standard radical	57	86	151	86	53	85
Extended radical	6	9	14	8	5	8
Modified radical	1	2	5	3	3	5
Total (simple)	2	3	6	3	1	2

* Post-operative radiation therapy was administered to 4 (6%) of patients with Stage I, 55 (31%) with Stage II and 30 (48%) with Stage III.

Table 8 Summary of end results at 10 years by TNM stage of breast cancer

(Reprinted by permission, Editor *Cancer*)

	Stage I		*Stage II*		*Stage III*		*Total*	
	No.	*(%)*	*No.*	*(%)*	*No.*	*(%)*	*No.*	*(%)*
Total number at risk	66	100.0	175†	100.0	62	100.0	303	100.0
Alive at end of interval	60	90.9 (3.5)*	100	57.1 (3.7)*	21	33.9 (6.0)*	181	59.7
1. Without clinical evidence of disease	59	89.4	92	52.6	18	29.0	169	55.7
2. With clinical evidence of disease	1	1.5	8	4.5	3	4.9	12	4.0
Died during interval	6	9.1	75	42.9	41	66.1	122	40.3
1. Of breast cancer	2	3.0	58	33.1	31	50.0	91	30.0
2. Of other causes	3	4.6	17	9.8	9	14.5	29	9.6
3. Unknown cause	1	1.5	—	—	1	1.6	2	0.7

()* Standard error of survival rate, expressed in per cent, as derived by the non-actuarial method.

† Corrected for 1 case lost to follow-up

readapting, similar to those of other patients undergoing major surgery (Atkins et al., 1972). We believe that longevity is far more important than the preservation of a major symbol of feminimity—the breast.

Dr. Frank Adair's 30 year report (Adair et al., 1974) is an example of standardized reporting of long-term survival in women who had quality control in their management. Only 6% of the patients were lost to follow-up. Both this report and that of Schottenfeld and Robbins (1970) noted a marked drop in survival of patients in all categories between 5 and 10 years after surgery. Credit for 30 year survival cannot be given to surgery alone, for there were surviving patients in each category except those with primary tumors larger than 5 cm and with metastatic apical nodes (Figure 2). One must relate prolonged survival in some cases to host resistance or other

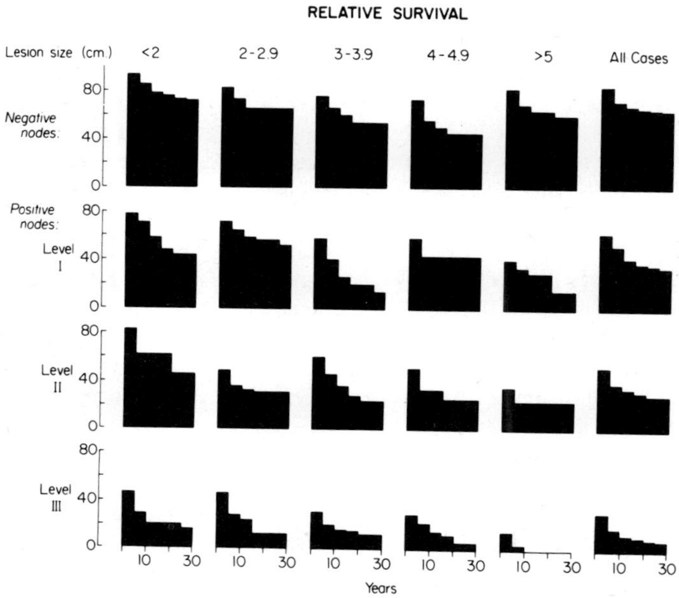

Figure 2. Thirty-year prospective study of potentially curable breast cancer treated by radical mastectomy in 1,458 patients (Memorial Hospital, 1940-73). (Reprinted by permission, Editor *Cancer.*)

Table 9 Survival at 5 and 10 years according to clinical tumor size and pathological extent of axillary disease
(Reprinted by permission, Editor *Cancer*)

	Primary tumor size											
	2 cm or less			*2-5 cm*			*5 cm +*			*Total†*		
		Survival (%)			*Survival (%)*			*Survival (%)*			*Survival (%)*	
Axillary nodes	*No.*	*5 yr.*	*10 yr.*	*No.*	*5 yr.*	*10 yr.*	*No.*	*5 yr.*	*10 yr.*	*No.*	*5 yr.*	*10 yr.*
Negative	55	90.0	81.8	72	87.3	65.1	20	66.7	44.4	147	86.2	71.5
Positive, Level I only	18	94.4	72.2	27	81.5	74.1	14	61.5	38.5	59	80.7	65.1
Positive, Levels II and/or III	7	—*	—*	63	46.9	28.1	28	43.3	36.7	98	45.8	30.6
Total	80	91.8	79.4	162	70.6	57.3	62	55.0	40.2	304	72.7	62.2

* Number of cases not adequate to provide reliable survival ratios

† If we apply the criteria of the TNM system but use the pathological node status, then survival at 5 and 10 years respectively was: Stage I (90.9%), 81.8%), Stage II (87.0%, 68.1%) and Stage III (50.9%, 34.5%). When compared with the statistics by clinical stage in Figure 2, survival by pathologic stage was less for Stage I, greater for Stage II and unaltered for Stage III.

Table 10 Relative survival according to extent of disease at the time of primary treatment

Extent of disease	*1940-43 (1,281)* 5 years	10 years	*1950-55 (2,168)* 5 years	10 years	*1960-65 (2,212)* 5 years	10 years
	(%)	(%)	(%)	(%)	(%)	(%)
Negative nodes	81.7	72.3	85.8	77.4	84.6	76.6
Positive nodes	45.5	35.1	51.2	34.9	57.7	51.7
Total	61.6	51.6	66.2	53.8	74.2	63.9

unexplained phenomena, but the size of the primary lesion and the extent of axillary metastasis seem to be the predominant factors in survival.

Some of the proponents of conservative treatment for patients with potentially curable breast carcinoma make much of reports that seem to indicate the lack of improvement of survival rates over the past 50 years (Crile et al., 1973). Our figures (Table 10) show that although control of the disease has not improved significantly among patients with negative axillary nodes, there has been an increased survival rate in those women with positive nodes treated in the sixties compared to those treated in 1940 and 1950. We have also noted that the proportion of primarily inoperable patients has dropped from 12% in 1940 to 6% in 1974 and that there has been a decrease in the extent of axillary node involvement found at the time of surgery.

The carcinogenic potential of gamma radiation is accepted, and the profession has been alerted to this by epidemiologists and radiation therapists. The radiation exposure resulting from the utilization of mammography for screening women for minimal breast carcinoma is not inconsiderable and although new techniques are under investigation we do not know the dangers from multiple mammographies over long periods of time, especially in young women. All agree that more information is necessary if we are to promote this valuable method of detecting pre-clinical breast carcinoma. If this is so, should we also question the risks involved in applying full therapeutic doses of gamma radiation to women with pre-clinical or small clinical (< 2 cm) breast carcinomas?

TWO STAGE SURGERY

It has been suggested that there may be some advantage in permitting a time interval of several days between a biopsy procedure in suspected breast cancer and the definitive surgery. Several reports have now confirmed that it makes no difference to the survival rate, provided that the time interval is less than 3 weeks and post-biopsy infection of the breast does not occur. We are sometimes forced to follow this procedure when the pathologist is uncertain of the diagnosis from the frozen section, and we have found that most of these patients come under emotional stress and their families are equally distraught.

A symposium was held recently under the auspices of the American Cancer Society and was attended by nearly 500 women who had undergone mastectomy. The vast majority had had the biopsy and definitive surgery as part of a single surgical procedure. After the two-stage concept had been explained, all but 20 of the 500 women voted in favor of the single procedure method, provided a definitive diagnosis had been established by the frozen section report.

Nevertheless, it is imperative that the health professionals involved in the management of women undergoing breast surgery recognize the emotional impact of the situation. Most of all, the procedures contemplated must be clearly understood by the patient and her family. To assist this we have produced a 5-minute phonograph record explaining what the patient can expect during her stay in the hospital. This is given to the patient at her initial visit and she takes it home where her family is able to hear what we have told her. This can avoid considerable misunderstanding later.

CONCLUSIONS

Our patients with Stage I breast carcinomas treated by radical, modified radical and extended radical mastectomies have between 70 to 80% 10 year crude survival rates. We will not revert to the regimens of partial mastectomy plus radiation therapy until we are satisfied that there is a reasonable probability that this form of treatment will provide a comparable length and quality of survival for those so treated.

Perhaps well controlled studies will disprove our beliefs, but data presented to date are not of sufficient depth. To be acceptable, survival times must be at least 10 years, not 5 years. The statistical methods of reporting must be identical, and adequate numbers of patients with similar stages of diseases must be compared. There must be "quality control" not only of the surgery, but also of the pathologic dissection of the specimens, and adjunct therapy.

Such controlled studies may well sacrifice a generation of women but scientifically it does have merit. Meanwhile we have found that women usually will accept conventional treatment, if their primary physician and surgeon take the time to explain the frequency of multicentric existence of breast cancer, the inadequacy of clinical diagnosis of the status of the axillary lymph nodes and the possibility of the carcinogenic properties of gamma radiation.

APPENDIX

Summary of TNM clinical classification for invasive breast cancer.*

T (Primary Tumor)

T0: No demonstrable tumor in the breast.

T1†: Tumor 2 cm or less in its greatest dimension.
(a) With no fixation to underlying pectoral fascia and/or muscle.
(b) With fixation to underlying pectoral fascia and/or muscle.

T2†: Tumor more than 2 cm but not more than 5 cm in its greatest dimension.
(a) With no fixation to underlying pectoral fascia and/or muscle.
(b) With fixation to underlying pectoral fascia and/or muscle.

T3†: Tumor more than 5 cm in its greatest dimension.
(a) With no fixation to underlying pectoral fascia and/or muscle.
(b) With fixation to underlying pectoral fascia and/or muscle.

T4: Tumor of any size with direct extension to chest wall or skin. (Note: Chest wall includes ribs, intercostal muscles, and serratus anterior muscle, but not pectoral muscle.)
(a) With fixation to chest wall.
(b) With edema (including peau d'orange), ulceration of the skin of the breast, or satellite skin nodules confined to the same breast.
(c) Both of above.

N (Regional lymph nodes)

N0: No palpable homolateral axillary nodes.

N1: Movable homolateral axillary nodes.
(a) Nodes not considered to contain growth.
(b) Nodes considered to contain growth.

N2: Homolateral axillary nodes considered to contain growth and fixed to one another or to other structures.

N3: Homolateral supraclavicular or infraclavicular nodes considered to contain growth or edema of the arm.

M (Distant metastasis)

M0: No evidence of distant metastasis.

M1: Distant metastasis present, including skin involvement beyond the breast area.

CLINICAL STAGE-GROUPING

Stage	Groups	
Stage I	T1a, N0 or $N1_a$ T1b, N0 or $N1_a$	M0
Stage II	T0, $N1_b$ T1a, $N1_b$ T1b, $N1_b$ T2a or T2b, N0, $N1_a$ or $N1_b$	M0
Stage III	Any T3 with any N Any T4 with any N Any T with N2 Any T with N3	M0
Stage IV	Any T, and N with M1	

* Clinical staging system for carcinoma of the breast. The American Joint Committee for Cancer Staging and End Results Reporting, September, 1973.

† Dimpling of the skin, nipple retraction, or any other skin changes except those in T4b may occur in T1, T2 or T3 without affecting the classification.

REFERENCES

Adair, F., Berg, J., Joubert, L. and Robbins, G. F. (1974). Long-term follow-up of breast cancer patients: The 30-year report. *Cancer 33,* 1145.

Atkins, H., Klugman, D. J. and White, A. B. (1972). Treatment of early breast cancer: A report after ten years of clinical trials. *British Medical Journal 2,* 423.

Berg, W. and Robbins, G. F. (1961). Modified mastectomy for older poor risk patients. *Surgery, Gynecology and Obstetrics 115,* 631.

Crile, G., Jr., Esselstyn, C. B., Jr. and Hoer, S. O. (1973). Partial mastectomy for carcinoma of the breast. *Surgery, Gynecology and Obstetrics 136,* 929.

Fisher, B. and Fisher, E. R. (1972). Studies concerning the regional lymph nodes in cancer: Maintenance of immunity. *Cancer 29,* 1496.

Gallager, H. S. and Martin, J. E. (1969). The study of mammary carcinoma by mammography and whole organ sectioning. *Cancer 23,* 855.

Hammond, W. G. and Rolley, R. T. (1970). Retained regional lymph nodes: Effect on metastasis and recurrence after tumor removal. *Cancer 25,* 368.

Huvos, A. G., Hutter, R. V. P. and Berg, J. W. (1971). Significance of axillary micrometastasis. *Annals of Surgery 44,* 173.

Mustakallio, S. (1972). Conservative treatment of breast carcinoma: Review of 25 years of follow-up. *Clinical Radiology 23,* 110.

Qualheim, R. E. and Gall, E. A. (1957). Breast carcinoma with multiple sites of origin. *Cancer 10,* 460.

Rissaner, P. M. (1969). Comparison of conservative and radical surgery combined with radiotherapy in the treatment of Stage I carcinoma of the breast. *British Journal Radiology 42,* 423.

Robbins, G. F., Lucas, J. C., Fracchia, A. A., Farrow, J. H. and Chu, F. C. H. (1966). An evaluation of post-operative prophylactic radiation therapy in breast cancer. *Surgery, Gynecology and Obstetrics 122,* 979.

Robbins, G. F. and Urban, J. A. (1972). Axillary and internal mammary lymph nodes in patients with potentially curable breast cancer. *Memorial Clinical Bulletin 1,* 127.

Robbins, G. F., Knapper, W. J., Barrie, J., Kripalani, I. and Lawrence, J. (1972). Metastatic bone disease developing in patients with potentially curable breast cancer. *Cancer 29,* 1702.

Robbins, G. F. (1974). The rationale for the treatment of women with potentially curable breast carcinoma. *Surgical Clinics of North America 54,* 793.

Rosen, P. P., Fracchia, A. A., Urban, J. A., Schottenfeld, D. and Robbins, G. F. (1975). "Residual" mammary carcinoma following simulated partial mastectomy. *Cancer 35,* 739.

Schmid, W., Kiss, M., Hilbert, L. (1974). The team approach to rehabilitation after mastectomy. *AORN Journal 19,* 821.

Schottenfeld, D. and Robbins, G. F. (1970). Quality of survival among patients who have had radical mastectomy. *Cancer 26,* 650.

Schottenfeld, D. and Robbins, G. F. (1971). Breast cancer in elderly women. *Geriatrics 26,* 121.

Schottenfeld, D., Nash, A., Robbins, G. F. and Beattie, E. J. (1975). Ten year results of the treatment of primary operable breast carcinoma: A summary of 304 patients evaluated by the T.N.M. System. *Cancer 38,* 1001.

Shah, J. P., Rosen, P. and Robbins, G. F. (1973). Pitfalls of local excision in the treatment of carcinoma of the breast. *Surgery, Gynecology and Obstetrics 136,* 721.

Shaw, R. E. (1968). Incidence of disability in long-term survivors following radical mastectomy. *Bulletin de la Société Internationale de Chirurgie,* 6.

Urban, J. A. and Baker, H. W. (1952). Radical mastectomy with en bloc resection of the internal mammary lymph node chain. *Cancer 5,* 992.

Urban, J. A. (1964). Surgical excision of internal mammary nodes for breast cancer. *British Journal of Surgery 51,* 209.

Urban, J. A. and Marjani, M. A. (1971). Significance of internal mammary lymph nodes metastasis in breast cancer. *American Journal of Roentgenology 111,* 130.

Urban, J. A., Rosen, P. P. and Mike, V. (unpublished data). Joint symposium on breast carcinoma with National Cancer Center Hospital of Tokyo.

Urban, J. A. (1969). Biopsy of the "normal" breast in treating breast cancer. *Surgical Clinics of North America 49,* 2; 291.

Wallace, I. W. J. and Champion, H. R. (1972). Axillary nodes in breast cancer. *Lancet 1,* 271.

Wanebo, H. J., Huvos, A. G. and Urban, J. A. (1974). Treatment of minimal breast cancer. *Cancer 33,* 349.

Winick, L., Robbins, G. F., Trachtenberg, J. and Holz, S. (1975, unpublished data). Physical and psychological readjustment after mastectomy, an evaluation of Memorial Hospital's program.

Chapter

4

GEORGE CRILE, Jr.

The Place for Partial Mastectomy in Selected Cases

INTRODUCTION

All *prospective* randomized trials between various treatments of clinical Stage I breast cancer have shown that, regardless of what treatment is used, there is no difference in survival. Ultraradical operations are no more effective than radical ones. Radical operations are no more effective than simple ones with radiation therapy added. Simple operations with radiation therapy added are no more effective than simple mastectomy alone with treatment of the axilla deferred until the nodes show signs of progressive enlargement. Radical mastectomy and radiation therapy give no better results than partial mastectomy and radiation therapy.

In the experience of the Cleveland Clinic, a retrospective matching of patients treated by partial mastectomy alone, with patients who had tumors of the same size and clinical stage treated by modified radical or total mastectomy, showed no differences in survival or in the incidence of local recurrence (Crile, 1975).

Because of this world-wide experience, the policy of the Cleveland Clinic has been to explain to the patient that in terms of survival, there is no proof that one method of treatment is better or worse than another. However, if any operation less than a mastectomy and axillary dissection is employed and if radiation therapy is not given, there is an 8% chance that the tumor will appear later in nodes and require an axillary dissection. There is also a 6% chance of local recurrence in the breast which will require mastectomy. This total 14% chance of requiring a secondary operation is about the same as that of developing local recurrence after radical mastectomy.

Since complete protection against the development of a new cancer in the same breast and nearly complete protection against axillary metastases can be provided by removing the breast and axillary nodes, this is recommended as the treatment of choice. But, if loss of the breast is an overpowering consideration, we feel that in selected cases the breast can be saved without diminishing the chance of cure. However, the cancer must be small, apparently

localized, and situated in the periphery of the breast. The absence of axillary involvement is determined by operative staging, i.e. palpation of the axillary nodes with the axilla open, and biopsy when in doubt.

Each patient is told that the partial mastectomy must be viewed as an excisional biopsy. The pathologist will examine the specimen and if there is no cancer scattered through the tissue, out to the lines of resection, nothing more need be done. But if there is cancer all through the specimen, as is found in nearly 15% of the cases, mastectomy will be advised at a later date.

CLINICAL BASIS FOR POLICY

Because of differences in the extent of the disease at the time of operation, the only valid comparisons that can be made are between scientifically controlled trials. After being examined and accepted into a trial, the patients are assigned at random to have one type of treatment or another. This method has been used extensively in Europe for nearly 20 years and recently has been used in this country under the auspices of the National Cancer Institute. The following is a resumé of the results of the trials to date.

1. Radical mastectomy vs. simple mastectomy and radiation therapy

There have been four trials comparing radical mastectomy and simple mastectomy and radiation therapy (Table 1). In none was there any advantage shown for the radical operation.

The next significant trial was that of Forrest (1974). In one group simple mastectomy was done with biopsy of the axillary nodes and radiation therapy was given only if the nodes showed cancer. In the other group, radical mastectomy was done and again radiation was given only if cancer was found in the nodes. So far, 243 patients are in the trial and to date (7 years) there is no difference in the survival of the two groups.

Table 1 **Reported trials comparing radical mastectomy with simple mastectomy and radiation therapy**

Series	*No. of patients*
Hamilton et al. (1974)	498
Burn (1974)	195
Kaae and Johansen (1968)*	404
Brinkley and Haybittle (1971)†	204

* Extended radical mastectomy.

† Stage II cases showed 10% better survival for simple mastectomy and radiation.

Perhaps the most dramatic of all the trials is a national study done under the auspices of the British Cancer Research Campaign (Murray, 1974). This trial is between simple mastectomy and radiation therapy, and simple mastectomy alone. Regardless of whether or not the axillary nodes are palpably involved, they may be given no treatment for at least four months. After that, if they persist and are growing, they can be removed or irradiated. Already 2,000 patients are in the trial, and at 5 years there is no difference in survival rates between the groups, although post-operative radiation reduces the local recurrence rate (see Chapter 7).

So far the trials have proven that radical mastectomy gives no better results than simple mastectomy with radiation therapy and that simple mastectomy alone, deferring treatment to such a time as nodes may appear, gives similar results to simple mastectomy and post-operative radiation. Since the results of simple mastectomy and radiation are the same as those of radical mastectomy, it is obvious that simple mastectomy alone, with treatment of the axilla deferred until the cancer appears, would be found to give at least as good results as radical mastectomy.

2. Results of partial mastectomy

Vera Peters (1975) at Toronto has compared the results of partial mastectomy and radiation therapy with those of radical mastectomy and radiation for periods of time up to 30 years. The survival curves of the 217 patients in each group are identical. Peters concludes "that radical methods are not in the best interest of the patient. Prophylactic radiation and prophylactic mastectomy could, with few exceptions, be eliminated in early breast cancer".

Similar results were reported by Taylor and his associates (1971) who found no difference in survival between patients treated by "sector mastectomy" and that of patients treated by radical mastectomy. The same conclusion was drawn by the distinguished British surgeon, Sir Arthur Porritt, who studied 156 patients treated by local excision (Porritt, 1964).

As early as 1954, Mustakallio in Finland reported results of treatment by local excision and radiation therapy that were comparable to those obtained by radical operations. Mustakallio (1972) subsequently reported these cases with a 25-year follow-up. Again the results were comparable to those after radical operations.

In a retrospective study of 96 patients treated by

local excision with or without radiation therapy, Drs. Leslie Wise, York-Mason and the distinguished American pathologist, Lauren Ackerman (1971), reached the same conclusion. The cases were matched by stage, age, size and histology with patients treated by radical mastectomy with or without radiation. The authors concluded that "There was no significant difference between the 5 year, 10 year and ultimate survival rates for the local excision and radical mastectomy series".

A similar but randomized study was made by Sir Hedley Atkins and his associates (1972) in 370 patients followed for 5 to 10 years. When the axillary nodes were not palpably involved the survival rate of the patients treated by partial mastectomy was similar. When nodes were involved, the survival of patients treated by partial mastectomy and radiation was worse. This may have been because the radiation therapy was given with older equipment and in low doses, because the results of Brinkley and Haybittle (1971) indicate that when nodes are involved, the survival rate, when treatment is by modern type of therapy, is no worse following simple mastectomy and radiation (see Chapter 7).

It is clear from these trials that in terms of survival there is no difference between the various methods of treatment. The same is true of the American trial now under the direction of Dr. Bernard Fisher and the National Cancer Institute. To date radical mastectomy has shown no advantage over simpler treatments that do not remove the axillary nodes (Fisher, 1975).

3. Experience at the Cleveland Clinic

The Cleveland Clinic experience, although not a randomized trial, has compared the survival rate of patients treated during the past 20 years by partial mastectomy with or without radiation therapy, with those matched for size and clinical evidence of nodal involvement, but treated by total mastectomy with or without axillary dissection or radiation. At both 5 and 10 years there were fewer patients dead of cancer in the group treated by partial mastectomy, and also fewer local recurrences (Crile, 1975).

Experience at the Cleveland Clinic with 355 Stage I and II patients seen between 1957 and 1963 and followed from 10 to 15 years was recently reported in detail (Crile, 1975). None were excluded because of age or debility. Radiation therapy was used mainly in patients with advanced disease but also in 13% of patients with Stage I disease because the tumours were large or in the medial quadrant. Of the total, 41% of the patients were treated by modified radical, 47% by simple mastectomy, 11% by partial mastectomy and 1% by radical mastectomy. Only 2% were lost to follow up before 10 years and counted as dead.

The 10 year survival rate was 45%, the same as that reported after radical mastectomy in the 30 or more cancer centers and university hospitals that are cooperating with Fisher and his associates (1975) in the National Surgical Adjuvant Breast Project. (They report that 45.8% of patients under age 70 survived for 10 years.) It is noteworthy that the 5 year survival rate for patients in Stage III and IV (inoperable) was only 14% at 5 years and 0% at 10 years.

Failure to remove or irradiate axillary nodes at the time of operation on the breast did not reduce the chances of survival (Crile, 1975). There were 28 patients who at operation were thought to have no nodes involved but were treated by modified radical mastectomy and the pathologist found nodal involvement. Eighteen of these lived for 5 years and eight lived 10 years (64% and 29% respectively). In 24 patients, who at the time of operation were thought to have no involvement of nodes and therefore had no axillary dissection or radiation therapy, node involvement appeared later and was treated by axillary dissection or radiation. Eighteen of these lived 5 years and eight lived 10 years (75% and 33% respectively).

The incidence of local recurrence was 5.6% after 10 years which is lower than in most reports of radical operations. Even after partial mastectomy the incidence of local recurrences was only 7%. (If the axilla had not been treated by surgery or irradiation the first appearance of cancer in the axilla was not counted as a recurrence.) This may be attributed to the fact that after simple operations there is no damage to the blood and lymph supply of the skin and hence no tendency to trap cancer cells in the field and to stimulate their growth by tissue damage (Crile, 1965).

Forty-two patients were treated by partial mastectomy. Nine had axillary dissections at the time of the mastectomy, usually in continuity with it, 11 had cobalt teletherapy while 22 had no treatment of the axilla at the time of the first operation. The 42 patients treated by partial mastectomy were matched by size and clinical evidence of nodal involvement with a similar number of patients treated by modified radical or total mastectomy. It was found that the 10 year survival rate of patients treated by total mastectomy was a little higher than that of the patients treated by partial mastectomy but this was presumably because of selection of older and debilitated patients for partial mastectomy. More

patients died of their cancer after total than after partial mastectomy (16 and 14 respectively).

The survival rates in two groups of patients seen in 1955, 1956 and 1959 were compared. One group of 69 patients was treated by simple mastectomy or local excision, and the other, with 62 patients, was treated by radical or modified radical mastectomy. Between 2 and 11 years later there was a clear advantage to the patients treated by the simple operations (33/69 being alive at 10 years compared to 21/62). But at 15 years the proportion of survivors was the same. This was because of several patients with small Stage I cancers treated by simple operations, who died of distant metastases between 10 and 15 years, but without evidence of local recurrence.

DISCUSSION

Because well educated and intelligent patients tend to use the most modern diagnostic tests, to pay attention to early signs and symptoms of disease, and to consult their doctors early, there is often a difference between the stage of the disease at presentation, depending on whether the patient is private or first seen in an out-patient clinic. The stage distribution of the disease also differs from one institution to another.

For example, Van Heerden and his colleagues report that the incidence of patients with axillary node involvement at the Mayo Clinic fell from nearly 70% in 1910 to 30% in 1974 and that as a consequence, using the same treatment, the 5 to 10 year survival rates have increased 10% in each decade. But at the Cleveland Clinic, the incidence of axillary node involvement is not 30% but more than 50%, a situation that makes it impossible to compare the results of treatment at the two institutions. By the same token, many of the high survival rates reported in private practice are due to the fact that most of the patients come earlier in the disease than do those who come to public institutions.

Perhaps the greatest difficulty in comparing the results of treatment in the hands of different surgeons is the selection of cases. No surgeon operates on all patients who consult him, because in at least 20% of the patients the disease has already spread out of the field of operation and cannot be cured by surgery. The selection of these cases introduces a problem that makes comparisons of results impossible.

One surgeon may operate on many patients that most surgeons would consider inoperable, and as a result his figures may show a very low 10 year survival rate. Another may consider inoperable many patients whose disease, although moderately advanced, most surgeons would consider operable. This surgeon will have an inordinately high 10 year survival rate—60% in the case of Dr. Haagensen, for example, as compared to 43% for patients in the cancer registries of Connecticut, Massachusetts and California, and 45% (45.8% in patients under age 70) for those in the National Surgical Adjuvant Breast Project (Fisher et al., 1975). The 10 year survival rate of the Cleveland Clinic is the same as that of the NSABP, namely 45%.

One way to judge how selective a surgeon has been in deciding which patients to operate on is by observing the survival rate of the patients he considers *inoperable*. If this is high, it means he has rejected many bad risk cases. If it is low, it means that the surgeon has accepted many high risk cases. For example, Dr. Haagensen's 5 year survival rate for patients judged inoperable after triple biopsy is more than 50% (Guttman, 1962) whereas the Cleveland Clinic's survival rate for inoperable patients is only 9%.

CONCLUSION

Since patients' survival depends less on the type of treatment than on the stage of the disease, it is urged that the Halsted type of radical mastectomy be abandoned, and that women be assured that a diagnosis of breast cancer does not inevitably imply surgical mutilation. The knowledge that in selected cases, diagnosed early, the breast can often be saved, should provide an incentive to women to examine themselves, have periodic mammograms and to consult their physicians at the first suspicion of disease. This in turn should result in a significant decrease in the incidence of death from breast cancer.

REFERENCES

Atkins, H. Hayward, J. L. and Klugman, D. J. (1972). Treatment of early breast cancer: ten years of clinical trial. *Brit. Med. J. 20,* 423.

Brinkley, D. and Haybittle, J. L. (1971). Treatment of stage 2 carcinoma of the female breast. *Lancet 2,* 1086.

Burn, J. I. (1974). Early breast cancer: the Hammersmith trial. *Brit. J. Surg. 61,* 762.

Crile, G., Jr. (1965). Rationale for cutting thick skin flaps in operations for cancer of the breast. *Cancer 18,* 795.

Crile, G., Jr. (1975). Results of conservative treatment of

breast cancer at 10 and 15 years. *Ann. Surg. 181,* 26.

Fisher, B., Slack, N., Katrych, D. and Wolmark, N. (1975). Carcinoma of the breast—evaluating surgical adjuvant chemotherapy. *Surg. Gyn. and Obst. 140,* 528.

Forrest, A. P. M., Roberts, M. M. and Preece, P. et al. (1974). The Cardiff–St. Mary's Trial *Brit. J. Surg. 61,* 766.

Guttman, R. J. (1962). Survival and result after 2 meV irradiation in the treatment of primary operable carcinoma of the breast. *Cancer 15,* 383.

Hamilton, T., Langlands, A. O. and Prescott, R. J. (1974). Treatment of operable cancer of the breast in S.E. Scotland. *Brit. J. Surg. 61,* 759.

Kaae, S. and Johansen, H. (1968). In *Prognostic Factors in Breast Cancer,* p. 93 (Eds A. P. M. Forrest and P. B. Kunkler). Edinburgh: E. & S. Livingstone.

Murray, J. G. (1974). Cancer Research Campaign breast study. *Brit. J. Surg. 61,* 772.

Mustakallio, S. (1954). Treatment of breast cancer by tumour extirpation and roentgen therapy. *J. Faculty of Radiology 6,* 23.

Mustakallio, S. (1972). Conservative treatment of breast carcinoma. Review of 25 years follow up. *Clinical Radiology 23,* 110.

Peters, V. (1975). Carcinoma of the breast. *Annals of the Royal College of Physicians and Surgeons of Canada,* 186.

Porritt, Sir Arthur (1964). Early carcinoma of the breast. *Brit. J. Surg. 51,* 214.

Taylor, H., Baker, R. and Windsor Fortt, R. (1971). Sector mastectomy in selected cases of breast cancer. *Brit. J. Surg. 58,* 161.

Wise, L., Mason, A. Y. and Ackerman, L. V. (1971). Local excision and irradiation; an alternative method for treating early mammary cancer. *Ann. Surg. 174,* 393.

Chapter

5

PAUL STRICKLAND

Radical Radiation Therapy for Locally Advanced Disease

INTRODUCTION

The statistics of survival after breast cancer are simply stated—even the "early" operated patients have a less than one in two chance of surviving 10 years: once the axillary nodes are microscopically involved, less than one in two will survive even 5 years. It is from such dissatisfaction that all attempts to improve matters derive.

Two parallel strands may be discerned: increasing disillusionment with the results of surgical treatment, and the increasing understanding that high doses of super-voltage irradiation can eradicate cancer both locally and in metastatic areas.

Most surgeons would regard Haagensen's "grave signs of locally advanced disease" as so grave that any *one* of them (let alone two), would automatically rule out surgery. Yet many patients with large primary tumours, or with skin oedema of marked extent, or with doubtful tumour mobility, are still being operated upon. These manifestations in the primary growth are almost always associated with regional lymph node infiltration, or with distant metastases, or with both.

Why then are many such cases subjected to surgery? It is because contemporary accounts stress repeatedly that in the absence of proven distant metastases, the patient must not be denied the *only chance of a cure*—and this is widely assumed to be surgical. Not only is this assumption false, but the decision to operate in such cases contravenes a primary rule of cancer surgery—that all affected tissue with a good margin of apparently normal tissue must be encompassed. If the rule is broken, the patient's condition will be made worse not better.

Halsted's response to the disappointing results of radical mastectomy was to increase the extent of the operation (Halsted, 1894, 1907). The results worsened (Eggers et al., 1941) and a swing to greater selectivity was inevitable. Thus, "The transfer of borderline operable patients into the inoperable group significantly improves response rates to different palliative measures" (Fracchia and Kaufman, 1973). It appears that 75 years after

Halsted, the inoperable is still equated with the palliative, and it is the aim of this chapter to show that this belief is incorrect.

CRITERIA OF INOPERABILITY

"All discussion of the suitability of breast cancer for one form of treatment against another must take one dominant fact into account, that prognosis is determined by the extent of haematogenous spread prior to the initial therapy" (Galasko, 1974). Scanning studies have repeatedly shown that up to 30% of women with early breast cancers have occult skeletal deposits when first seen (see Chapter 2). Thus case selection is often the choice of the best *local* method of treatment, if the disease has disseminated before the patient has presented.

Haagensen and Stout (1943a, b) tried to identify clinical factors that were unfavourable for radical mastectomy: in all, 21 were considered and eight were selected as so significant that the presence of any two was deemed to be an absolute contraindication to surgery. "It is distressing to note that in cases with the smallest tumour (under 20 mm in diameter) the incidence of axillary metastases is high, to be exact 43.8%." They add that had they observed their own criteria of operability in a series of 640 cases, 109 would not have been operated upon, "yet the number of cures would not have been decreased by a single one".

In the 32 years that have passed since publication of Haagensen and Stout's monumental papers, their conclusions have not been shaken, only refined. It is clear that the presence of axillary nodes 2.5 cm or more in diameter, or the presence of high axillary nodes of whatever size, carries such grave prognostic overtones that the patient should not be treated even by simple mastectomy, however small the primary may be.

The size of the primary tumour also is almost certainly more important than has been appreciated. Very few patients whose tumours are larger than 5 cm survive even 5 years; they are therefore best spared irrelevant surgery. Yet as indicated earlier, many such patients are still operated upon, with disastrous results.

Inner quadrant primaries present a more difficult problem. The work of Urban (1959) and Dahl–Iversen and Tobiassen (1963) indicates how often the internal mammary nodes are infiltrated, and Haagensen (1972) would classify as inoperable any case with a positive apical axillary or internal mammary node biopsy. He carried out internal mammary node biopsies in all cases with medium size primaries or inner quadrant primaries of whatever size; 16% were positive even with the smallest primary tumours. With the 5-8 cm primary, 40% of these nodes were positive, and this rose to 57% in tumours bigger than 8.0 cm. Bearing in mind that mammographic size is much more accurate and nearly always smaller than size determined by caliper measurement, the true size of Haagensen's measured tumours was almost certainly less than the sizes quoted by him, and this reinforces his point.

As a result of multiple node biopsy, 50% of "operable" breast cancers (using the usually agreed criteria of operability) were deemed inoperable on the grounds that no surgical procedure could remove all the disease. These patients were referred for radiotherapy as the definitive treatment.

If these rigid rules of selection were universally obeyed, patients would be spared the irrelevance and psychic trauma gross of mastectomy for the wrong reasons. It is not suggested that multiple biopsies should be performed on all cases: merely that conclusions based on the natural evolution of the disease be properly taken into account. If this were done, the results of radical radiotherapeutic techniques would improve because a more hopeful group of cases would be referred for treatment. The ultimate gain to the patient in terms of survival would be great.

CAN RADIOTHERAPY ERADICATE BREAST CANCER?

There are almost as many radiation techniques as there are radiotherapists and yet there is little to choose between them. All follow the principles of homogeneous dose distribution and all do their best with the irregularities of human geometry. There is basic agreement that the breast itself should be sandwiched between two large opposing fields: some would use a further field to cover the internal mammary nodes, other would include these nodes within the medial tangential breast field. The axillary contents and supraclavicular and infraclavicular zones are covered by two or sometimes three fields.

There is, however, far less general agreement on dose and time relationships. Although "tumour doses" of 5,000 rads in about 5 weeks may still be considered the norm, some give a higher dose in a longer time, and others like Mustakallio (1945, 1954, 1972) favour about one half of the conventional dose. Most radiotherapists give five fractions a week while others believe that two or three larger fractions

a week do as well. In the absence of properly controlled trials to settle the matter, there is insufficient knowledge to specify the best radiotherapeutic method in attempting radical treatment. Until further evidence is available, most radiotherapists will continue to judge dose in terms of macroscopic (and occasionally microscopic) tumour response, tissue reactions (insofar as these can be assessed), and early and late morbidity.

It is agreed that the beam quality used in treatment should be in the supervoltage range, but it is immaterial whether it derives from an X-ray generator, such as a linear accelerator, or from a massive isotope source, such as a cobalt unit.

The French school of radiotherapists (Calle et al., 1973a, b) follow the pioneering work of Baclesse (1949, 1965). Baclesse had only orthovoltage radiation (250 kV) available with an extremely low output (20 röntgens per minute), but using a prolonged fractionation technique, he was able to show in his earlier (1949) report that lymph nodes 3-5 cm in size responded well to irradiation. In 26 of 52 such cases (50%) the nodes were clinically eradicated at the end of treatment, and 10 remained absent for periods of 3 to 5 years. Baclesse's cautious conclusions were that "radiotherapy alone can cause the disappearance of the primary, of the supraclavicular nodes and to a lesser extent, of the axillary nodes" and that "it may be compared here to a Halsted operation extended to the supraclavicular fossa".

In Baclesse's later (1965) report, the 5 year results in treating 431 breast cancers solely by röntgen rays are reported. Cases were treated twice weekly using 200 kV beams and prolonged fractionation over 2 to 3 months. A 5 year "cure" rate of 61% was reported (53 out of 86 patients) in the group with positive lymph nodes, a most remarkable achievement. Such results showed that even with the imperfect technical resources then available, radiotherapy could eradicate breast cancer both locally and in lymph nodes, but that high doses would be needed. This is consistent with the limited radiosensitivity of most breast cancers.

Calle et al. (1973b) used the 5,000 rads tumour dose in 5 weeks as a reasonable point of departure and assert that doses of this order will control nearly all "subclinical" lesions. They believe, however, that the sterilizing dose required for the main tumour mass increases with tumour size and this is in accord with the experimental radiobiological evidence which will be described later. Calle's group sometimes uses doses of 6,000 rads in 6 or 7 weeks, but in T3 lesions (primaries greater than 5.0 cm) a minimum dose of 8,000 rads is recommended.

Radiation of the axilla to high dosage level is, however, a problem; firstly, because of the high complication rate and secondly because of the inaccuracy of clinical classification. About 20 to 30% of clinically suspicious lymph nodes contain no tumour and about 30 to 40% are microscopically invaded though impalpable. Invasion of only the lower axillary nodes is associated with a 5 year "cure" rate of the order of 50% but once the highest nodes are invaded, radiotherapy is of curative value only if the invasion is microscopic. In that case "5,000 rads in 5 to 6 weeks seems a sufficient dose to us and higher doses are useless and dangerous" (Calle et al., 1973b).

In this respect Calle's experience is broadly in line with that of Fletcher (1972) who showed convincingly that 5,000 to 6,000 rads in 6 to 7 weeks given to low axillary nodes proven positive by biopsy, eradicated all but 7 of 161 cases. Node control is judged by their total disappearance at 5 years or by negative histology at later salvage surgery. Parasternal recurrences normally found in approximately 5% of patients, occur in 1% or less after high dose radiotherapy which includes this area.

These important papers show that with proper case selection, and a technique which takes into consideration what we know of the spread of breast cancer, determined high dose radiotherapy can eradicate both the primary and early lymph node metastases. But chances of success when the axilla is grossly involved or the supraclavicular fossa involved, are negligible and attempts to cure will increase morbidity but not the cure rate.

In breast cancer the term "cure" should be used sparingly. While conceding that 5 year disease-free rates are highly fallible guides to the ultimate survival of a group, they are valuable pointers. It is still too early to produce 10 year results from radiation therapy in large patient groups because our present supervoltage methods are still too young. Strickland's (1973) series with *advanced* disease showed a disease-free survival rate of 21% at 10 years. This figure is by no means negligible and is capable of improvement by better case selection.

Ruth Guttmann (1975) has completed long term follow up on a group of 174 patients treated by irradiation exclusively, because of proved evidence of disease in the internal mammary chain, apex of axilla or both. She is able to show a 5 year survival of 57% and a 10 year, or longer, survival of 28%. She adds that "14 patients died between 6 and 17 years of other causes with no evidence of disease at autopsy. If these patients had been taken statistically into account the percentages would be higher". These very important findings show how excellent the results of

radiotherapy can be, provided the therapy is determined enough and the case selection is good.

CONTROL OF LOCALLY ADVANCED DISEASE

The value of radiotherapy will continue to be judged by surgeons by its ability to control locally advanced disease for a period of years. How effective is it?

Griscom and Wang (1962) treated 97 patients with 4,000-5,000 rads in 35 to 40 days and obtained a "local response rate" of 87% lasting for 18 months on an average. This represents a poor response to moderate orthovoltage dosage. Atkins and Horrigan (1961) treating a fairly hopeful group of 39 women with 4,250 rads in 4 weeks noted that 34 (87%) had recurred locally in 3 to 5 years after good initial regression. This again indicates a disappointing response to conventional orthovoltage radiation dosage. Bouchard (1965) using a prolonged fractionation technique inspired by Baclesse obtained 61 complete regressions out of 109 inoperable cases treated. However, an orthovoltage technique taking up to 75 days for completion is not likely to find favour nowadays.

The work of Sarrazin and Fajbisowicz (1970) represented a new departure. Though their 190 advanced cases treated by radiotherapy alone were given 4,500 rads in a month using a conventional telecurie machine, they understood that if good local control was to be achieved, supplementary radiation had to be given. Selected tumours were therefore given either 6,500 rads (large primaries) or 8,500 rads (small primaries) and they achieved a sustained local control rate of 75%.

In Strickland's (1973) group of 285 mainly advanced cases, the whole breast was treated with 6,500 rads in 5 weeks using a 4 MeV linear accelerator beam. This is a substantially greater dose than those cited, but it usually held the primary clinically until the patient died, either of metastatic disease or other causes. The number of certain local recurrences within 5 years of treatment was only 5% (14 cases) but, of course, patient morbidity was higher than usual.

It is therefore certain that high dose radiotherapy can control primary breast cancer in the vast majority of cases and for an indefinite time. With proper case selection, morbidity can be reduced to levels acceptable to patient and physician.

SELECTION OF CASES FOR RADICAL RADIOTHERAPY

If the argument outlined in the opening paragraph on the principles of case selection for surgical treatment is correct, then certain clinical groups of patients should be treated by radiotherapy instead. These groups will include those whose primary is of only doubtful mobility, all carcinomas larger than, say, 6.0 cm whatever their degree of mobility, and all primaries in the inner half of the breast, other than very small ones.

Although signs of locally advanced disease in the breast will automatically contraindicate surgical treatment, they do not necessarily mean that *radical* radiotherapy should be given. Strickland (1973) reporting the treatment by high dose radiotherapy of 385 consecutive cases of advanced breast cancer showed a "disease free" rate of 36% at 5 years for all T2 and T3 cases, but not one patient with a primary larger than 8.0 cm survived 5 years. The outlook in the case of very large malignant masses is so bad, however they are treated, that such patients should be excluded from any rigorous radiotherapy technique that extends over many weeks.

It would generally be agreed that lymph nodes adherent to skin or to each other are by definition inoperable, wherever they are situated in the axilla. Again, even if the nodes are mobile but palpable as high as the examiner can reach, the results of surgery are so bad that intervention should be limited to biopsy. Both groups of cases may, however, be suitable for radical radiotherapy. This principle does not apply to supraclavicular nodes. In the Strickland (1973) series, 39 cases had obviously palpable supraclavicular node on presentation. These cases were, at the time, thought suitable for a radical course of radiotherapy but not one survived 5 years. The presence of palpable supraclavicular nodes is so clearly evidence of a poor prognosis that such cases should be excluded from any radical attempt at cure.

Radical radiotherapy is a physical strain even for the fit: patients who are aged or whose general condition is poor should obviously be excluded. They may best be helped by a simpler radiotherapy technique lasting perhaps 2 or 3 weeks in all, the intention being palliative from the outset. The ideal type of case for radical treatment is that in stage T2a or T2b (TNM classification) and most T3 cases may also be treated despite their generally poor outlook. On the other hand, most T4 cases are best treated palliatively because they do not survive long enough or in sufficient numbers to justify the endeavour.

LOCAL EXCISION AND RADICAL RADIOTHERAPY

Radical radiotherapy has been used for small tumours too, and the work of Calle et al. (1973a, b) repays careful study. The combined surgical/radiotherapy team have treated 1,000 cases of histologically verified breast cancer by wide local removal and radiotherapy or by radiotherapy alone. More extensive surgery is reserved for late recurrence. Of the total, 287 patients have been followed up for at least 5 years and they include 75 treated by local removal and radiation and 212 treated by radiotherapy alone.

Their indications for "tumourectomy" are the apparently solitary tumour focus not exceeding 3.0 cm in the absence of axillary node enlargement. Radiotherapy is started soon after excision, is free of complications, and produces a satisfactory aesthetic result. Sixty-one of these 75 cases were free of disease 5 years later (80%) with 53 of the 61 having kept their breast. In contrast to the findings of Mustakallio (1972) and Papillon et al. (1972), the under 35 group fared badly and of 16 such patients, 13 recurred and nine of them died.

In Mustakallio's earlier report (1954), local tumour removal is reserved for those tumours "not bigger than a hen's egg, and those where no lymph nodes are palpable". Radiotherapy was given soon afterwards to a dose of no more than 2,100 rads in about 3 weeks. Of 127 patients treated, 107 (84%) were free of disease 5 years later. Radiotherapy dosage is low yet his 1972 results are strictly comparable to the best surgical results: "for patients under 50, the 5 year relative survival rate was 90% and the 10 year survival rate 81%, whereas the corresponding rates for patients over 65 were 83% and 58% respectively".

These results of the treatment of early cases of breast cancer by local excision and radiotherapy are so consistent and good that further evaluation of the technique is vital. The value of radiotherapy in deliberately chosen low-dose schedules is open to criticism. It may be suggested that in the region of the excision or elsewhere in the breast, multiple "sub-clinical" foci of carcinoma may persist at the clinically undiagnosable stage. However, if these foci are no bigger than 10^6 cells (1 cu mm of tumour), we will see later that the burden of radiobiological evidence is that low doses of radiation should be sufficient to kill the majority. This hypothesis is by definition clinically unprovable, but if long term survival figures continue to confirm the 5 and 10 year results already published, it will be given strong reinforcement.

It may also be argued that combined local excision and radiotherapy does not prove the value of radiotherapy per se, and that excision alone might provide as good a result. This may be, but if it were proved, it would provide an argument at least as strong against the use of mastectomy in Stage I cases as against the case for radiotherapy in the same group.

RADICAL RADIOTHERAPY–DOSAGE CONSIDERATIONS

The tolerance of normal tissues was established empirically in the very early days of radiotherapy using energies of about 200 kV (orthovoltage irradiation). The earliest X-ray machines were often poorly calibrated and an estimate of the dose actually given to the irradiated parts was often wildly wrong. Thus, the biological action of radiation was observed first and only later was it accurately quantified in terms of dose and time. The limiting factor clinically was moist desquamation of the skin and, in general, this was roughly equivalent to a dose of 5,000 röntgens in 5 weeks.

The experimental work of Puck and Marcus (1956) showed that for a given dose of radiation to a cell population that was uniformly well oxygenated, the same proportion of cells is sterilized whatever the total number of cells irradiated. It follows that the total dose required to sterilize a cell population completely will increase with tumour volume. In other words, tumour dose must increase with tumour size. Conversely, the smaller the tumour, the smaller the dose of radiation needed for its total sterilization.

We also know that the centre of a tumour is less well oxygenated than its periphery and that it is the hypoxic cell component of a tumour that is the least radiosensitive. As tumours grow beyond a few dozen cells, regions develop in which the oxygen tension may fall so low as to render the cells relatively insensitive to radiation injury. Local recurrence may result if the cells survive not only the effect of radiation but also the adverse environmental conditions which lead to hypoxia.

Experimental evidence on the dose of radiation required to prevent local recurrence has been obtained for very small tumours in mice (Suit and Maeda, 1966). The dose needed to cure 50% of the animals bearing tumours of 0.001 cu mm, 0.6 cu mm and 250 cu mm volume (that is with mean diameters of 0.124 mm, 1.0 mm and 7.8 mm respectively) was

determined under three conditions in each case; firstly when the tumours were made wholly anoxic by local occlusion of the circulation, secondly when the circulation was free and the animals were breathing air, and thirdly when air was replaced by hyperbaric oxygen. In tumours of each size the dose required was found to be markedly different under conditions of anoxia and hyperbaric oxygen. With the smallest tumours the dose needed in the air-breathing conditions was similar to that with hyperbaric oxygen, with the middle sized tumour it was intermediate, and with the largest tumour it was nearly as great as that needed under anoxic conditions.

These experiments indicate that in this rapidly growing carcinoma in the mouse, hypoxic cells affecting the response to irradiation were present in tumours of *only* 1 mm diameter, and increased progressively till the tumour size reached 7.8 mm. Compared with the dose required under hyperbaric oxygen conditions an increase by a factor of about 2.7 was needed under anoxic conditions.

For air-breathing, on the other hand, the required dose increased by a factor of 1.7 for the intermediate and 2.2 for the largest tumours, i.e. 61% of the "anoxic" increment for the intermediate group and 85% for the largest. This is not, of course, equivalent to saying that 61% and 85% of the cells were hypoxic; no such value can be calculated from the data.

Similar conclusions for human tumours result mainly by extrapolating from experimental observations, but the fundamental response to radiation of animal tumours is fairly constant, irrespective of host. The whole burden of clinical experience supports the view that there are vast numbers of hypoxic cells in every palpable breast tumour. This accounts for the comparative "radioresistance" and increase in dose that is required as tumour size increases, and justifies the application of a supplementary radiation field to the primary tumour after treatment to the main tumour bearing volume has been completed.

It is interesting to compare these conclusions with criteria used for staging cancer. "It is now recognized that tumours more than 5 cm in diameter all carry much the same prognosis. It is therefore necessary to have only three size groups, 2 cm or less, between 2 cm and 5 cm and more than 5 cm" (TNM Classification, 1974). The prognosis is increasingly bad from the point of view of local recurrence and distant metastases, as tumour size increases. Treatment is made more difficult by the increasing importance of hypoxia and therefore radio-resistance as tumour size increases.

It is not practical to treat patients with breast cancer in a hyperbaric oxygen chamber, and in practice, radiotherapy must seek to eradicate every cancer cell by giving the maximum possible dose to the affected tissues. The classical work of Strandqvist (1944) showed that dose levels could be roughly equated not only with local recurrence and cure rates but also with the necrosis rate; as dose rises, so clearly does the complication rate, and a balance must be struck between the greatest likelihood of tumour sterilization and a minimal radiation morbidity.

The average sized lesion can be controlled by a dose of about 5,000 rads in about 5 weeks, using any conventional supervoltage machine, and the tolerance of the axillary contents is about the same level of dose. This dose, however, is insufficient to sterilize the large majority of bulky tumours and supplementary radiation may need to be given to the centre of such a tumour. This is sometimes applied by a direct radiation field and sometimes by electron therapy.

The aim of radiotherapy is to deliver a uniform dose of radiation to the whole of the tumour volume and to the lymph drainage areas, that is to say, the axillary, the supraclavicular and infraclavicular regions and the internal mammary chain on the homolateral side. The practical difficulty in achieving this lies in the physical shape of the parts. The areas mentioned cannot be thought of as part of a simple geometrical figure; the breast and axilla are roughly at right angles to each other and the parasternal region is not in the same plane as either.

Moreover, certain vital structures such as the brachial plexus, the head of the humerus and (as far as possible) lung parenchyma, must be excluded from the beams for fear of high dose effects. It is not, of course, possible to exclude these structures completely, so they must be shielded from the full effect of radiotherapy without at the same time shielding foci of tumour in their vicinity. These matters complicate accurate geometrical planning, and impose a series of compromises on the radiotherapist. He must accept areas of non-homogeneous dose distribution including in practice doses lower than the optimum.

"VIABLE" TUMOUR CELLS AFTER RADIOTHERAPY

Histological studies of invaded lymph nodes before and after radiation show that it is possible to destroy all metastatic deposits, provided the dose is high enough (Guttman, 1963, 1966). The critical factor is the size of the lymph node: control is possible in a

substantial proportion of nodes under 3.0 cm in size, but it becomes increasingly difficult with increasing size of node. The reporting of apparently "viable" cancer cells does not mean that local recurrence is inevitable, or, for that matter, that distant metastases are inevitable. Unfortunately, there is sometimes a tendency for the clinician to nudge the histologist into occupying a position that he cannot defend.

The histologist reports what he sees and when he reports viable or non-viable cells, he is using agreed histological criteria only. Thus an irradiated cancer cell, whose form is bizarre, whose nucleus is densely pyknotic and whose degree of differentiation appears greater than the host tissue that gave origin to it, is likely to be non-viable. That is to say, it will grow old without further mitosis and will ultimately be treated by the organism as a foreign body.

The likelihood of "viability" is a very different matter. The histologist indicates that future life of the cell is possible, but no opinion on future cell *behaviour* is implied. Some cells which appear fully viable never undergo further cell division; their intimate biochemistry has been so deranged by the insults they have suffered—by radiation for example—that they take on the characteristics of non-viability *if observed for long enough.* So the report of "viable malignant cells seen" does not necessarily indicate that local recurrence of disease is inevitable, or even likely.

The milieu in which the apparently viable malignant cell is observed must also be considered. Though apparently active cancer cells can be seen in a breast removed many years after high dose radiation therapy, the cells are characteristically buried in strata of dense mature fibrous tissue, representing a long-term healing process and providing an environment quite different to any normal stromal reaction. It does not follow that viable cancer cells reported in these circumstances will ever "escape".

In an important paper by Paterson Ross (1939) simple removal of the breast was carried out routinely in 50 patients whose carcinomas had been treated by a radium implant of the Keynes type. "About half of them contained carcinoma cells, the remainder showed only dense scar tissue, and we noted that among the latter group there were several in which a heavy dose of radium had been used."

The precise radiation dose received by these cases will never be known but it was certainly less than that used routinely nowadays in radical supervoltage radiation techniques. As there is a rough linear relationship between applied dose and likelihood of tumour cell death, it is not surprising that such autopsy material as becomes available after high dose radiotherapy repeatedly shows no local evidence of active cancer.

MORBIDITY OF HIGH DOSE RADIATION

Statements about radiation damage that do not specify the quality of the radiation beam, the "tumour dose" achieved and its distribution, and the overall time in which this tumour dose was delivered, have little value. However, useful generalizations are firstly, that as the penetration of the treatment beam increases, the brunt of tissue damage is borne increasingly by tissues deep to the skin; and secondly, that there is a very rough linear relationship between dose/time (thought of as a single parameter) and radiation injury.

Strandqvist (1944) showed that low dose/time ratios cured few cases and caused negligible tissue damage, but that while high dose/time ratios gave good cure rates, this was counterbalanced by a high and therefore unacceptable morbidity. Useful cure rates with tolerable morbidity were best secured within the 5,000 röntgen in 5 weeks dose range and this, in fact, has proved to be the point of departure for those who have investigated the effect of prolonged fractionated or very high dose techniques.

Very few centres now use "conventional" X-ray beams (250 kV or less) for the radical treatment of breast cancer but, as patients so treated have survived into this decade, some consideration of their problems is needed. The limiting factor in the use of conventional radiotherapy was moist desquamation of the skin, affecting principally the axillary folds, the inframammary region and the thin tissue overlying the clavicle. Limitations of skin tolerance often precluded the giving of high tumour doses so that the local results, even in the hands of a determined radiotherapist (Baclesse, 1949, 1965), were indifferent. Mucosal reactions were relatively unimportant and damage to skeletal and nervous tissues only followed errors of technique (e.g. too high a dose or field overlap).

Moist desquamation sometimes took weeks to subside but healing was ultimately complete, leaving an atrophic pigmented skin surface. Telangiectases developed within a few months, increased in severity for a year or two and then remained static. Late tissue necrosis was rare, even when the whole breast became progressively shrunken. These changes were seen occasionally at the 5,000 röntgen in 5 weeks dose range but with lower doses or longer times, reactions were generally negligible.

The advent of supervoltage radiation transformed the preconceived ideas of the radiotherapist, because maximum doses were now delivered to tissues lying 0.5-2.0 cms below the skin (that is, to the soft tissues). The use of skin reactions as a guide to tolerance was no longer possible and radiotherapists were therefore tempted into giving higher tumour doses, with a consequent increase in morbidity. Whether this is accompanied by an improved local and regional node cure-rate is still not proved.

During the first few weeks of a radical supervoltage treatment for breast cancer there may be no reaction at all, apart from a "tickle" in the throat due to early mucosal swelling. Towards the end of treatment mild dysphagia is commonplace and some cases may take up to 3 months to settle down. Barium swallow investigation—even for this group—shows only minimal oesophageal narrowing, and post radiation stricture of the oesophagus is very rare.

At the end of a radical treatment course, the irradiated tissue of the breast often looks deceptively normal. However, within a few months, progressive thickening of subcutaneous tissues occurs and may continue fairly steadily for 2 or 3 years. The end-result depends on the dose/time ratio used. In the more conservative treatment schedules moderate soft tissue fibrosis is all that is encountered: the breast feels thickened and leathery, but it moves freely. The overlying skin is slightly dusky and there may be a few telangiectases.

With the higher dose/time ratios these changes are magnified. The whole breast is replaced by dense fibrous tissue which contracts gradually, leaving a shrunken organ densely plastered on to the chest wall. The breast skin is sometimes paler than normal, sometimes duskier, and telangiectases are often numerous. Irradiated breasts of this type are usually painless and their possessors are grateful for them, poor as they may look. They are less grateful if pain occurs, as it does from time to time for no apparent reason and in the absence of injury.

Though trauma to an irradiated breast may cause local pain, massive tissue breakdown is very rare. In 393 consecutive cases treated by the writer with tumour doses of the order of 6,500 rads in 6 weeks, it occurred only once. Occasionally the whole breast becomes pink and somewhat tender, due, presumably, to low grade cellulitis affecting devitalized tissues.

As a result of minor trauma, or of none, rib fractures occur not uncommonly. Most post-radiation rib fractures are chance findings but some are painful and may first be seen many years after irradiation. Often several ribs are found to be broken but all heal eventually with normal callus formation. Fractures of the clavicle, body of the sternum or neck of the humerus may occur in rare cases when errors of technique have failed to shield the bone correctly during treatment.

Despite the use of tangential fields angled specifically to exclude as much lung tissue as possible from the irradiated volume, damage to the lungs is inevitable, but it is surprising how infrequently it produces severe symptoms. Temporary cough or mild dyspnoea on exertion is common after radical radiation dose levels; X-ray changes may include plaques of pleural thickening or evidence of increased lung striation with slight deviation of the mediastinum towards the fibrotic side. Some patients with severe dyspnoea have minimal abnormal physical signs and X-ray changes while on the other hand, some show evidence of severe fibrothorax with only the mildest symptoms.

By far the worst damage by radiation may occur in the brachial plexus. Pain down the arm due to "brachial neuritis" presumed due to radiation damage to the nerve trunks in the axilla or above it, is an intractable condition. Pain may be very severe and persistent and there is no effective treatment. It is presumably due to vascular damage in the perineural tissue and leads to a strangling of nerve tissue by dense fibrosis. The tolerance of the axillary tissues is undoubtedly less than that of the breast itself and Calle and his co-workers (1973b) advise against doses of more than 5,000 rads in 5 weeks. Very large fixed masses high in the axilla or above the clavicle should be regarded as palliative propositions from the outset and such patients should be spared the possibility of post-radiation morbidity in addition to that of their advancing disease.

Radiation damage to the myocardium is rare but is well recorded. High dose radiation may cause changes in the electrocardiograph, but this is seen mainly with primary tumours of the left breast treated with poorly planned fields. The myocardium consists of a highly radioresistant cell population and the electrocardiographic changes are far more likely to be due to the primary effect of radiation on small blood vessels, with secondary ischaemic change in the heart muscle. Pericardial thickening is common but symptomless. The whole range of radiation-induced cardiac damage and an attempt to correlate it with the applied dose has been fully described elsewhere (Stewart and Fajardo, 1972).

Late radiation-induced soft tissue sarcoma is likely to become an increasing risk as more patients survive their high dose treatment. A number of cases are recorded in the literature and the writer has three

unpublished cases. It is possible that some may masquerade as late local recurrences and if a local recurrence has unusual clinical features, a further biopsy is warranted.

Radiation-induced lymphoedema of the arm is due to progressive fibrosis of the lymphatic channels in and above the axilla. Mild cases are very common and do not greatly affect the patient's welfare but gross swelling due to radiation is rare. Management is discussed fully in Chapters 11 and 21. Rarely lymphangiosarcoma may develop. Radiation lymphoedema is best prevented by using the same principles outlined for the prevention of radiation nerve injury.

It will be seen that the morbidity following high dose radiotherapy may be considerable. It can only be justified by a high local cure rate as defined by control of the primary growth and of its immediate lymph node extension. It is not possible at present to express quantitatively what a high local cure rate should mean but with proper case selection and dose/time levels appropriate to different tissue regions, radical radiation therapy of breast cancer will have little difficulty in justifying itself.

LOCAL CARCINOGENIC EFFECTS OF RADIOTHERAPY

It is sometimes stated that radiotherapy to the breast area is carcinogenic and this, largely anecdotal, statement needs critical analysis.

When moderate doses of radiotherapy—mostly of the order of 500 rads—were given to a group of 606 women suffering from acute post-partum mastitis (Mettler et al., 1969) there was an apparent increase in late breast cancer and a much more striking increase in the incidence of benign breast tumours. As the authors point out "we cannot exclude the possibility that this selected group of women with breast disease, as is suggested by the apparently high incidence of chronic cystic mastitis, may be pre-disposed to develop breast tumours". This must therefore preclude direct causal relationship to the irradiation.

This cannot be said about the development of breast cancer in female patients with pulmonary tuberculosis treated by artificial pneumothorax controlled by repeated fluoroscopy (Mackenzie, 1965; Myrden and Hiltz, 1969; Cook et al., 1974). Radiation exposure increased breast cancer risk two or three times compared with a matched group treated without pneumothorax and fluoroscopy. The exposed group were screened up to several hundred times using soft X-rays impinging more or less directly on the skin of the front of the chest. "Radiodermatitis" consistent with high overall doses of soft radiation given over a long period of time was repeatedly observed.

This group of patients developed breast cancer after an average latent interval of 17 years and at an average age of 39. The type of insult suffered by these tissues has no bearing whatever on the type of dose/time relationships used in treating breast cancers, primarily or postoperatively. These groups need *high* doses given in *short* overall times, using a radiation quality totally different to the fluoroscopy cases. Comparisons, in the presence of multiple variables, are meaningless and though the fate of the over-irradiated fluoroscopy group is interesting and important, it is totally irrelevant to what happens in the usual clinical situation.

In the tens of thousands of women who formerly suffered intense skin damage following the post-operative use of orthovoltage radiotherapy, there is not an iota of hard evidence to suggest that the local or general risks of malignancy are increased. Some observers (Freund et al., 1976) think that scar tissue and surgical trauma to the chest wall are as likely as radiation to predispose to breast malignancy.

CONCLUSION

Breast cancer is a disease of moderate radiosensitivity only: a few cases will respond rapidly, a few will barely respond at all. Most will need doses close to the tolerance of normal tissues. It follows that radiation morbidity is inevitable if a "reasonable" local cure rate is to be attained. What is reasonable and what unreasonable is ultimately a matter of opinion; it is certain that the majority of women are glad to retain their breasts, even if these are deformed or of unusual texture.

REFERENCES

Atkins, H. L. and Horrigan, W. D. (1961). Treatment of locally advanced carcinoma of the breast with roentgen therapy and simple mastectomy. *American Journal of Roentgenology 85,* 860.

Baclesse, F. (1949). La Roentgenthérapie seule employée dans le traitement des cancers du Sein opérables et inopérables. *Journal de Radiologie et d'Electrothérapie 30,* 323.

Baclesse, F. (1965). Five year results in 431 breast cancers treated solely by Roentgen rays. *Annals of Surgery 161,* 103.

Bouchard, J. (1965). Advanced cancer of the breast treated primarily with irradiation. *Radiology 84,* 803.

Calle, R., Pilleron, J. P. and Schlienger, P. (1973a). Thérapeutique "a visée conservatrice" des Epitheliomas Mammaires. *Bulletin du Cancer 60,* 217.

Calle, R., Fletcher, G. H. and Pierquin, B. (1973b). La base de la radiothérapie curative des epitheliomas mammaires. *Journal de Radiologie et d'Electrologie 54,* 928.

Cook, D. C., Dent, O. and Hewitt, D. (1974). Breast cancer following multiple chest fluoroscopy: the Ontario experience. *Canadian Medical Association Journal 111,* 406.

Dahl-Iversen, E. and Tobiassen, T. (1963). Radical mastectomy with parasternal and supraclavicular dissection for mammary carcinoma. *Annals of Surgery 157,* 170.

Eggers, C., de Cholnoky, T. and Jessup, D. S. D. (1941). Cancer of the breast. *Annals of Surgery 113,* 321.

Fletcher, G. H. (1972). Local results of irradiation in the primary management of localised breast cancer. *Cancer 29,* 545.

Fracchia, A. A. and Kaufman, R. J. (1973). Management of advanced breast cancer. *Proceedings National Cancer Conference 7,* 303.

Freund, S., Biran, S., Laufer, N. and Eyal, Z. (1976). Breast cancer arising in thoracotomy scars. *Lancet 1,* 97.

Galasko, C. S. B. (1974). The significance of occult skeletal metastases. Surgical Research Society meeting.

Griscom, N. T. and Wang, C. C. (1962). Radiation therapy of inoperable breast carcinoma. *Radiology 79,* 18.

Guttmann, R. J. (1963). Radiotherapy in treatment of primary operable carcinoma of the breast with proved lymph node metastases. *American Journal of Roentgenology 89,* 58.

Guttmann, R. J. (1966). Role of supervoltage irradiation of regional lymph node bearing areas in breast cancer. *American Journal of Roentgenology 96,* 560.

Guttmann, R. J. (1975). Personal communication.

Halsted, W. S. (1894). Results of operations for the cure of cancer performed at Johns Hopkins Hospital, June 1889–January 1894. *Annals of Surgery 20,* 497.

Halsted, W. S. (1907). The results of radical operation for the cure of carcinoma of the breast. *Annals of Surgery 46,* 1.

Haagensen, C. D. and Stout, A. P. (1943a). Carcinoma of the breast. *Annals of Surgery 118,* 858.

Haagensen, C. D. and Stout, A. P. (1943b). Carcinoma of the breast. *Annals of Surgery 118,* 1032.

Haagensen, C. D. (1972). *Diseases of the Breast,* 2nd edition. Philadelphia: W. B. Saunders Co.

Mackenzie, I. (1965). Breast cancer following multiple fluoroscopies. *British Journal of Cancer 19,* 1.

Mettler, F. A., Hempelmann, N. L. H., Dutton, A. M., Pifer, J. W., Toyooka, E. T. and Ames, W. R. (1969). Breast neoplasms in women treated with X-rays for acute postpartum mastitis; a pilot study. *Journal National Cancer Institute 434,* 803.

Mustakallio, S. (1945). Uber die Möglichkeiten der Röntgentherapie bei der Behandlung des Brustkrebses. *Acta Radiologica 26,* 503.

Mustakallio, S. (1954). Treatment of breast cancer by tumour extirpation and roentgen therapy instead of radical operation. *Journal of Faculty of Radiologists 6,* 23.

Mustakallio, S. (1972). Conservative treatment of breast carcinoma. *Clinical Radiology 23,* 110.

Myrden, J. A. and Hiltz, J. E. (1969). Breast cancer following multiple fluoroscopies during artificial pneumothorax treatment of pulmonary tuberculosis. *Canadian Medical Association Journal 100,* 1032.

Papillon, J., Montbardon, J. H. and Ingels, J. (1972). Le traitement conservateur du cancer du sein per l'association tumorectomie et irradiation. *Journal Belge de Radiologie 55,* 1, 129.

Puck, T. T. and Marcus, P. I. (1956). Action of X-rays on mammalian cells. *Journal of Experimental Medicine 103,* 653.

Ross, J. Paterson (1939). An investigation into the effects of radium upon carcinoma of the breast. *British Journal of Surgery 27,* 211.

Sarrazin, D. and Fajbisowicz, S. (197[illegible]). Evolution de rôle et des techniques de la Radiothérapie dans le cancer du Sein. *Annales de Radiologie 14,* 631.

Stewart, R. and Fajardo, L. F. (1972). Radiation induced heart disease. In *Radiation Effects & Tolerance of Human Tissue* (Ed. J. M. Vaeth). Baltimore: University Park Press.

Strandqvist, M. (1944). Studien uber die kumulative Wirkung der Rontgenstrahlen bei Fraktionierung. *Acta Radiologica,* supplement 55.

Strickland, P. (1973). The management of carcinoma of the breast by radical supervoltage radiation. *British Journal of Surgery 60,* 569.

Suit, H. and Maeda, M. (1966). Oxygen effect factor and tumor volume in the C_3H mouse mammary carcinoma, a preliminary report. *American Journal of Roentgenology 96,* 177.

T.N.M. Classification of Malignant Tumours. U.I.C.C., Geneva, second edition 1974, page 51.

Urban, J. A. (1959). Clinical experience and results of excision of the internal mammary lymph node chain in primary operable breast cancer. *Cancer 12,* 14.

Chapter

6

BERNARD FISHER

Attempts at Combined Modality Therapy

Most, if not all, patients with primary breast cancer have disseminated disease at the time of diagnosis. Operation alone is too frequently inadequate to effect a cure and extension of surgery has not produced any noteworthy gains in patient survival and freedom from disease during the past three or four decades. There is increasing receptivity to the suggestion that improvement in survival is likely to result only from the employment of effective systemic therapy in conjunction with those modalities which control loco-regional disease, that is surgery and radiation.

The use of chemo- immuno-, or hormonal therapy in conjunction with operation has been inappropriately designated "adjuvant" therapy. But, on the contrary, as a result of recent advances in our understanding of the disease, it may be suggested that an operation and/or radiation may actually serve as "adjuvant" to systemic treatment! Consequently, the term "combined modality" therapy seems more appropriate to describe such conglomerate treatment regimens. This report will provide a brief overview of the rationale for the use of such therapy; what has been and is being accomplished with it, and what the prospects for the future seem to be.

RATIONALE FOR THE USE OF COMBINED MODALITY THERAPY

The most compelling justification for the use of combined modality therapy is that breast cancer is a systemic disease at the time of operation. This is not at all surprising when it is appreciated that a 1 cm tumor, which is usually the minimal size capable of physical diagnosis in the breast and which is looked upon as an "early" tumor, has already progressed through 30 of the 40 doublings which are lethal to a patient. Considering that relatively few tumors are detected when they are less than 1 cm, it is appropriate that breast cancer be considered "advanced" at the time of diagnosis.

Data have been recently reported (Fisher et al., 1975b) on treatment failure 10 years following radical mastectomy for what were considered to be clinically "curable" breast cancers, and strikingly emphasize the systemic nature of that cancer (Table 1). The finding of treatment failure in three of four patients with positive axillary nodal involvement, and almost nine of ten with four or more of such nodes containing tumor, indicates the inadequacy of loco-regional surgery. Even that one of four

Table 1 Treatment failures 5 and 10 years post radical mastectomy according to histologic nodal status

	5 years	10 years
	(%)	(%)
All patients	40	50
Negative nodes	18	24
Positive	65	76
1-3 nodes	50	65
⩾ 4 nodes	79	86

patients with negative axillary nodes succumbed to a recurrence is significant in that regard.

Skipper (1974) correlated information concerning the fate of patients having breast cancer with what is known about its growth rate and other features of its cell kinetics. Employing certain assumptions, he has provided estimates of the residual tumor cell burden that might be expected to be present in a host following primary tumor removal, i.e. the number of viable cancer cells that are beyond the reach of surgery (Table 2). Zero viable tumor cells in that

Table 2. Residual tumor cell burden following primary tumor burden (Skipper, 1974)

Viable breast cancer cells beyond the reach of surgery	% of operable patients bearing the numbers of tumor cells indicated presuming an overall median doubling time of 30 or 40 days (and other stated assumptions): Negative nodes 30-day	Negative nodes 40-day	1 or more positive nodes 30-day	1 or more positive nodes 40-day	4+ positive nodes 30-day	4+ positive nodes 40-day
0 or "1" slow cell	65*	65*	36*	36*	14*	14*
"1" (with median DT) or <	80	74	56	47	22	17
10^1 or <	82	77	59	51	26	18
10^2 or <	85	80	63	56	30	22
10^3 or <	88	82	69	59	39	26
10^4 or <	90	86	73	65	45	33
10^5 or <	93	89	78	70	52	42
10^6 or <	95	93	83	78	63	53
10^7 or <	97	96	89	85	76	67
10^8 or <	99	99	94	92	88	85
10^9 or <	"100"	"100"	"100"	"100"	"100"	"100"

* 5 year tumor-free survivors *observed.*

Table 3 Seemingly reasonable estimates of the body burden of tumor cells at detection of recurrence (Skipper, 1974)

No. of tumor cells	*Weight*	*If in a single spherical clone or mass:* *Diameter (mm)*	*Palpable (depending on site)*
10^1	0.01 μg	0.025	No
10^2	0.1 μg	0.06	No
10^3	1 μg	0.12	No
10^4	10 μg	0.25	No
10^5	100 μg	0.6	No
10^6	1 mg	1.2	No
10^7	10 mg	2.5	No
10^8	100 mg	6	?
10^9	1 gm	12	Yes*
10^{10}	10 gms	25	Yes*
10^{11}	100 gms	60	Yes
10^{12}	1 kilo	120	Yes

The volume of a sphere = $0.5236d^3$

Subcutaneous solid animal tumors are usually first palpable and measurable at about 60 mg

* Reasonable range: the average is likely to be somewhere between 1 and 10 grams.

chart refers to none above some relatively small number with which host immune mechanisms may be able to cope.

He has also provided some "reasonable" estimates of the body burden of tumor cells present at detection of a recurrence (Table 3). As a result of such "modeling" there arises some insight into the prevalence of cancer as a systemic disease at diagnosis, and the number of cells which need to be eradicated by systemic therapy in order to enhance the curability of surgery.

The fact that some patients are apparently "cured" by operation alone is no indication that the surgical procedure eradicated every last cancer cell, that the disease was completely loco-regional in extent, and that dissemination had not taken place. Such a concept is most difficult for the surgeon to accept. There is failure to appreciate that the residual tumor cell burden may have been small enough for its eradication by host factors which play a significant role in the success or failure of the operative procedure. It is impossible to estimate the number of micrometastases which may have been aborted by removal of a primary tumor.

Another justification for the use of adjuvant therapy has to do with the effect of removal of a primary tumor on residual (metastatic) tumor cell kinetics. Numerous studies have demonstrated that as tumors increase in mass there is a slowing of their growth rate. According to Schabel (1969) there is a decrease in the growth fraction of viable tumor cells in cell division cycle. Large tumors are apt to contain a preponderance of resting cells, i.e. those with a prolonged G_1 time. Slowing of the rate of growth of an implanted tumor as well as of its metastases (even though the latter were microscopic) has been reported (DeWys, 1972). With removal of the primary tumor there resulted an increase in the growth fraction and shortening of the generation time in the metastases, making them more vulnerable to chemotherapeutic agents. Other investigations of a similar nature suggest to Simpson–Herron et al. (1974) that metastases may display greater sensitivity than a primary tumor to chemotherapeutic agents, and that the use of a large primary tumor as an index of drug effectiveness may be misleading.

Results from investigations in a variety of experimental animal systems have helped formulate principles which supply a rationale for the use of systemic agents in conjunction with surgery. That the effectiveness of chemotherapy can be increased through reducing the tumor burden of a host by operation has been repeatedly documented (Chirigos et al., 1962; Karrer et al., 1967; Martin et al., 1962; Schabel, 1975; Straus et al., 1975). Since a given course of chemotherapy consistently destroys the same proportion of tumor cells present and not identical absolute numbers (thus obeying first order kinetics), the fewer the number of tumor cells subjected to chemotherapy the greater is the likelihood that they will be reduced to a number small enough to be eliminated by host factors such as immunity.

Since chemotherapy, just as surgery or radiation, may by itself fail to destroy every cancer cell, the ultimate success of treatment may relate to the capability of host immunity to eradicate the residual tumor cell burden. As a consequence there is increasing emphasis on the evaluation of therapeutic regimens combining immuno- and chemotherapy. Our own investigations (Fisher et al., 1975c, d, 1976b), utilizing an animal model system, have demonstrated the efficacy of such combined modality therapy. When *C. parvum* was administered in combination with cyclophosphamide, a tumor growth inhibitory effect was achieved which was greater than that resulting from the use of either agent alone.

A variety of ablative and additive hormonal treatments have been employed in the management of advanced breast cancer. With the demonstration that the cells of some breast cancers are capable of binding estrogen and that responsiveness to hormonal manipulation in patients with extensive tumor burden is related to this quality, there has been a resurgence of interest in the employment of endocrine therapy in combination with other modalities for the treatment of primary tumors.

EARLY EVALUATIONS OF COMBINED MODALITY THERAPY

In 1957, under the auspices of the National Institutes of Health, Cancer Chemotherapy National Service Center, representatives of 23 institutions in the United States adopted a common protocol which was to determine the efficacy of administering chemotherapy in conjunction with "curative" cancer surgery to decrease recurrence and extend survival of patients with cancer of the breast. The impetus and rationale for that undertaking resulted primarily from laboratory observations (Cruz et al., 1956; McDonald et al., 1956, 1957) of favorable effects by chemotherapeutic agents on disseminated tumor cells in experimental animals, as well as from reports of the frequent presence of cancer cells in the circulating blood of patients with tumor (Engel, 1955; Fisher et al., 1955).

It was anticipated that such a therapeutic regimen could destroy tumor cells dislodged into the blood and lymph during surgical manipulation and/or destroy minute metastatic foci of tumor which defied detection. That effort became known as the National Surgical Adjuvant Breast Project (NSABP) and it has for almost 20 years carried out clinical trials to evaluate a variety of treatment modalities in the management of patients with primary breast cancer. The group has expanded over the years so that at present it consists of almost 400 surgeons, radiation and medical oncologists as well as pathologists from 70 institutions in the United States, Canada and other countries.

THIO-TEPA TRIAL

Triethylenethiophosphoramide (Thio-TEPA; TSPA), because of its effectiveness in palliation of advanced mammary cancer, was the first drug chosen for evaluation and the first patient was entered on study in 1958. Women were randomized in double-blind fashion between two treatment groups: (a) conventional Halsted radical mastectomy and TSPA, and (b) radical mastectomy with or without placebo (control).

Patients received TSPA intravenously in a dose of either 0.8 or 0.6 mg/kg of body weight—0.2 or 0.4 mg/kg at the time of operation and 0.2 mg/kg on each of the first two postoperative days. Since subsequent analysis of data revealed no difference in those receiving one or the other dose, results were combined. Recurrence and survival rate calculations were obtained from 826 acceptable study patients grouped according to nodal and menopausal status, and the results have been reported in detail (Fisher et al., 1968). Positive node patients were further subdivided into those having one to three, or four or more such nodes.

At the end of 5 years, there was no significant difference in recurrence rate between patients receiving TSPA or placebo in any of the six principal categories. If, however, recurrence rates for TSPA and placebo groups were plotted against time following surgery (similar to a plot of life table values), significant information was revealed which was not obtained by examination of data only at the end of 5 years.

There was a significant difference between the two treatment groups in premenopausal patients who had four or more positive nodes. TSPA-treated patients in that category demonstrated a recurrence rate between the 18th and 36th postoperative months which was approximately 40% less than in the placebo group. After that time, the number of recurrences in the TSPA-treated patients gradually increased, so that by 48 months the groups were no longer significantly different.

The effect of TSPA in this particular category was best demonstrated by the observation that 50% of patients in the placebo series had recurrences by the 13th month after surgery, whereas recurrences did not occur in half of the TSPA patients until the 45th month of follow-up. While the difference between the treated and control groups relative to treatment failure was no longer statistically significant after 5 years, it was nevertheless 20%. Moreover, there was at that stage a 33% difference in the survival rate ($p < 0.05$) between the TSPA treated and control groups: 56.5% for the former vs. 24.3% for the latter.

Ten-year follow-up of the patients entered into the TSPA study has recently been reported (Fisher et al., 1975b). Only 0.7% of the initial 826 patients evaluated were lost to follow-up at 5 years, and only 4.7% of patients had no 10 year follow-up information. Contrary to expectations, the 10 year findings revealed persistence of the difference in treatment failure and survival rates. After 10 years, 21% fewer patients in the specific TSPA group were treatment failures and 21% more of them survived. Thus, it would seem that the initial suppression of recurrences had a lasting effect that was reflected in patient survival.

The data also suggested that the limited chemotherapy employed was more effective in patients having smaller tumors. Such a finding is in keeping with experimental observations and with modern concepts of chemotherapy which suggest that a therapeutic regimen should be more effective in a host with a minimal tumor burden.

5-FLUOROURACIL TRIAL

With completion of the TSPA study in 1961 a new protocol was begun. It evaluated the worth of 5-fluorouracil (5-FU) compared to TSPA as an adjunct to operation and again, only a short course of chemotherapy was employed. TSPA-treated patients received a total dose of 0.8 mg/kg—0.4 mg/kg on the day of operation and 0.2 mg/kg on each of the next 2 days. Those who were administered 5-FU received 15 mg/kg intravenously on each of four consecutive days, beginning 7 days postoperatively for a total of 60 mg/kg.

Of patients who received 5-FU, 52% suffered local complications and significantly more patients receiv-

ing that drug demonstrated systemic complications. Moreover, 42% of patients administered 5-FU became leukopenic and almost half of those had counts < 2,500 per cu mm. Of 16 deaths occurring within 60 days following operation in the 1,725 patients, eight were in the recipients of 5-FU, and all demonstrated drug toxicity.

As in the first study, TSPA-treated premenopausal patients with ⩾ 4 positive nodes had less recurrences than did untreated patients. Results with 5-FU were not improved, and recurrence rates were the same as in patients receiving placebo.

In retrospect the findings with TSPA must be considered remarkable in view of the small amount of drug employed for only a brief interval. Skipper had commented (1971) that if such an amount of TSPA given in split doses over 3 days "can significantly delay recurrence and death after surgery in premenopausal patients with ⩾ 4 positive nodes, the odds are good that we might do much better in this patient category (and others) with surgery followed by an optimal regimen of this drug, or better yet, a more effective alkylating agent or combination of drugs".

At the time, however, the results were considered by many to be disappointing. Despite that climate, in 1968 the NSABP began a feasibility study with methotrexate (MTX) in patients having positive axillary nodes. That drug was administered orally (0.2 mg/kg body weight) twice a week, no less than 3 and no more than 5 days apart beginning 1 month after mastectomy. Because of the high incidence of severe toxic manifestations encountered early, the effort was aborted.

OTHER EARLY TRIALS

Until recently only a few other adjuvant chemotherapy trials had been carried out and the findings had not been consistent. A report by Nissen-Meyer of a study by the Scandinavian Adjuvant Chemotherapy Study Group is of interest (Nissen-Meyer et al., 1971). Eleven hospitals in Finland, Norway, and Sweden began a cooperative clinical trial in 1965, to evaluate the effect of a short course of chemotherapy after mastectomy for breast cancer.

Patients were randomized for chemotherapy, but each hospital was permitted to employ its own standard method of surgical, radiologic, and endocrinologic treatment of such tumors. Thus, variations in management were allowed between hospitals but within each hospital the initially established treatment schedule was to be followed. Operations varied from radical mastectomy to simple mastectomy, with combinations thereof. Postoperative radiation therapy varied between conventional and cobalt-60 treatment. In most, but not all, of the hospitals, surgical or radiologic castration was performed in Stage II cases. The organizers were of the opinion that all these variations were of minor importance, since each hospital was providing an equal number of patients to the chemotherapy and control groups. Cyclophosphamide (Cytoxan; CTX), 30 mg/kg body weight, was given for 6 days with one daily i.v. injection.

In 10 of the hospitals, patients were randomized immediately after surgical treatment and the patients received injections on the day of operation and on each of the next 5 days. This "surgical subseries" consisted of 621 patients at time of reporting. In the 11th institution, patients were admitted for postoperative radiotherapy after surgical treatment in other hospitals. In that institution, the randomization and administration of chemotherapy took place 2 to 4 weeks after surgical treatment. That group became known as the "radiologic subseries" and was composed of 108 patients.

According to the authors, results from this heterogeneous patient population indicated a trend in favor of those patients in the surgical subseries who received chemotherapy (i.e. a higher proportion free of disease). No such trend was noted in the "radiologic" subseries. The data presented for the surgical subseries showed that the control group of 323 patients had 71 recurrences and 45 deaths, and the chemotherapy group of 298 patients had 50 recurrences and 40 deaths. These results indicate a 5% difference in recurrence rates between the groups and no difference in survival rates.

In another study Mrazek and McDonald (1970), between 1956 and 1964, divided 156 patients into treated and control groups. Mechlorethamine hydrochloride (nitrogen mustard) was given to the treated patients—one half the "usual" dose at operation and the remainder on the first and second postoperative days. Every 3 months after operation, treated patients received courses of nitrogen mustard to bone marrow tolerance for a mean of 2.9 courses/patient. All patients were followed for 8 to 13 years. No patient who received chemotherapy had a recurrence, and all deaths in that group were unrelated to cancer. There was a recurrence of cancer in 36% of the control group, and only 57% survived.

Donegan (1970) instituted a prospective trial in 1962, to determine the value of prolonged treatment with TSPA as an adjuvant to radical mastectomy. After an initial course of therapy begun on the day of surgery (0.4 mg/kg) and for two successive days

(0.2 mg/kg/day), patients received 0.2 mg/kg/week for a minimum of 1 year. Forty-one control and 55 treated patients comprised the study. The author found that the overall recurrence rate was higher among treated patients than among controls, prompting him to suggest that prolonged systemic adjuvant chemotherapy may interfere with host resistance.

In 1974 he updated his findings (Donegan, 1974) and reported results from 75 controls and 90 treated patients observed from 1 to 10 years. It was not possible to establish that TSPA was of value as a surgical adjuvant. Local recurrence was reduced but recurrence overall was not altered, either in its frequency or time of appearance. A notable trend associated with treatment was improved disease-free survival among treated patients without axillary metastases. This led him to suggest that the adjuvant may be most effective when residual cancer is minimal.

Finney (1971) reported results of a trial in England in which all patients were treated by surgery and postoperative irradiation, but half of them also received pre- and postoperative chemotherapy. CTX was administered (2-3 mg/kg i.v.) daily for 4 days preoperatively, on the day of operation, and for 5 days postoperatively. After 3 years, results in the group receiving chemotherapy were worse than those in the control group. It is only fair to state that the number of patients was few, and information concerning comparability of patient groups was lacking.

Between March 1964 and March 1967 91 patients under 50 years of age with Stage I or II carcinoma were entered into a trial carried out at Guy's Hospital, London, to assess the value of postoperative testosterone therapy (Meakin et al., 1968). They were randomized, either receiving no further treatment after operation and irradiation, or having 200 mg of testosterone implanted subcutaneously on the 12th postoperative day and at 9-month intervals until recurrence. Urinary steroid excretion patterns were obtained. Preliminary data at 12 months following mastectomy from 46 patients implanted and 45 controls indicated a frequency of recurrence in patients with positive discriminants not significantly different from the rates in previous studies. The frequency of recurrence for patients with negative discriminants was lower in the testosterone-treated group than in the controls, but the number of patients was too few for the data to be statistically significant.

Because of ambiguity concerning the worth of prophylactic castration (i.e. oophorectomy following operation) for Stages I and II breast cancer, the NSABP began a randomized prospective trial in 1961 to obtain specific information to support or deny its value. Results of that trial failed to demonstrate an advantage for patients so treated (Ravdin et al., 1970).

This was the state of affairs in late 1971 when it was decided to set up a trial utilizing prolonged chemotherapy following surgery in women with clinically "curable" breast cancers. For the concept of using prolonged chemotherapy had experimental and clinical justification.

CURRENT CLINICAL TRIALS

As a consequence of increasing awareness of the rationale for combined modality therapy a large number of clinical trials have recently begun around the world. Alterations in protocol design make it impossible to ensure complete documentation and accuracy, but the following summarizes information about them that is known to this reviewer. Only a few have as yet produced data concerning the efficacy of the regimens being tested. They are not presented to supply the reader with a complete "registry" of all trials but to indicate the spectrum of investigations that are currently being carried out.

NSABP protocol #5 (L-PAM versus placebo)

Despite our recognition of the need for trials of prolonged combined modality therapy there was no unanimity as to the best agent, combination of agents or schedule of administration to employ. There was general agreement, however, that if a single agent were to be used, an alkylating agent–because of its cycle phase nonspecificity–offered the best chance for success. In choosing such an agent, it seemed reasonable also to select one which demonstrated effectiveness in patients with advanced disease. Of the several alkylating agents which have displayed that property–CTX, nitrogen mustard, L-phenylalanine mustard (L-PAM), chlorambucil, or TSPA–there was little difference in terms of their accomplishment. Each produced a 20-30% objective response rate.

However, in the extensive quantitative studies of Schmidt et al. (1965) in which 59 alkylating agents were evaluated against 20 animal neoplasms, CTX and L-PAM demonstrated the highest therapeutic indices. Because L-PAM can be administered orally at high intermittent doses for a prolonged period without causing alopecia or undue gastrointestinal toxicity, and because it had been noted (Sears et al., 1966) to produce regression in breast cancer at all sites in patients of all ages, it was the drug selected for use.

There were many who felt that it was a great mistake to employ only a single agent when there "is so much convincing evidence" (Cooper, 1969; Greenspan, 1966; Shingleton et al., 1971) to indicate that combination chemotherapy in patients with advanced disease results in a significantly greater remission rate than is provided by single agents. Others, however, had reservations concerning this approach for adjuvant treatment and noted that there have been virtually no concurrently controlled studies in man to determine whether drugs in combination would be of greater value than agents used alone under such circumstances (as "adjuvants").

Because of the interest generated by its preliminary report (Fisher et al., 1975a), a detailed account of this trial is presented. Data were obtained from women undergoing treatment at 37 institutions in the United States and Canada. All women having a radical mastectomy (conventional or modified) for potentially curable breast cancer, and having one or more axillary nodes proved histologically to contain tumor, were considered eligible for inclusion in the study provided they fulfilled specific criteria described in the protocol. These included tumors confined to the breast or breast and axilla; tumors movable in relation to the underlying muscle and chest wall; axillary nodes movable in relation to the chest wall and neurovascular bundle; no arm edema; white-cell count $\geq$ 4,000; platelet count $\geq$ 100,000; blood urea nitrogen $\leq$ 25 mg per 100 ml; geographic accessibility for follow-up observation; absence of psychiatric or addictive disorders prohibiting the attainment of informed consent; and patient's consent to participate.

Women were considered to be ineligible for inclusion if they were over 75 years of age; were pregnant or lactating; had previously been treated for their current neoplasm or had a prior or concomitant cancer other than an effectively managed basal or squamous-cell skin tumor; had a bilateral breast cancer or a tumor other than a carcinoma; the tumor was inflammatory; there was skin ulceration $>$ 2 cm, or peau d'orange involving more than one third of the skin of the breast. They were also ineligible for participation if satellite or parasternal nodules were present; there was fixation of axillary lymph nodes (over 2 cm); there were lymph nodes elsewhere suspected of containing tumor and unproved by biopsy to be negative. If they were poor surgical risks precluding their being subjected to any of the treatment options, or if nonmalignant systemic disease made prolonged follow-up study unlikely, they were also unacceptable.

After stratification according to age ($\leq$ 49 and $\geq$ 50 years), patients in each age group within each participating institution were randomized so that one-half received L-PAM, and the other placebo. Neither the physician nor the patient was aware of the treatment administered so as to ensure lack of bias in subsequent observations. Initially, only patients having four or more tumor-positive axillary nodes were placed on protocol but after study had progressed for 3 months, those having one to three positive nodes were also included. Consequently, patients were also stratified according to their nodal status (one to three, four or more positive nodes). The first patient was entered into the evaluation on September 22, 1972.

Patients assigned to L-PAM therapy received 0.15 mg/kg/day for five consecutive days every 6 weeks. Dosage was determined according to the patient's actual or ideal body weight, whichever was less. The entire daily dose was taken by mouth at bedtime. Treatment was begun no sooner than 2 weeks and not later than 4 weeks after operation and was to be continued until there was documented evidence of treatment failure, or for 2 years, whichever occurred first. Placebo was similarly administered.

Drug dosage was modified according to the presence and degree of toxicity. The latter was categorized according to a drop in white-cell or platelet count (or both) obtained before the onset of each course of therapy. If no toxicity had occurred, the patient received 100% of her calculated dose. If Grade 1 toxicity occurred, as evidenced by a decrease either in white-cell count to between 2,500 and 3,999, or in platelet count to between 75,000 and 99,999 per cu mm, 50% of the calculated dose was given. In the presence of Grade 2 toxicity, when the white-cell count was $<$ 2,500 or the platelet count was $<$ 75,000 per cu mm, the drug was discontinued and resumed only upon evidence of increase in those counts. If after three consecutive courses of therapy no toxicity was observed, the drug dosage was increased to 0.2 mg/kg of actual or ideal body weight per day, whichever was less.

A progress report of findings has been recently presented (Fisher et al., 1975a). At that time it was observed that treatment failures had occurred in 22% of 108 patients receiving placebo and 9.7% of 103 women given L-PAM ($p = 0.01$). A statistically significant difference ($p = 0.02$) existed in favor of L-PAM relative to disease-free interval. In premenopausal women, the difference with respect to disease-free interval between treated and control groups was highly significant ($p = 0.008$). Treatment failure occurred in 30% of premenopausal patients receiving

placebo and in 3% in those treated with L-PAM ($p = 0.008$). Whereas a similar trend was observed in postmenopausal patients, the difference was not statistically significant. Results were achieved with minimal upset of the well-being of patients despite the fact that 60% of women demonstrated myelosuppression (Grades 1 and 2 toxicity).

At that time it was pointed out that many questions were raised by the findings which only time could resolve. Would the differences in disease-free rates be sustained or would they be only transient? Would such differences be manifested in survival rates? Might undesirable sequelae of L-PAM therapy such as lymphoproliferative neoplasms become apparent only after prolonged follow-up study? Those questions remain to be answered.

NSABP protocol #7 (L-PAM versus L-PAM plus 5-FU)

In general, combination chemotherapy results in response rates in patients with advanced breast cancer which are better than those produced by single agents (Carter, 1972). By itself, CTX produces a 35% response rate, L-PAM 23%, Thio-TEPA 30% and nitrogen mustard 35%. Since Cooper (1969) first reported a 90% response rate utilizing a five-drug combination, numerous investigations have been reported with a variety of combinations. None have equalled his claimed response rate but most have demonstrated greater effectiveness than single agents alone. For example, in an Eastern Cooperative Oncology Group (ECOG) protocol employing CTX, 5-FU and MTX, a 50% remission rate was observed (Carter, 1973). An Acute Leukemia Cooperative Group B (ALGB) protocol using 5-FU, vincristine and prednisone, produced a 52% remission in advanced breast cancer. The Mayo Clinic reported 50% remission rates when CTX, vincristine and prednisone were used. Such findings justify the employment of drug combinations in protocols for the management of primary operable breast cancer.

Consequently, with completion of patient entry into NSABP Protocol #5 (placebo vs L-PAM), NSABP Protocol #7 was implemented. Utilizing the same criteria of patient acceptability and keeping all other aspects of the protocol compatible with Protocol #5, patient entry began in February, 1975. At the time of writing, over 500 patients have been randomized between L-PAM and L-PAM plus 5–FU. The L-PAM is administered as the only agent at a dose of 6 mg/M^2 by mouth. When combined with 5-FU, 4 mg/M^2 is given orally. The 5-FU dosage is 300 mg/M^2, i.v. Drugs are given on five consecutive days every 6 weeks for 2 years. To date, the toxicity of this two-drug combination is only a little greater than L-PAM alone, and is entirely acceptable. Since patients have been entered into this protocol for only a year, no data are as yet forthcoming.

Trial of the Cancer Institute of Milan (No treatment versus CMF)

In 1973, Bonadonna and his associates at the National Cancer Institute in Milan, Italy embarked upon a clinical trial to evaluate the effectiveness of CTX, MTX, and 5-FU (CMF) as an adjuvant. The patient selection and experimental design were essentially similar to those outlined for the NSABP Protocol #5 above. Patients were randomized following radical mastectomy so as to receive either 12 cycles of CMF or no treatment. Each cycle of drug therapy consisted of CTX (100 mg/M^2 po from day 1 to 14), MTX (40 mg/M^2, i.v. on days 1 and 8), and 5-FU (600 mg/M^2, i.v. on days 1 and 8). There was a 2-week rest period between cycles.

Whereas 24% of 179 control patients showed treatment failure by 14 months following operation, only 5.3% of 207 CMF treated patients demonstrated a recurrence (Bonadonna, 1976). In contrast to the minor toxicity obtained with the single agent L-PAM, greater side effects were noted. Alopecia occurred in more than 50% of patients, cystitis in 30%, and nausea and vomiting in almost all. About one-third of patients showed a repeated tendency to discontinue treatment or diminish the dose because of prolonged nausea and loss of appetite. Although 68% demonstrated leukopenia, only 4% had WBCs below 2,500 per cu mm. Similarly 66% had thrombocytopenia but in only 12% was this below 75,000 per cu mm.

NSABP Protocol #8 (L-PAM plus 5-FU versus L-PAM plus 5-FU plus MTX)

To test the hypothesis that a three-drug combination is better than two or one, the following trial will be implemented shortly. It will compare L-PAM (4 mg/M^2, po) plus 5-FU (300 mg/M^2, i.v.), with L-PAM (4 mg/M^2, po) plus 5-FU (300 mg/M^2, i.v.) plus Methotrexate (MTX; 25 mg/M^2, i.v.). As in previous protocols the L-PAM and 5-FU will be given on 5 consecutive days every 6 weeks and the MTX on days 1 and 5 of each cycle.

NSABP Protocol #9 (L-PAM or L-PAM plus 5-FU with and without tamoxifen)

Tamoxifen (ICI 46474, Nolvadex) is a synthetic non-steroidal compound with potent anti-estrogen

activity demonstrated in several mammalian species (Harper et al., 1967). Its mode of action is by blockade of estrogen receptors (see Chapter 8). It has been shown to yield a high response rate in metastatic breast cancer with a low incidence of troublesome side effects. This is discussed fully in Chapter 13.

Because of its demonstrated effectiveness in advanced disease, a trial of its effect on early disease seems warranted. Patients with surgically "curable" breast cancer who have one or more positive axillary nodes will be randomized into four groups: L-PAM, L-PAM plus 5-FU, L-PAM plus tamoxifen, and L-PAM plus 5-FU plus tamoxifen. Dosage of L-PAM and of 5-FU is identical to that in Protocol #8, and tamoxifen will be administered 10 mg by mouth twice a day.

NSABP Protocol #10 (L-PAM or L-PAM plus 5-FU with and without *C. parvum*)

Since increasing evidence implicates the role of immunity in a variety of aspects of tumor biology, a third clinical trial (NSABP Protocol #10) will compare chemotherapy, with and without *C. parvum*, in the management of patients with surgically "curable" breast cancer who have one or more positive axillary nodes.

The rationale for the employment of immunotherapy in combination with chemotherapy is sound and there are several reasons for utilizing non-specific immune stimulation in combination with surgery in the treatment of primary breast cancer. A correlation has been established between immuno-depression and cancer and it has been shown both experimentally and clinically that non-specific immune stimulants may increase or restore the general immune status in cancer patients. While manipulation of "specific" immune mechanisms may be more appropriate, this is unlikely to take place in a state of non-specific immune deficiency.

The reasons for employment of *C. parvum* are its reputed relatively high degree of effectiveness and its reputed relatively low toxicity as compared to BCG. *C. parvum* has repeatedly been demonstrated to stimulate RES function in various experimental tumor systems (Halpern et al., 1963; Scott, 1972; Smith et al., 1968). It has also been demonstrated to enhance resistance of mice to infection (Adlam et al., 1972), and to augment both delayed hypersensitivity and antibody production (Neveu et al., 1964). *C. parvum* can inhibit tumor growth in animal tumor systems (Halpern et al., 1966; Woodruff and Boak, 1966; Woodruff et al., 1971), and has been shown to augment the effectiveness of cytostatic chemotherapeutic agents (Currie et al., 1970; Fisher et al., 1975d).

It has been shown that the use of *C. parvum* prolongs survival to a greater degree in metastatic lung cancer when administered together with combined chemotherapy (Israel et al., 1973), than does chemotherapy alone. In patients with disseminated epidermoid bronchogenic carcinoma, 39 cases treated by chemotherapy alone were compared by random allocation to 43 cases receiving, in addition to the same combination chemotherapy (5-drug), a weekly injection of *C. parvum*. In the *C. parvum* group, there was a survival rate of 85% at 1 year and 41% at 2 years. The chemotherapy control group had a 41% and 16% survival respectively. It has been similarly employed against a variety of other solid tumors with significant benefit. Recently, tumor regressions have been noted when *C. parvum* was used intravenously even in the absence of chemotherapy (Israel et al., 1975).

Side effects with the use of *C. parvum* administered subcutaneously have been uncommon. Significant local inflammation has occurred in only three of more than 400 cases treated by Israel and Edelstein (1973), and no allergic reactions were encountered. An increase in the conversion of skin test negative to positive has been reported with the use of *C. parvum* (Israel et al., 1972). Accelerated tumor growth has not been observed in patients given *C. parvum*.

Due to the paucity of specific information available on *C. parvum* toxicity, a Phase I study was recently carried out by us in patients with advanced disease (Fisher et al., 1976c). From 273 injections of *C. parvum* (5 mg/M^2) in 40 patients it was observed that following intravenous infusion of *C. parvum*, (a) a febrile response and chills occurred in almost all patients and did not appreciably diminish in intensity following repetitive administrations; (b) nausea, vomiting and headache were observed; (c) a "flu-like" syndrome lasting 24 to 48 hours occurred following almost all courses of *C. parvum*; (d) blood pressure elevations occurred on occasion and were related to the severity of other side effects; hyper- or hypotension was not a problem; (e) no anaphylactic reactions or other untoward side effects were observed.

Pretreatment with a single administration of 100 mg (or 50 mg) of hydrocortisone prior to *C. parvum* infusion markedly, and in some instances dramatically, diminished the toxicity and made acceptable the use of intravenous *C. parvum* on an outpatient basis. The use of intravenous *C. parvum* in patients with cerebral metastases may be hazardous. Subcutaneously administered *C. parvum* resulted in a

significant number of undesirable local reactions. Evaluation of delayed cutaneous hypersensitivity response, immunoglobulins, complement, E and EAC rosette forming cells during *C. parvum* administration failed to demonstrate significant change from pre-injection values. Results were similar whether hydrocortisone pretreatment was or was not employed.

It must be pointed out, however, that those measurement were made on patients having advanced disease who had received a variety of therapeutic regimens which could depress host immune responses. More recently, it has been observed by us in further Phase I trials that 50 mg of hydrocortisone (SoluCortef) also diminishes the side effects. From accumulating data (Fisher, 1976; Fisher et al., 1976a) there is no evidence to suggest that such a dose of cortisone would interfere with *C. parvum* effectiveness. A base of information has accumulated from animal models (Fisher et al., 1975c; Fisher et al., 1976b) to provide guidelines for the timing, frequency and dose of *C. parvum* to be employed.

Patients will be randomized so that they receive L-PAM or L-PAM plus 5-FU in doses and schedules as described in the other NSABP studies. One-half the patients receiving L-PAM and one-half those getting L-PAM plus 5-FU will receive *C. parvum* (2.5 mg/M^2, i.v. every 3 weeks for 1 year).

SWOG Trial (L-PAM versus a five-drug combination)

The Southwest Oncology Group (SWOG) under the leadership of Dr. Barth Hoogstraten has begun a trial to compare combination chemotherapy with a single agent in patients with operable breast cancer who have one or more positive axillary nodes. Patients are stratified according to number of nodes involved, whether or not they receive postoperative radiation, and according to menopausal status. They are randomized so that they receive either (a) L-PAM (5 mg/M^2/day x 5 q 6 weeks); or (b) combination of 5-FU (300 mg/M^2, i.v. weekly), MTX (15 mg/M^2, i.v. weekly), vincristine (VCR) (0.625 mg/M^2, i.v. weekly), CTX (60 mg/M^2, po daily) and prednisone (30 mg/M^2 from 1-14 days, 20 mg/M^2 from 15-28 days, 10 mg/M^2 from 29-42 days and then discontinued). Following 10 weeks of the five-drug therapy the VCR and prednisone are discontinued and the CMF combination is given weekly. All therapy is discontinued after 1 year. No results are as yet available.

ALGB Trial (five-drug combination versus three drugs with and without MER)

The Acute Leukemia Cooperative Group B (ALGB) under the chairmanship of Dr. James Holland has begun a trial to evaluate long term systemic adjuvant chemotherapy with or without MER. Patients with positive axillary nodes are stratified according to age, tumor size and nodal status. They are then randomized into one of three treatment groups. They either receive (a) CTX (80 or 10 mg/M^2, po daily), 5-FU (500 mg/M^2, i.v. weekly), MTX (40 mg/M^2, i.v. weekly; 30 mg if over age 60), VCR (1.0 mg/M^2, i.v. weekly) and prednisone (40 mg/M^2, po daily); (b) CMF as in (a) above; or (c) CMF as in (a) or (b) plus MER (200 mg i.d. in each of five sites q 2nd week).

An induction phase of therapy from the 1st through the 6th week is followed by a 3-week rest period. The therapy is resumed utilizing a 4-week cycle. The drug is given for 2 weeks and the patient is rested for 2 weeks. After the first year of therapy patients in all groups receive CMF for an additional year. No information concerning results has been reported.

COG Trial (L-PAM versus a four-drug combination)

The Central Oncology Cooperative Group (COG) under the chairmanship of Dr. Robert Johnson has initiated a trial in which breast cancer patients with positive axillary nodes are randomized into two groups. They receive either (a) L-PAM (0.15 mg/kg, po daily x 5, q 6 weeks for 1 year); or (b) 5-FU (10 mg/kg, i.v. weekly x 7; days 1, 7, 14, 21, 28, 35 and 42), MTX (0.5 mg/kg, i.v. weekly x 7 on the same days as the 5-FU), VCR (0.025 mg/kg, i.v. weekly x 4 days, 1, 7, 14, 21), and CTX (2 mg/kg, po; days 1-42).

The drugs are given in 6 week cycles followed by 4 week rest periods for 1 year.

Case-Western Reserve Trial (three-drug combination plus anti estrogen with and without subsequent BCG versus no treatment)

Dr. Charles Hubay and associates in Cleveland, Ohio are carrying out a trial in which patients with positive axillary nodes are stratified according to whether or not their tumors displayed estrogen receptor sites. They are randomized to either a "no treatment" control group or to a treatment group. The patients in the latter group receive 5-FU (400 mg/M^2, i.v. on days 1 and 8 of each month), MTX (25 mg/M^2, i.v. on days 1 and 8 of each month), CTX (60 mg/m^2, po on days 1-14 each month), and tamoxifen (20 mg bid every day of the month.

A cycle of treatment consists of 2 weeks of therapy and 2 weeks of rest (except for tamoxifen). After 1 year of therapy, half of the patients in the

treatment group continue treatment for an additional year with BCG (Tice strain). They receive 1 ampoule (2 to 8 x 10^8 organisms), via the tine technic, weekly for four consecutive weeks and subsequently once a month.

Mayo Clinic Trial (L-PAM versus a three-drug combination with and without radiation)

Under the direction of Dr. David Ahmann, patients with positive axillary nodes are randomized into three treatment groups at the Mayo Clinic, Rochester, Minnesota. They receive either (a) L-PAM (6 mg/M^2, po daily x 5); (b) CTX (150 mg/M^2, po daily x 5), 5-FU (300 mg/M^2, i.v. daily x 5) and prednisone (300 mg daily x 7); or (c) CTX, 5-FU, prednisone as in (b) plus postoperative radiation.

Additional Clinical Trials Employing Immunotherapy

In addition to those trials already mentioned which employ immunotherapy as adjuvants following surgery for primary operable breast cancer, the International Registry of Tumor Immunotherapy of the National Cancer Institute, Bethesda, Maryland, under the direction of Dr. Dorothy Windhorst, lists the following studies.

A clinical trial has been begun under the supervision of Dr. Frank Sparks of the University of California at Los Angeles to determine the effect of CMF and BCG, with or without a tumor cell vaccine, on recurrence and survival of women with Stage II breast cancer. Patients are accepted into the study whether or not they have had postoperative radiation. They are randomized into three groups—CMF, CMF plus BCG, and CMF plus BCG plus allogeneic tumor cells.

At Duke University in Durham, North Carolina, a study under the direction of Dr. S. A. Wells, Jr., is comparing immunotherapy and chemotherapy as adjuvant treatment in the surgical management of early breast cancer. Patients with disease limited to the breast and ipsilateral axilla are being randomized so that they receive either CMF plus prednisone, or CMF plus prednisone plus irradiated allogeneic tumor cells plus *C. parvum.*

Dr. Jordan Gutterman at M.D. Anderson Hospital, Houston, Texas, is evaluating the efficacy of chemotherapy and immunotherapy in the prevention of metastatic disease, and in prolongation of survival of Stage II breast cancer patients. They are randomized into three treatment groups; those receiving Adriamycin alone, those getting Adriamycin plus BCG by scarification, and those treated with BCG alone.

Dr. J. Hermon-Taylor of the London Hospital, London, England, is principal investigator of a randomized trial to determine whether oral BCG administration for 3 years has any effect on the length of remission and survival of Stages I and II patients having simple mastectomy with no postoperative radiotherapy. Patients receive either no further treatment, or BCG orally.

Dr. Edward Scanlon of Northwestern University, Evanston, Illinois, is principal investigator of a trial to evaluate chemotherapy and immunotherapy in patients with Stages II and III breast cancer. They are randomized so that they receive either L-PAM or CTX, 5-FU and prednisone, or CTX, 5-FU, prednisone and BCG.

Dr. J. P. Stephens of Norwich, England, is indicated as principal investigator of a trial to study the efficacy of BCG in the treatment of early breast tumors. Following initial treatment patients are randomized so they receive either no further therapy or percutaneous BCG.

At the Sloan Kettering Institute for Cancer Research, Dr. H. F. Oettgen is conducting a trial on patients with operable breast cancer having either four or more positive nodes, any number of positive nodes at level III, any number of macroscopically positive nodes at levels II or III, or three or more macroscopically positive nodes at level I. Patients receive either (a) L-PAM, (b) CTX, adriamycin, 5-FU or (c) levamisole.

Dr. F. Lacour at Institute Gustave Roussy, Villejuif, France, has been evaluating the nonspecific adjuvant immunotherapeutic agent Poly A Poly U in patients having T2 and T3 tumors less than 7 cm in greatest diameter and regional lymph nodes NO or N1. Following operation patients are randomized so that they receive either (a) no further therapy, (b) radiation alone, (c) radiation plus Poly A Poly U, or (d) Poly A Poly U.

COMMENTS, CONCLUSIONS AND SPECULATIONS

The next decade may well represent the most critical and significant period in the history of breast cancer therapy. The present spectrum of combined modality trials, added to those which are proliferating at an ever more rapid pace throughout the world, is setting the stage for that crisis situation. Should many or most of those trials fail to be continued to a point where meaningful data are obtained (or even worse, because of their improper design or implementation,

produce information of questionable credibility) valuable time will have been lost, patient resources will have been squandered and above all, therapeutic confusion and disenchantment will prevail.

On the other hand, should a sufficient number of the protocols be impeccably carried to completion and meaningful data obtained, the next 10 years could be even more crucial. For, there will result verification or repudiation not only of the concepts and principles upon which the use of adjuvant therapy is based, but also of the very worth of those modalities which, at present, represent our total therapeutic resources and hopes for cure of breast cancer.

If, for example, from the multiplicity of trials evaluating different chemotherapeutic combinations, we fail to observe significant prolongation of freedom from disease which is reflected in a major improvement in survival, the entire chemotherapeutic approach to the treatment of breast cancer will be subject to challenge. The present regression of metastases for 6 to 18 months following combination chemotherapy in up to 85% of patients should not obscure the dismal fact that control for three or more years after the onset of chemotherapy is achieved in less than 15% of those treated for recurrence, and 5 year survival in less than 5%, despite the best efforts. Consequently, if adjuvant chemotherapy fails to make a dramatic impact on the disease-free survival of patients with "minimal" disease, the outlook is indeed bleak for those with advanced tumors—unless, of course, new agents become available.

Similar considerations relate to the use of immunotherapeutic and hormonal agents. Obviously, unless they can aid in the "cure" of more "early" lesions, their worth in advanced disease will be nil.

More optimistically, it is likely that from the multiplicity of trials there will come information as to the regimens most effective against a particular subset of breast cancer patients, with a minimum of toxicity. It is not unreasonable to predict that the same magnitude of chemotherapy employed in patients with ⩾4 positive nodes having a highly unfavorable prognosis will not be required for the patient with one positive node. Most urgently needed for the proper synchronization of our available therapeutic modalities is a biological assay which can indicate with precision the amount and the location of residual tumor present following operation.

It may be predicted that, as information becomes available from more of the trials currently in progress, the physician caring for such patients will be faced with a disturbing situation worse than the surgical dilemma of the last decade or two. A debate for example, that CMF is categorically better than L-PAM or that CAMP (CTX, adriamycin, MTX, prednisone) is better than CMF, could well rival the simple vs radical mastectomy polemic. Hopefully, since results are being obtained from carefully controlled studies, in contrast to the method by which the surgical data were generated, such controversies will be avoided.

This reviewer has pointed out that the most important aspect of the findings achieved with L-PAM, and more recently with CMF, is not the statistical magnitude of the differences, or even that the results could be obtained with acceptable toxicity, but that it has been demonstrated that the rationale for using prolonged chemotherapy as an adjunct to operation is a sound one. Different agents in various combinations, refinements of administration, sequences of drugs, etc. will undoubtedly produce increasingly better results.

One of the pressing decisions to be made is whether or not systemic therapy should be employed at the present time in patients with negative axillary nodes. Since, as has been pointed out, 25% of these patients show treatment failure by 10 years, it is this reviewer's opinion that a trial of such therapy should be begun at once. Obviously such a trial will require significantly greater numbers of patients followed for much longer times than those utilizing women with a more unfavorable prognosis.

As systemic therapy becomes more effective, the more likely it becomes that lesser operative procedures could be practised. As a consequence, increased disease control could be accomplished together with better cosmesis and quality of life. It is not unreasonable to anticipate that when diagnostic methodology has so improved that earlier cancers are detected, and when there is better understanding regarding the proper use of anticancer agents in concert so as to maximize effectiveness, surgery may play a subsidiary role in the management of solid tumors and may be entirely supplanted by other modalities.

At present there would seem to be justifiable reason for optimism concerning the future of women who develop breast cancer. Paradoxically, however, in the foreseeable future there will be no permanent prescription or recipe for the management of this disease simply because progress will proceed in various directions with increasing momentum and it is impossible to predict the ultimate nature of the next plateau.

In conclusion, the answer to the universal question, "Should *all* women with primary breast cancer receive systemic therapy in addition to

surgery?", must be a qualified one. The answer can, for the present, only be "yes" if this is carried out in a clinical trial situation. Since it has not yet been shown that any therapeutic regimen cures *more* (let alone *all*) patients, a multiplicity of additional trials carried out in a *coordinated* fashion are necessary to make further gains. Where will patients for those trials come from if each is treated by her physician without making a contribution to our knowledge? How will it be possible to resolve the plethora of new questions raised by each additional piece of information? In this reviewer's opinion as of the time of writing, adjuvant therapy for breast cancer is still a component of clinical research in oncology.

REFERENCES

Adlam, C., Broughton, E. S. and Scott, M. T. (1972). Enhanced resistance of mice to infection with bacteria following pretreatment with *C. parvum. Nature New Biology 235,* 219.

Bonadonna, G., Brusamolino, E. and Valagussa, P. et al. (1976). Combination chemotherapy as an adjuvant treatment in operable breast cancer. *New England Journal of Medicine 294,* 405.

Carter, S. K. (1972). Single and combination non-hormonal chemotherapy in breast cancer. *Cancer 30,* 543.

Carter, S. K. (1973). Reported at NSABP Group Meeting, Bethesda, Maryland.

Chirigos, M. A., Colsky, J., Humphreys, S. R., Glynn, J. P. and Goldin, A. (1962). Evaluation of surgery and chemotherapy in the treatment of mouse mammary adenocarcinoma 755. *Cancer Chemotherapy Reports 22,* 49.

Cooper, R. (1969). Combination chemotherapy in hormone resistant breast cancer. *Proceedings of the American Association of Cancer Research 10,* 15.

Cruz, E. P., McDonald, G. O. and Cole, W. H. (1956). Prophylactic treatment of cancer; the use of chemotherapeutic agents to prevent tumor metastasis. *Surgery 40,* 291.

Currie, G. H. and Bagshawe, D. (1970). Active immunotherapy with *C. parvum* and chemotherapy in marine fibrosarcomas. *British Medical Journal 1,* 541.

DeWys, W. D. (1972). Studies correlating the growth rate of a tumor and its metastases and providing evidence for tumor related systemic growth retarding factors. *Cancer Research 32,* 274.

Donegan, W. L. (1970). Prolonged surgical adjuvant chemotherapy with Thio-TEPA for mammary carcinoma: a progress report, p. 500. Abstracts of the *Tenth International Cancer Congress,* Houston, Texas.

Donegan, W. L. (1974). Extended surgical adjuvant Thio-TEPA for mammary carcinoma. *Archives of Surgery 109,* 187.

Engel, H. C. (1955). Cancer cells in the circulating blood. *Acta Chirurgica Scandinavica,* Supp. 201.

Finney, R. (1971). Adjuvant chemotherapy in the radical treatment of carcinoma of the breast—a clinical trial. *American Journal of Roentgenology 111,* 137.

Fisher, B. (1976). Unpublished data relative to *C. parvum* and macrophage colony production and macrophage cytotoxicity.

Fisher, B., Ravdin, R. G., Ausman, R. K., Slack, N. H., Moore, G. E. and Noer, R. J. (1968). Surgical adjuvant chemotherapy in cancer of the breast: results of a decade of cooperative investigation. *Annals of Surgery 168,* 337.

Fisher, B., Carbone, P. and Economou, S. G. et al. (1975a). 1-Phenylalanine mustard (L-PAM) in the management of primary breast cancer; a report of early findings. *New England Journal of Medicine 292,* 117.

Fisher, B., Slack, N., Katrych, D. and Wolmark, N. (1975b). Ten year follow-up of breast cancer patients in a cooperative clinical trial evaluating surgical adjuvant chemotherapy. *Surgery, Gynecology & Obstetrics 140,* 528.

Fisher, B., Wolmark, N., Rubin, H. and Saffer, E. (1975c). Further observations on the inhibition of tumor growth by *C. parvum* with cyclophosphamide: I. Variation in administration of both agents. *Journal of the National Cancer Institute 55,* 1147.

Fisher, B., Wolmark, N., Saffer, E. and Fisher, E. R. (1975d). Inhibitory effect of prolonged *Corynebacterium parvum* and cyclophosphamide. administration on the growth of established tumors. *Cancer 35,* 134.

Fisher, B., Rubin, H., Saffer, E. and Wolmark, N. (1976a). Further observations on the inhibition of tumor growth by *C. parvum* with cyclophosphamide. II. Effect of cortisone acetate. *Journal of the National Cancer Institute, in press.*

Fisher, B., Rubin, H., Saffer, E. and Wolmark, N. (1976b). Effect of *C. parvum* in combination with 5-Fluorouracil, 1-Phenylalanine mustard or Methotrexate on the inhibition of tumor growth. *Cancer Research, in press.*

Fisher, B., Rubin, H., Sartiano, G., Ennis, L. and Wolmark, N. (1976c). Observations following *C. parvum* administration to patients with advanced malignancy: a phase I study. *Cancer, in press.*

Fisher, E. R. and Turnbull, R. B., Jr. (1955). The cytologic demonstration and significance of tumor cells in the mesenteric venous blood in patients with colorectal carcinoma. *Surgery, Gynecology & Obstetrics 100,* 102.

Greenspan, E. M. (1966). Combination cytotoxic chemotherapy in advanced disseminated breast carcinoma. *Journal of Mount Sinai Hospital, New York 33,* 1.

Greenspan, E. M. (1975). *Clinical cancer chemotherapy,* p. 171. New York: Raven Press.

Halpern, B. N., Prevot, A. R., Biozzi, G., Stiffel, C., Mouton, D., Morard, J. C., Bouthillier, Y. and Decreusefond, C. (1963). Stimulation of the phagocytic activity of the RES provoked by *C. parvum. Journal of the Reticuloendothelial Society 1,* 77.

Halpern, B., Biozzi, G., Stiffel, C. and Mouton, D. (1966). Inhibition of tumor growth by administration of killed *C. parvum. Nature 212,* 853.

Harper, M. J. K. and Walpole, A. L. (1967). A new derivative of triphenylethylene: Effect on implantation and mode of action in rats. *Journal of Reproduction & Fertility 13,* 101.

Israel, L. and Halpern, B. N. (1972). *C. parvum* in advanced cancers: initial evaluation of therapeutic activity. *La Nouvelle Presse Medicale 1,* 19.

Israel, L. and Edelstein, R. (1973). *Nonspecific immunostimulation with* C. parvum *in human cancer,* p. 485. Baltimore, Maryland: Williams and Wilkins Company.

Israel, L. and Edelstein, R. (1975). A phase II study of daily intravenous *Corynebacterium* in 33 disseminated cancers. *Proceedings of the American Association of Cancer Research 16,* 67.

Karrer, K. and Humphreys, S. (1967). Adjuvant chemotherapy given before or after surgery. *Proceedings of the American Association of Cancer Research 8,* 35.

Martin, D. S., Fugmann, R. A. and Hayworth, P. (1962). Surgery, cancer chemotherapy, host defenses and tumor size. *Journal of the National Cancer Institute 29,* 817.

Meakin, J. W., Allt, W. E. C. and Beale, F. A. et al. (1968). A preliminary report of two studies of adjuvant treatment of primary breast cancer. In *Prognostic Factors in Breast Cancer,* p. 157 (Eds A. P. M. Forrest and P. B. Kunkler). Edinburgh: E. & S. Livingstone, Ltd.

McDonald, G. O., Cruz, E. P. and Cole, W. H. (1956). The effect of cancer inhibitor drugs on the "take" of Walker carcinosarcoma 256 in rats. *Surgical Forum 7,* 486.

McDonald, G. O., Livingston, C., Boyles, C. F. and Cole, W. H. (1957). The prophylactic treatment of malignant disease with nitrogen mustard and triethylenethiophosphoramide (Thio-TEPA). *Annals of Surgery 145,* 624.

Mrazek, R. G. and McDonald, G. O. (1970). Surgery and adjuvant chemotherapy in treatment for breast carcinoma, p. 501. Abstracts of the Tenth International Cancer Congress, Houston, Texas.

Neveu, T., Branellec, A. and Biozzi, G. (1964). Adjuvant effect of *C. parvum* on antibody production and delayed hypersensitivity conjugated proteins. *Annales de l'Institut Pasteur 106,* 771.

Nissen-Meyer, R., Kjellgren, K. and Mansson, B. (1971). Preliminary report from the Scandinavian adjuvant chemotherapy study group. *Cancer Chemotherapy Reports 55,* 561.

Ravdin, R. G., Lewison, E. F. and Slack, N. H. et al. (1970). Results of a clinical trial concerning the worth of prophylactic oophorectomy for breast carcinoma. *Surgery, Gynecology & Obstetrics 131,* 1055.

Schabel, F. M., Jr. (1969). The use of tumor growth kinetics in planning "curative" chemotherapy of advanced solid tumors. *Cancer Research 29,* 2384.

Schabel, F. M., Jr. (1975). Animal models as predictive systems, p. 323. *Cancer Chemotherapy—Fundamental Concepts and Recent Advances.*

Schmidt, L. H., Fradkin, R., Sullivan, R. and Flowers, A. (1965). Comparative pharmacology of alkylating agents. *Cancer Chemotherapy Reports,* Suppl. *2,* 1.

Scott, M. T. (1972). Biological effects of adjuvant *C. parvum.* I. Inhibition of PHA, mixed lymphocytes and GVH reactivity. *Cellular Immunology 5,* 459.

Sears, M. E., Haut, A. and Eckles, N. (1966). Melphalan (NSC-8806) in advanced breast cancer. *Cancer Chemotherapy Reports 50,* 271.

Shingleton, W. W., Sedransk, N. Johnson, R. O. (1971). Systemic chemotherapy of mammary carcinoma. *Annals of Surgery 173,* 913.

Simpson-Herron, L., Sanford, A. H. and Holmquist, J. P. (1974). Cell population kinetics of transplanted and metastatic Lewis lung carcinoma. *Cell and Tissue Kinetics 7,* 349.

Skipper, H. E. (1971). Some thoughts on surgery-chemotherapy trials against breast cancer. In *Monograph,* p. 1. Birmingham, Alabama: Southern Research Institute.

Skipper, H. E. (1974). Combination therapy, Booklet 13, p. 1. Birmingham, Alabama: Southern Research Institute.

Smith, L. H. and Woodruff, M. F. A. (1968). Comparative effect of 2 strains of *C. parvum* on the phagocytic activity and tumor growth. *Nature 219,* 197.

Straus, M. J., Sege, V. and Chor, S. C. (1975). The effect of surgery and pretreatment or post-treatment adjuvant chemotherapy on primary tumor growth in an animal model. *Journal of Surgical Oncology 7,* 497

Woodruff, M. F. A. and Boak, J. L. (1966). Inhibitory effect of injection of *C. parvum* on the growth of tumor transplants in isogeneic hosts. *British Journal of Cancer 20,* 345.

Woodruff, M. F. A. and Inchley, M. P. (1971). Synergistic inhibition of mammary carcinoma transplants in A-strain mice by antitumor globulin and *C. parvum. British Journal of Cancer 25,* 584.

Chapter

7

DIANA BRINKLEY

The Role of Post-operative Radiotherapy

Policy on the routine use of post-operative radiotherapy after mastectomy for breast cancer has changed during the last ten years. Such treatment was often used routinely in the past with the aim of lessening the risk of recurrence in the scar and draining node areas. It was assumed that the prognosis was improved as a result, and therefore that damage which might ensue from such treatment was a price that had to be paid for the benefits. As more information on the results of treatment and on the natural behaviour of the disease has become available, these facts must be taken into account when selecting patients for post-operative radiotherapy.

AIMS OF POST-OPERATIVE X-RAY THERAPY

With the development of modern surgical techniques, the radical mastectomy became the operation of choice for many surgeons who were attempting to cure breast cancer. This operation involves resection of the breast, pectoral muscles and axillary tissues in one block but leaves untreated any possible metastases in the supraclavicular, infraclavicular and internal mammary nodes. Post-operative X-ray therapy was then given to destroy any malignant cells which had escaped the surgeon's knife in the area of the pectoral scar and axilla, and to destroy any cancer cells which had spread to the lymphatics in the supra- and infraclavicular areas or in the internal mammary chain of glands.

The type of treatment that was recommended often lasted six weeks, gave a high dose and could result in considerable morbidity. It might be expected that such post-operative treatment would be a standard procedure but it is not so. Such fundamental issues as when to give treatment, which areas to irradiate, the total dose to be used, the length of time the treatment should take, the spacing of the treatment fractions and the type of radiation to be used are still undecided.

In understanding the role of post-operative radiotherapy in the treatment of breast cancer, it is helpful to consider the action of irradiation on living tissues

and the development of X-ray therapy since the discovery of X-rays by Röntgen in 1895.

All types of radiation used in the treatment of cancer are ionising radiations and are destructive. They produce damage to the nucleus and cytoplasm of cells which, if severe, may result in cell death or if less severe, may prevent the cell from successful replication or cause damage from which the cell may never recover. Cancer cells, for reasons which are not fully understood, are more sensitive than normal cells to the effects of irradiation, and normal cells and tissues although damaged by irradiation have greater powers of recovery and repair. It is this difference between malignant cells and normal cells in sensitivity to irradiation and power of recovery from irradiation which makes treatment of cancer with X-ray therapy possible. However, the difference is not standard; it varies between one type of cancer and another and between one type of normal tissue and another, so that the planning of a successful treatment which will eradicate malignant cells and not leave irreparable damage to normal tissue is a matter requiring considerable knowledge, skill and experience.

To undertake such treatment a radiotherapist must take into account the extent of the area to be covered, the nature of the cancer, the structure of the various normal tissues he will inevitably have to irradiate, the age and condition of the patient and the equipment he has available. He will then decide how to apply the treatment, over what period of time, and how many doses or fractions should be used.

Radiotherapists are still uncertain of the optimum treatment method and of the role of post-operative radiotherapy after mastectomy. High dosage irradiation may produce some of the serious reactions which are listed in Table 1. It is perhaps misleading to list *all* the possible complications of post operative radiotherapy but there is no doubt that the courses of treatment recommended are demanding and debilitating, and mild degrees of the complications described are not uncommon.

Fears have been expressed that as radiation is known to be carcinogenic, the routine use of radiotherapy in the treatment of breast cancer may result in the development of radiation-induced malignancy many years later. There is well documented evidence that radiation exposure can cause cancer, and in particular breast cancer, when repeated small doses have been received, as in fluoroscopy in patients with tuberculosis (Cook et al., 1974; Myrden and Hiltz, 1969; Mackenzie, 1965). However, there is not a single report in the literature of radiation-induced carcinoma developing after treatment for breast cancer and in our study of 704 patients followed up in Cambridge for 25 years, no such cases occurred (Brinkley and Haybittle, 1975).

Table 1. Serious reactions and complications which may follow high dose irradiation after mastectomy

Skin changes	Immediate erythema, proceeding to desquamation followed by pigmentation. Late telangiectasia and sometimes skin necrosis. Rarely squamous cell carcinoma many years later. Subcutaneous tissues may develop induration and atrophy.
Bone	Ribs may fracture because of impaired blood supply.
Lungs	Pheumonitis a few weeks after treatment but usually resolves. Lung fibrosis 18-24 months or more after treatment is irreversible and may be disabling.
Nerves	Damage to brachial plexus may cause intractable pain.
Shoulder and arm	Shoulder joint may become stiff. Arm may develop oedema due to lymphatic damage.
General reactions	Lowering of local and general immunity. Damage to local immunity may be reflected in extensive local recurrence just within irradiated area. Lowering of general immunity reflected by prolonged lymphopenia.

Malignancy occurring many years after X-ray therapy for chronic mastitis and puerperal mastitis has been reported in a few women (Mettler et al., 1969). It may be that in patients with a normal life expectation the risk is greater because they are more likely to survive through the long latent period required for the carcinoma to develop. Therefore while it is impossible to quote a figure indicating the risk of radiation-induced cancer following routine post-operative radiotherapy in treating breast cancer, it must be a very small risk indeed and should not be allowed to influence clinicians in their choice of treatment. In most cases, the breast will have been removed in any case and the irradiation will be given only to the scar and axillary node area.

In the past clinicians had no doubt that post operative radiotherapy was capable of dealing with local residual malignancy and decreasing local recurrence in a proportion of cases. They therefore assumed that this improved the long term survival rate, and under these circumstances the risk of undesirable side effects had to be taken. Some large series of patients were studied over long periods but they were of highly selected groups of patients and therefore could not prove or disprove the suggestion that post-operative X-ray therapy was really improv-

ing the survival rate. The high frequency of early dissemination in breast cancer was not appreciated and all efforts were channelled into developing more and more radical treatment.

CLINICAL TRIALS AND RETROSPECTIVE SURVEYS

The certainty of many clinicians about the soundness of their treatment policy in patients with breast cancer was disturbed in Britain when McWhirter (1948) published the results of a survey he undertook on patients treated in Edinburgh. His work showed that patients treated by simple mastectomy and post-operative radiotherapy survived as well as did those patients treated by radical surgery. This result, suggesting that radical surgery was not essential, caused many surgeons and radiotherapists to reconsider their treatment policy; further retrospective studies were undertaken and a number of prospective clinical trials set up to try and clarify the situation. A brief description of these studies and of the published results will perhaps help to clarify the role of post-operative radiotherapy.

Retrospective surveys have been undertaken by reviewing the results of treatment in groups of patients from one centre or hospital. Information has been extracted from hospital records and death certificates, but in many cases the information is incomplete and sometimes inaccurate. Other surveys on a larger scale have been undertaken by examination of regional and national cancer registration bureau statistics. Again the information available may be incomplete and inaccurate, but the advantage of this type of survey is the very large numbers of cases which may be reviewed and analysed.

RETROSPECTIVE STUDIES

(1) The U.S.A. Health Department (1960) produced survival figures on over 37,000 women. Those who underwent some type of operation for breast cancer without irradiation were compared with those having some type of operation followed by irradiation. The 5 year survival rates for Manchester Stage I and Stage II patients who did not have irradiation were 10% and 7% higher respectively than for those who were irradiated.

(2) Lipworth (1965) published figures from the cancer registries in England and Wales for 1952 and 1953. The records of about 13,000 patients with breast cancer were analysed according to age group and expressed in terms of 5 year survival. In all groups except in those over 65 years of age with non-localised disease, the patients who did not have irradiation fared better; in those under 45 with localised disease, the difference between the irradiated and non-irradiated groups was 14.4%.

(3) Bond (1967) reported results in over 6,000 patients with breast cancer and showed that those without axillary metastases treated by simple mastectomy alone had a 5 year survival rate 9% higher than those in whom simple mastectomy was followed by irradiation. Similar differences were found between patients who had radical mastectomy alone and those with radical mastectomy followed by irradiation.

(4) Crile (1968) reported on a small series of patients with operable breast cancer treated by simple mastectomy with or without cobalt irradiation, or by radical mastectomy with or without cobalt irradiation. He concluded that in patients with Stage I disease (the axilla at the time of operation contained no palpably involved nodes), the 5 year survival rate was 13% higher if the nodes were left and not irradiated than if they were removed with the breast. He also concluded that if the axillary nodes were involved, the different methods of treatment employed seemed to give comparable results as far as survival was concerned.

(5) Hamlin (1968) reassessed 272 patients treated between 1935 and 1945 and found 15 year survival rates to be higher in those patients with Stage I, II and III disease who had surgery alone, than in those who had surgery followed by irradiation.

(6) Cutler and Connelly (1969) reported on survival figures in 50,000 patients treated in the U.S.A. whose data were published by the End Results Group. In one group of patients with Stage II disease, those who had surgery alone showed 59% 5 year survival, while the group who had surgery followed by irradiation showed 49% 5 year survival. The type of surgery was not specified.

The use of retrospective studies to assess the merits of different forms of treatment is however open to criticism. Many factors may have influenced the selection of treatment and the records are often inadequate. It is likely that X-ray therapy was selected for those patients with more advanced disease and this would bias long term results against the groups having radiotherapy.

However, it is interesting that all these surveys,

some of them very large, report the same trend in favour of surgery alone without irradiation. A better understanding of the role of post-operative radiotherapy requires study of prospective controlled clinical trials.

PROSPECTIVE CONTROLLED CLINICAL TRIALS

In such trials two or more types of treatment are selected prospectively, and attempts are made to compare the results of one form of treatment against another in groups of patients who are comparable in as many respects as possible. Every effort is made to avoid bias in the selection of treatment for any patient or group of patients, and to adhere strictly to the rules of the trial both in the primary selection and treatment of the patients and also in their aftercare and follow-up. A clinician who considers he already knows which of two treatments is better should not agree to participate in such a trial. Expert advice from medical statisticians on the design of a trial and on the analysis of the results is of prime importance.

A number of controlled, prospective clinical trials have been undertaken in the treatment of early breast cancer, comparing various types of surgery associated with radiotherapy. The results of these trials give some guidance on the role of post-operative radiotherapy.

(1) Easson (1968) reviewed the 10 year results of trials conducted at the Christie Hospital in Manchester. These compared the results of treatment of patients with operable breast cancer who had either radical mastectomy and routine post-operative radiotherapy, or else radical mastectomy and radiotherapy given only if and when local recurrence of the disease occurred.

Their studies showed no difference in survival between the two groups of patients at any point during the 10 years follow-up period, and in each group 55% of patients died from distant metastases within 10 years. In the group not having routine post-operative radiotherapy, 35% died from distant secondaries without ever developing local recurrence and were thus spared radiation morbidity. When local recurrence did occur, local irradiation controlled the disease until death in a similar proportion of cases as did prophylactic irradiation. Two different X-ray techniques yielded similar results.

These trials showed no advantage for post operative radiotherapy in terms of survival. Post-operative irradiation did prevent local recurrence, but such recurrences were as well controlled by "on demand" radiotherapy. Easson concluded that it was an advantage to patients to avoid routine post-operative radiotherapy after radical mastectomy.

(2) Kaae and Johansen (1968) reported the 10 year results of a clinical trial comparing treatment in two groups of patients. One group was treated by extended radical mastectomy (including excision of the internal mammary lymph nodes) without post-operative radiotherapy, and the other group was treated by simple mastectomy followed by post-operative irradiation, including the pectoral scar and the peripheral nodes. The 5 and 10 year survival and local recurrence figures were similar in the two groups, but morbidity in terms of oedema and weakness of the arm was higher in the group having radical mastectomy. In view of these findings it appeared reasonable to give preference to simple mastectomy and routine post-operative radiotherapy.

(3) Fisher (1970) reported the results of a controlled trial conducted at a number of centres in the United States. All patients had a radical mastectomy and were then allocated to groups receiving radiotherapy, Thiotepa or a placebo. Different protocols were used for pre- and post-menopausal patients. Five year figures for survival and recurrence rates showed no significant differences between the groups.

(4) Brinkley and Haybittle (1971) reported the results of a trial carried out at Cambridge, which compared the results of radical mastectomy and routine post-operative irradiation with those of simple mastectomy and routine post-operative radiotherapy in patients with Stage II disease. In both groups the radiotherapy was similar. The survival rates and recurrence rates at 10 years were similar, but the morbidity in terms of delayed healing after operation and arm oedema, was higher in the group having the radical operation. They concluded that in this group of patients, simple mastectomy with post-operative radiotherapy was preferable to radical mastectomy with post-operative radiotherapy.

(5) Atkins (1972) reported from Guy's Hospital the 10 year results of a prospective clinical trial in early breast cancer. One group of patients was treated by radical mastectomy followed by radiotherapy to the axilla, supraclavicular triangle and internal mammary chain. The second group of patients had a wide local excision of the primary tumour followed by radiotherapy to the breast, axilla, supraclavicular area and internal mammary chain.

In patients with clinically involved nodes, there was a higher incidence of local and distant recurrence in those treated by local excision, and this group had a poorer survival rate. In patients with clinically uninvolved nodes there was again a higher local recurrence rate in the group having the less extensive operation, but there was no increase in the distant recurrence rate and no difference in survival rate. (The early intake of patients in the trial had Thiotepa as an adjunct to surgery). This trial indicated that only a small highly selected group of patients is suitable for local excision and post-operative radiotherapy.

(6) Roberts (1973) reported the result of a trial carried out in Cardiff on two treatment groups. One group had radical mastectomy or modified radical mastectomy and the other simple mastectomy. In both groups adjuvant local radiotherapy was given only if the pectoral or axillary node histology indicated metastatic disease. The initial results showed nothing to suggest that the radical approach was superior to the simple one, and confirm that simple mastectomy and post operative radiotherapy is a suitable treatment for patients with Stage II disease.

ASSESSMENT OF RESULTS

Various criticisms are levelled at these trials. Were there sufficient numbers of patients in the groups being compared? Were the groups strictly comparable in terms of stage of disease and histology? Were the doses of irradiation effective and comparable? However, the trials were carried out carefully and without bias and it would seem reasonable to accept their results with perhaps some reservation, and to consider what light they throw on the role of post-operative radiotherapy.

One interesting result which has emerged is that with the exception of the Guy's trial, all the various treatment methods tested give similar results in terms of survival and in terms of distant recurrence. It should also be noted that the prospective clinical trials have not shown the same disadvantage for post-operative radiotherapy as the retrospective surveys suggested.

The results seem to provide no justification for routine post operative radiotherapy after radical mastectomy but on the other hand, they demonstrate no harmful effects from post-operative radiotherapy on the survival rate after ten years follow-up. After less radical surgery, post-operative radiotherapy seems to have played a useful role in cutting down the incidence of local recurrence and again no serious damage is reported.

Mention must be made of Stjernswärd (1974) who has reviewed the results of six prospective clinical trials of treatment in early breast cancer, in which one group had surgery and the other group had surgery and X-ray therapy. When assessed separately the results of the trials after 5 years follow-up showed no statistical difference between the survival rates of the two groups of patients. However, when he summated the results (using a mathematical formula) he found that overall, the patients having X-ray therapy did less well. This applied especially to the pre-menopausal group although the difference was lost if the patients were castrated by irradiation at the same time. He also comments on the prolonged lymphopenia after post operative radiotherapy and suggests that X-ray therapy may endanger an already failing immune surveillance.

The possibility that a course of X-ray therapy after a mastectomy for breast cancer may lower the patient's resistance (so that she is less able to suppress micro-foci of disseminated disease) challenges the role of treatment which has just been clarified—that is, that radiotherapy reduces the incidence of local recurrence and does no serious damage. Stjernswärd's analysis has recently been criticised by Levitt and MacHugh (1975) who find his conclusions unjustified and are unable to accept his statistical methods. Many clinicians also find Stjernswärd's analysis unconvincing and would require more clear cut results before abandoning post-operative radiotherapy completely. The ten year results in the clinical trials so far reported would not support such a policy.

There therefore remain a number of questions unanswered regarding the role of post-operative radiotherapy.

(1) Post-operative radiotherapy lowers the incidence of local recurrence, but does it also lower the patient's resistance to malignant disease so that distant recurrence is more frequent and survival rates lower?
(2) In patients with enlarged axillary nodes, what is the optimum treatment of the axilla? Should the nodes be dissected, should they be treated with X-ray therapy or should they be watched and treated only if they are obviously the site of active growth?
(3) Does post-operative X-ray therapy to the supraclavicular and internal mammary nodes offer any advantage or disadvantage in terms of morbidity or prevention of local and/or distant recurrence?
(4) What is an acceptable dose level of X-ray therapy

after mastectomy which will decrease the incidence of local recurrence without excessive morbidity and with minimal depression of the patient's immunity?

CLINICAL TRIALS IN PROGRESS

There are two controlled clinical trials in progress which may throw some light on these as yet unanswered questions.

The Cancer Research Campaign

This trial was started in 1970 and in 1975 completed its intake with over 2,000 patients entered. The first 5 year results are now available (Cancer Research Campaign, 1976). The trial compares the results of treatment by simple mastectomy alone with those of simple mastectomy combined with routine post-operative radiotherapy, both in Stage I and Stage II disease. The radiotherapy covers the pectoral scar, axillary, supraclavicular and internal mammary node areas.

After 5 years follow up there are no differences in the survival rates between the two groups or in the rates of distant recurrence. There is however, a statistically significant difference in the local recurrence rates. The group who have simple mastectomy alone have 28% of patients with local recurrence, and the group who have routine post-operative radiotherapy have 12% with local recurrence.

Follow-up on patients having simple mastectomy alone who have their local recurrences treated later indicate that the "on demand" treatment is successful in about 75% of cases and the delay does not apparently expose the patients to a greater risk of developing distant disease.

The five year results help to answer some of the questions listed earlier:

(1) Post-operative radiotherapy lowers the incidence of local recurrence but does it also lower the patient's resistance to malignant disease so that distant recurrence is more frequent and survival rates lower?

The C.R.C. trial has confirmed that post-operative radiotherapy lowers the incidence of local recurrence but it does not appear to lower the patient's resistance as reflected in the development of distant secondaries and the survival rate.

(2) In patients with enlarged axillary nodes, what is the optimum treatment of the axilla? Should the glands be dissected, should they be treated with X-ray therapy or should they be watched and treated only if they are obviously the site of active growth?

In the C.R.C. Trial, Stage II patients with enlarged axillary nodes manifest a higher percentage of local recurrences than the Stage I patients. Routine post-operative radiotherapy reduces the incidence of local recurrence in Stage II patients by 40%. Although the survival rates and distant recurrence rates are unaffected for Stage I and Stage II patients, it would seem prudent to reduce the risk of local recurrence in patients with enlarged axillary nodes by giving routine post-operative radiotherapy to this group. Previous trials indicate that dissecting the axillary nodes would give the same result. However, giving the treatment only if and when it is required, and not using it initially, does not appear to lower the survival figures.

(3) Does post-operative radiotherapy to the supraclavicular and internal mammary nodes offer any advantage or disadvantage in terms of morbidity or prevention of local and/or distant recurrence?

The C.R.C. Trial suggests that X-ray therapy which includes the supraclavicular and internal mammary nodes helps prevent local recurrence. It does not as yet appear to produce any morbidity, or influence the development of distant secondaries.

(4) What is an acceptable dose level of X-ray therapy after mastectomy which will decrease the incidence of local recurrence without excessive morbidity and with minimal depression of the patient's immunity?

The C.R.C. Trial protocol suggested the regimes shown in Table 2 and these doses yield from 1,320 to 1,510 rets using the NSD formula (Ellis, 1967). However, a number of radiotherapists used higher or lower doses and their cases have been separately assessed from the point of view of survival and distant and local recurrence rates.

At 5 years follow-up there is no significant difference in the survival rates or distant and local recurrence rates in the three groups. Most of the dosages in the high and low dose groups were only just outside the suggested range, and so it seems reasonable to accept that these dose levels are acceptable for reducing the number of local recurrences. They have not produced any change in morbidity or obvious depression of the patient's immunity.

Table 2. The C.R.C. Trial protocol regimes of radiotherapy

	(18 days) *3 weeks*	*(25 days)* *4 weeks*	*(32 days)* *5 weeks*	*(39 days)* *6 weeks*
three fractions per week	2,850-3,150*	3,200-3,500	3,450-3,850	3,700-4,050
five fractions per week	3,250-3,600	3,650-4,000	3,950-4,350	4,200-4,600

* Dose in rads but multiply by 1.1 for supervoltage therapy.

The trial has already been of great value in helping to answer some of the questions regarding the optimum treatment of early breast cancer, but further long term follow up must be awaited.

The National Surgical Adjuvant Breast Project (Protocol No. 4)

Fisher (1973) is comparing radical mastectomy and simple mastectomy in Stage I and Stage II disease. Patients with Stage I disease either have radical or simple mastectomy followed by radiotherapy only if and when significant axillary nodes develop, or they have simple mastectomy and immediate post-operative radiotherapy. Patients with Stage II disease have either radical mastectomy, or simple mastectomy and routine post-operative radiotherapy. This trial should again help to determine if post-operative radiotherapy offers advantages to patients with clinically uninvolved axillae at the time of primary treatment but, as yet, results are not available.

RADIOTHERAPY TECHNIQUES

There are as many different opinions about radiotherapy techniques as there are about the place of post-operative radiotherapy. X-ray therapy can include irradiation of the skin flaps and the surrounding lymph nodes (pectoral, axillary, infra- and supraclavicular and internal mammary), or any one of a combination of these groups. Opinions vary on the advisability of different regimes but there is little real evidence to support claims for the advantages of any one system.

Clinical trials show that post-operative radiotherapy can reduce the incidence of local recurrence by 60% (Easson, 1965) Such recurrences occur either in the skin flaps, or in the axillary and supraclavicular nodes. There is however no evidence to show whether irradiation of the internal mammary chain offers any benefit to patients. As these nodes are known to be involved in 20% of patients with Stage I or II disease (Handley, 1975) and are not removed surgically by the majority of surgeons, one might expect irradiation of the internal mammary nodes to reduce the incidence of recurrence in this area, and possibly also the incidence of intrathoracic secondaries. This has not been demonstrated.

If post-operative radiotherapy is given, it would seem appropriate to include the pectoral scar (or the breast) and all the immediately adjacent nodes. Such treatment can be given without too much morbidity and is within the scope of most radiotherapy departments. Treatment programmes vary greatly from centre to centre and may also vary in the same centre. In the United Kingdom the courses of radiotherapy used to consist of 5 to 6 weeks of daily treatment and doses of 5,000 to 6,000 rads were prescribed. In recent years, work on fractionation and dose-time relationship has shown that treatments given over a shorter period in fewer fractions can also give satisfactory results. Such treatments are less demanding on the patients and may produce no more morbidity.

The result of post-mastectomy radiotherapy has to be assessed indirectly as there is no certainty as to whether or not there is malignant disease present to treat. Records are therefore kept of the local recurrences occuring after radiotherapy and of the morbidity attributable to the treatment. Any tendency to give very high radiation doses to prevent local recurrence is held in check by the increase in serious long term side effects which such high dose treatment may produce.

Bates (1975) reports work from St. Thomas' Hospital comparing the results of treatment with either two or three fractions a week over a period of 3 or 4 weeks. At 5 years the results showed no difference in survival, incidence of local recurrence or morbidity, but she finds that management of a treatment technique using a total of only six fractions is critical if overdose effects are to be avoided. Many radiotherapists in the United Kingdom have now adopted techniques which treat patients with three fractions a week, all areas being treated on each visit. Minimum doses range from 3,000 to 4,500 rads varying with the type of radiation used and with the overall time of the course. The doses are calculated so

that they are the minimum received at the target area, whether it is an axillary node or the skin over the chest wall.

For treating the deeper structures, gamma rays from a cobalt source are selected, or high energy X-radiation from a Linear Accelerator. More superficial tissues are usually treated with radiation of lower energy, and tangential fields are selected to treat the breast and chest wall and thus avoid the normal tissues of the lung. The axilla and supraclavicular areas are often treated with an anterior field, which may be supplemented posteriorly or from the axilla. The internal mammary nodes are treated separately or may be included in the tangential fields used for treating the chest wall; in some centres both the internal mammary nodes and chest wall are covered by two large tangential fields.

In spite of carefully planned and executed treatments local recurrence occurs in 9% of cases and one must assume that some malignant breast growths are not sensitive to radiation at a dose that can be given without unacceptable morbidity (See Chapter 5).

CONCLUSIONS

The place of post-operative X-ray therapy is still not clear but some useful information has come from the clinical trials already completed and from studies of the natural behaviour of breast cancer.

The results of the C.R.C. trial at 5 years show that radiotherapy reduces the number of local recurrences and does not apparently lower the patient's immunity so as to allow an increase in the number of distant secondaries and lower survival rates. In Stage II patients with a high risk of local recurrence, it would seem prudent to give post-operative radiotherapy routinely after simple mastectomy and so avoid the complications of locally recurrent or persistent disease. If the axilla appears clear clinically and where histological information is available, a wait-and-see policy seems justified and perhaps 60-70% of women will be spared X-ray therapy with its unpleasant immediate side effects and possible long term hazards.

In planning a treatment programme for patients with early breast cancer a careful assessment must be made not only of the extent and type of the disease but also of the patient and her general condition. Such an assessment is made initially by clinical examination and by X-rays, blood tests and bone scans, and post-operatively by histological indentification of the type and extent of the tumour and of the node involvement.

(1) In a few highly selected cases local excision may be considered the treatment of choice. In such cases post-operative X-ray therapy to the breast will usually be considered essential. There will be no histological information on the state of the nodes, and whereas some c inicians will be prepared to adopt a wait-and-see policy and give X-ray therapy only if local recurrence occurs, others will prefer a prophylactic course of X-ray therapy to all the nodes draining the breast.

(2) Radical mastectomy with routine post-operative X-ray therapy shows no advantage in terms of survival, over radical mastectomy with X-ray therapy "on demand", so that many clinicans will be prepared to follow a watching policy and treat only if and when local recurrence develops. Others may prefer prophylactic X-ray therapy aiming to reduce the number of local recurrences but realizing that the treatment will contribute nothing to the risk of distant recurrence or to the survival rate to justify the extra burden of X-ray therapy.

(3) A simple mastectomy with axillary dissection involves the same arguments for or against post-operative radiotherapy as does radical mastectomy. If a simple mastectomy *alone* is performed there may either be no histological information on the axillary node state or a pectoral node biopsy may be taken. The long term results of the Cancer Research Campaign trial should help to answer questions on the use of routine post-operative X-ray therapy after simple mastectomy alone as opposed to "on demand" treatment.

Radiotherapy will undoubtedly reduce the number of local recurrences in the treatment area but will it also reduce the patient's immunity and possibly lead to lower survival times? At this stage the answers are not clear and clinicians must back their own judgement on the advisability of post-operative X-ray therapy or of a wait-and-see policy. If the axillary nodes are known to be involved, most clinicians feel the likelihood of local recurrence is so high that treatment with post-operative X-ray therapy is to be advised. If the axilla appears clear, either clinically or on what histological information is available, a wait-and-see policy seems justified and perhaps 65-70% of women will be spared X-ray therapy with its unpleasant immediate side effects and possible long-term hazards.

Evidence is accumulating that in patients with apparently early breast cancer, the use of a bone scan will identify those patients with a bad prognosis

(Blair, 1975). Tests of immune competence also indicate that patients with depresssed immune reactions may have a poor prognosis. If such techniques are available for assessing patients before a treatment plan is agreed, it may well be that post-operative X-ray therapy should be avoided in those with positive scans and depressed immune reactions. It must be remembered that X-ray therapy is a local treatment and can contribute nothing to the control of already disseminated disease. It may in fact decrease a patient's resistance to the development of metastases particularly if this resistance is already depressed.

In these assessments, the quality of the patient's life must not be overlooked. Figures measure only quantity in terms of years and numbers and sites of recurrence. Post-operative radiotherapy may contribute to quality of life by diminishing the likelihood of local recurrence. Undoubtedly, the development of a local recurrence is a matter of great concern to the patient, and although the clinician may accept a local recurrence as a manifestation of persistent disease which can be treated, the patient will regard it as a treatment failure. Her hopes of being "cured" of her disease will be destroyed and her confidence will be lost.

To sum up, the advantages of using post-operative radiotherapy in suitable patients to diminish the incidence of local recurrence must be weighed against the disadvantages of both short-term morbidity and possible longer-term risks. For this reason, there can be at present no clear cut recommendation either for or against post-operative X-ray therapy in all patients. Each patient must be assessed individually using as many tests as are available and her treatment designed in the light of present knowledge to give her the best chance of a long and disease-free survival.

Appendix

Throughout the text the Manchester Staging has been used as this was the staging quoted in the studies reviewed and information was not available to re-stage the groups in the T.N.M.* classification.

MANCHESTER STAGING

Stage I. Tumour of any size confined to the breast. Skin dimpling but no skin or muscle infiltration. Nipple retraction. No axillary or supraclavicular nodes.

Stage II. As above but with palpable mobile homolateral axillary nodes.

Stage III. Tumour of any size with skin and/or muscle involvement. Homolateral axillary nodes present or absent.

Stage IV. Distant secondaries or skin metastases beyond the area of the breast. Fixed axillary nodes. Supraclavicular nodes.

* U.I.C.C. T.N.M. Classification of Malignant Tumours (1974) 2nd Edition. Geneva.

REFERENCES

Atkins, H. et al. (1972). Treatment of early breast cancer; a report after ten years of a clinical trial. *British Medical Journal 2,* 423.

Bates, T. D. (1975). A prospective trial of post-operative radiotherapy delivered in three fractions per week versus two per week in breast carcinoma. *Clinical Radiology 26,* 297.

Blair, S. G. (1975). Does early detection of bone metastases by scanning improve prognosis of breast cancer. *Clinical Oncology 1,* 185.

Bond, W. H. (1967). The influence of various treatments on survival rates in cancer of the breast. In *The Treatment of Carcinoma of the Breast,* p. 24 (Ed. A. S. Jarrett). Amsterdam: Excerpta Medica Foundation.

Brinkley, D. and Haybittle, J. L. (1971). Treatment of Stage II Carcinoma of the female breast. *Lancet 2,* 1086.

Brinkley, D. and Haybittle, J. (1975). The curability of breast cancer. *Lancet 2,* 95.

Cancer Research Campaign (1976). Management of early cancer of the breast. Cancer Research Campaign Study; An International Multicentre Trial. *British Medical Journal 1,* 1035.

Cook, D. C., Dent, O. and Hewitt, D. (1974). Breast cancer following multiple chest fluoroscopy; The Ontario experience. *Canadian Medical Association Journal 111,* 406.

Crile, G. Jr. (1968). Results of simple mastectomy without irradiation in the treatment of operative Stage I cancer of the breast. *Annals of Surgery 168,* 330.

Cutler, S. J. and Connelly, R. R. (1969). Mammary cancer trends. *Cancer 23,* 767.

Easson, E. C. (1968). In *Prognostic Factors in Breast Cancer,* p. 118. Edinburgh: E. and S. Livingstone Ltd.

Ellis, F. (1967). Fractionation in radiotherapy. In *Modern Trends in Radiotherapy,* p.34 (Eds T. Deeley and C. Wood). *Vol. 1.* London: Butterworths.

Fisher, B., Slack, N. H., Cavanagh, P. J. et al. (1970). Post-operative radiotherapy in the treatment of breast cancer. *Annals of Surgery 172,* 711.

Fisher, B. (1973). Co-operative clinical trials in primary breast cancer. A critical appraisal. *Cancer 31,* 1271.

Hamlin, I.M.E. (1968). Possible host resistance in carcinoma of the breast. *British Journal of Cancer 22,* 383.

Handley, R. S. (1975). Carcinoma of the breast. *Annals of*

the Royal College of Surgeons of England 57, 59.

Kaae, S. and Johansen, H. (1968). Simple versus radical mastectomy in primary breast cancer. In *Prognostic Factors in Breast Cancer*, p. 93. Edinburgh: E. and S. Livingstone.

Levitt, S. H. and McHugh, R. B. (1975). Early breast cancer and post-operative irradiation. *Lancet 2*, 1258.

Lipworth, L. (1965). Survival of cases of surgically treated mammary carcinoma with and without radiation therapy. *Lancet 2*, 231.

McWhirter, R. (1948). Simple mastectomy and radiotherapy in the treatment of breast cancer. *British Journal of Radiology 21*, 599.

Mackenzie, I. (1965). Breast cancer following multiple fluoroscopies. *British Journal of Cancer 19*, 1.

Mettler, F. A. Jr. et al. (1969). Breast neoplasms in women treated with X-rays for acute postpartum mastitis. A pilot study. *Journal of the National Cancer Institute 43*, 803.

Myrden, J. A. and Hiltz, J. E. (1969). Breast cancer following multiple fluoroscopies during artifical pneumothorax treatment of pulmonary tuberculosis. *Canadian Medical Association Journal 100*, 1032.

Roberts, M. M., Forrest, A. P. M. et al. (1973). Simple versus radical mastectomy. *Lancet 2*, 1073.

Stjernswärd, J. (1974). Decreased survival related to irradiation post operatively in early operable breast cancer. *Lancet 2*, 1285.

United States Department of Health, Education and Welfare (1960). Survival experience of patients with malignant neoplasms. Public Health Service Publication No. 789.

Chapter

8

BASIL A. STOLL

Prospects for Anti-oestrogen Adjuvant Therapy

The administration of intensive cytotoxic chemotherapy following surgery has been shown to increase the cure rate of certain experimental tumours in animals. Although most of these tumours are monoclonal and genetically homogeneous, similar principles are being hopefully applied to human mammary cancer, which is on the other hand, almost certainly a multiclonal tumour.

Again, while the declared intention of adjuvant treatment is "to increase the overall cure rate and not just delay the appearance of detectable metastases" (Hill and Price, 1977), it must be admitted that there is considerable doubt whether there is such a distinction between these two criteria in the case of human mammary cancer (see Chapter I).

For many years it was assumed that 5 or 10 year survival after radical treatment in breast cancer represented a high likelihood of "cure"; now there is good evidence that year by year after "curative" treatment, the patients die from the disease at a constant rate, and that by 20 years, about 70% of patients in Stages 1 and 2 have died of the disease (Bond, 1968; Brinkley and Haybittle, 1975; Mueller and Jeffries, 1975). Even *after* 20 years, these radically treated patients continue to die of breast cancer. It is very likely therefore, that in the case of breast cancer, "cure" merely means that the clinical appearance of metastases is delayed to the extent that the patient may ultimately die of old age or intercurrent disease.

In the past, four prospective randomised trials have proved that the use of ovarian ablation after mastectomy can delay the onset of recurrence or metastases for up to four years or even longer (see p. 83), although 5 year survival rates are apparently not improved. In recent years, anti-oestrogenic agents have been introduced into therapy and have two major advantages over ovarian ablation; not only do they appear to inhibit oestrogenic stimulation of target tissues but they can also sustain inhibition for a prolonged period. Even more promising is the observation that those patients unlikely to be sensitive to their action can be recognized by assay of hormone receptor protein in the tumour.

BASIS FOR TRIAL OF ENDOCRINE ADJUVANT THERAPY

(1) Randomized trials of cytotoxic adjuvant therapy have, to date, shown evidence of delayed recurrence only in premenopausal node-positive patients, and with the possible exception of Bonadonna's preliminary report (1976), not in postmenopausal women (see Chapter 6). Such cytotoxic regimes depress ovarian secretion in pre-menopausal women (Bulbrook, 1976), and it will be shown later that randomised trials of adjuvant castration in such women have produced a similar delay in recurrence for up to 4 years after primary treatment. These are good reasons to set up multicentre randomized trials, to assess the value in adjuvant therapy of new anti-oestrogens which have been shown to cause regression of advanced mammary cancer both in premenopausal and in postmenopausal women.

It is now possible to assay not only the oestrogen receptor content of the patient's tumour, but in addition, other hormonal receptors in the tumour cell. It will be seen later that these should permit even more accurate selection of those tumours suitable for adjuvant anti-oestrogen therapy.

(2) All of the commonly used cytotoxic agents are likely to depress the immune response in the human, including both the cell-mediated and the antibody reactions. This seems to apply especially if the drugs are given in small repeated doses (Berenbaum, 1975). Therefore, if in spite of this a cytotoxic agent shows evidence of being able to inhibit the growth of a tumour, it is presumably because its cell-kill rate is of more consequence than its immunosuppressive activity.

Carcinogenic danger from cytotoxic chemotherapy may or may not be related to its immunosuppressive action. Acute myeloid leukaemia has been shown to develop in some patients with breast cancer some years subsequent to treatment with thioTEPA or cyclophosphamide (Sieber and Adamson, 1975). Other agents used widely in adjuvant chemotherapy such as methotrexate and fluorouracil, have also been shown to exert carcinogenic effects in experimental animals when used in doses corresponding to the dose/weight ratios used in humans (Schmahl, 1974).

When cytotoxic chemotherapy is used in the treatment of *advanced* disease, the carcinogenic dangers are of little importance. In addition, it is assumed that the immunological response of the host to the tumour is depressed in any case, and the immunosuppressive effect of the cytotoxic agent may be of little importance. However, in the patient with minimal disease, her immunological defence may be of the greatest importance, and immunosuppression may be dangerous. While the effect of cytotoxic agents is to depress the immune system, the effect of most sex hormones used in the treatment of breast cancer is to stimulate the reticuloendothelial system (Stoll, 1972; Baum, 1975).

(3) While endocrine therapy is selective for breast cancer cells, cytotoxic therapy is selective for all proliferating cells. Until we can measure the tumour burden in the patient, we have no evidence during treatment as to whether cytotoxic therapy is having an effect on the tumour growth or whether it should be abandoned. At any time, a resistant population of cells may have emerged requiring a change in treatment, or on the other hand, it may be that all the tumour cells have been eradicated. In either case, the continuation of cytotoxic therapy leads to a risk of immunosuppression and myelosuppression without the compensation of a possible controlling effect on tumour growth. Such an objection does not apply to hormonal agents.

(4) It has been too readily assumed on too little evidence that the effect of adjuvant endocrine treatment is, by its very nature, transient. However, in the case of carcinogen induced mammary cancer in rats which responds to endocrine manipulation similarly to the human tumour, it has been shown that under certain circumstances a proportion of tumours can be extinguished completely. The tumours showing the most complete response to castration, androgen or anti-oestrogen therapy are those treated *early* in their development (Griswold and Green, 1970; De Sombre and Arbogast, 1974), and the longer the delay in instituting such treatment, the lower the response rate.

In other words, the phenomenon of first order kinetics (i.e. a constant percentage of cells is killed whatever the size of the population) applies to endocrine therapy in mammary cancer just as much as it does to cytotoxic chemotherapy. This means that endocrine therapy will be more efficacious earlier in the disease, and for greatest effect, it should be given immediately after the primary treatment.

(5) The evidence available suggests that only a small proportion of breast cancers are likely to show long term control from adjuvant use of those cytotoxic modalities which are at present available. There are two reasons for this.

Firstly, by the time a primary tumour is detected, it is already three quarters of the way through its life cycle (Schabel, 1975) and the tumour burden is in most cases almost certainly too large for control by presently available cytotoxic agents. This is illustrated by the early results in the widely quoted adjuvant trial of CMF by Bonadonna et al. (1976); patients

with four or more involved axillary nodes showed a higher percentage of relapses than those with only 1-3 nodes involved.

The second reason is that human mammary cancer is likely to be multiclonal or genetically heterogenous and this is possibly associated with the fact that it is usually multicentric (Qualheim and Gall, 1967; Gallager and Martin, 1969). Reactivation of tumour activity after temporary inhibition by cytotoxic therapy is presumably because resistant clones proliferate and replace the tumour after the sensitive clones have been eliminated by treatment. That is why, in some cases, a second response may be obtained from crossover to Adriamycin/Vincristine after progression or relapse from CMF treatment (Brambilla et al., 1976).

Thus, the tumour, even at the stage of microdissemination, is likely to contain different clones with different genetic cytotoxic sensitivity. On the other hand, most of the experimental mammary cancers established by transplant or carcinogens are monoclonal tumours (Schabel, 1975), and this may explain why they can be cured by intensive cytotoxic chemotherapy given after surgery. It is the multiclonal nature of the human mammary cancer which makes cure by either cytotoxic or endocrine methods difficult, but it is possible that a combination of hormonal and cytotoxic agents may eventually prove to be the best.

In order to decide on the most suitable agent for endocrine adjuvant therapy it is necessary to consider in more detail the mechanisms by which endocrine manipulation may exert control over the growth of breast cancer.

MECHANISMS IN ENDOCRINE MANIPULATION

A large number of methods of endocrine manipulation have shown an ability to cause regression of advanced breast cancer. Their mechanisms may be quite different. Following oophorectomy, Gullino et al. (1974) have shown lysis in occasional cells in specimens of mammary cancer. It is presumed that the effect is autophagic and involves release of lysosomal enzymes, because neighbouring cells are not affected and there are no specific effects on the vessels or stromal round cell infiltration. Following oestrogen therapy on the other hand, Huseby and Thomas (1954) have shown well marked stromal infiltration with round cells in specimens of human mammary cancer. Sometimes there is a tendency for the tumour to become more mature and differentiated.

It may be useful to list the possible mechanisms by which endocrine manipulation may cause a change in the growth of mammary cancer (Stoll, 1972).

Deprivation mechanism. It has been postulated that oophorectomy, adrenalectomy or hypophyseal ablation can deprive the tumour of oestrogen and that this explains why response to endocrine ablation is correlated with the level of oestrogen receptors in the tumour. A parallel mechanism is ascribed to orchidectomy in the case of prostatic cancer, although correlation with androgen receptors has not yet been shown in that case.

Antagonist mechanism. The use of androgen or anti-oestrogen comes under this heading. It is thought that they may inhibit cell proliferation in mammary cancer by competing with oestrogen for receptor sites. A parallel is the use of oestrogen therapy in prostatic cancer.

Maturation mechanism. It is possible that in some cases mammary cancer can be made to differentiate by the effect of high dosage of oestrogen or by progestogen therapy. A parallel is the tendency to differentiation sometimes observed in endometrial cancer following progestogen therapy.

Lympholytic mechanism. High dosage of corticosteroids may result in partial shrinkage of mammary cancer. The mechanism is probably by reduction of peripheral oedema and round cell infiltration, and not by a so-called "medical adrenalectomy".

Immunological mechanism. It has been suggested that one of the effects of high dosage of oestrogen in mammary cancer may be to increase the reticulo-endothelial response to the presence of the tumour.

OESTROGEN RECEPTORS IN BREAST CANCER

Certain target tissues in the body such as the breast, uterus, vagina, hypothalamus and anterior pituitary gland, which respond to the presence of oestrogen, also show a special affinity for oestradiol. This applies also to some of the tumours which arise in these tissues and it was shown that those carcinogen-induced rat mammary cancers which fail to regress after oophorectomy or adrenalectomy have a lower capacity to retain oestradiol (Mobbs, 1966). This led to the suggestion that in human mammary cancer also, oestradiol might be necessary to maintain the growth of those tumours which show the presence of specific oestrogen receptor protein.

It is now known that there are receptors for *several* steroid and polypeptide hormones, situated respectively in the cytoplasm and cell surface

membrane of hormone target cells. Most of our knowledge so far on the mechanism of primary interaction of hormones with the cell, is in connection with the uptake of oestradiol. It has been shown that circulating oestradiol becomes bound to a specific cytoplasmic receptor protein. After binding, the complex is transformed, and translocated to the nucleus where it attaches to the nuclear DNA. RNA synthesis is then affected through an effect on the RNA polymerase system.

Characteristic of the oestrogen receptor is the fact that it can be occupied by relatively simple non-steroidal agents such as diethyl stilboestrol, and some oestrogenic effects are therefore seen following the administration of such agents. At the same time they block the uptake of oestradiol by the receptors and this may be an important factor in the response of breast cancer to high dosage of diethyl stilboestrol. It has recently been shown that the uptake of oestradiol by target tissues can also be inhibited by the administration of specific oestrogen antagonists such as tamoxifen, nafoxidine and clomiphene which are presumably also taken up by the oestrogen receptor.

Ten years ago it was first suggested that the hormone dependence of some mammary cancers could depend to a large extent on the presence in the tumour cells of high affinity binding protein (Jensen et al., 1967). Although most reports suggest that only about 70% of human mammary cancers possess oestrogen receptor protein (ER+), it is more likely that *all* have it, but it cannot be measured accurately below a certain level (Korenman and Dukes, 1970; Leclerq et al., 1975). The ER is thought to be confined to the epithelial cells of the tumour and the receptor level recorded in the tissue therefore depends partly on the proportion of the epithelial cells to stromal tissue. Thus the receptor level in normal mammary tissue is relatively low because of its large content of fat relative to glandular tissue.

The level of ER found in breast cancer is not related to the size of the tumour or its staging at diagnosis or to its histopathology (Feherty et al., 1971; Spaeren et al., 1973). There is some difference of opinion whether in the presence of metastases, the ER level is related to the recurrence-free interval or to the location of the metastases.

Assay of the ER level is most accurately carried out by the sucrose density method. Tritiated oestradiol is added to the supernatant of the cytosol factor after homogenization of the tissue, and the mixture is then centrifuged in a sucrose gradient. It is said that as little as 200 mg of tissue can be accurately assayed by this technique (Block et al., 1975).

It may appear surprising that the level of ER in breast cancer is generally found to be lower in premenopausal than in postmenopausal women. Minimum significant levels are taken as 250 femtomoles per G of tumour in the former but 750 femtomoles per G in the latter (Block et al., 1975). It is probable that some of the receptors are already bound to endogenous oestrogen in premenopausal women and are therefore not available to take up the tritiated oestradiol.

It has been reported that when biopsy for ER assay is repeated in both primary and secondary tumours, or in the same patient after an interval of time, the level is found to be similar in over 80% of cases (Block et al., 1975). This means that if metastases are inaccessible for biopsy at the time of recurrence, the receptor characteristics of the primary tumour may be used as a reliable guide to endocrine therapy. It also suggests that ER assays should be carried out whenever possible on all primary tumours at the time of mastectomy.

OESTROGEN RECEPTORS AND HORMONAL SENSITIVITY

A large multicentre report (McGuire, 1975) provides reliable figures for the correlation between the level of ER in the tumour and the clinical response to presently used methods of endocrine manipulation. In 436 cases monitored by extramural clinical review, ER+ cases showed a 55% regression rate, and ER– cases a 8% regression rate, to endocrine ablation. For treatment by oestrogen, androgen or anti-oestrogen, the corresponding figures were 55% and 9% respectively (Table 1). There was no correlation between the ER level and either the duration of remission after treatment or the length of survival after treatment.

The report suggests that those mammary cancers which most resemble the parent tissue histopathologically (i.e. the more differentiated tumours) showed a higher proportion with ER+. Yet, in the literature there is no evidence that well differentiated tumours show a higher response rate to endocrine manipulation and in this respect mammary cancers seem to differ from cancers of the prostate, endometrium and thyroid. It must however be taken into account that the histopathological pattern of human mammary cancer is notoriously heterogenous.

The presence of ER has been shown in 70% of primary tumours and in 58% of metastatic deposits (McGuire, 1975), and there is a difference of opinion as to whether ER levels are similar at all tumour sites

Table 1. Presence of tumour regression (confirmed by external review) in relation to oestrogen receptor assay and type of endocrine therapy in patients with breast cancer. (After MacGuire, 1975.)

Therapy	*ER +*	*ER –*
Adrenalectomy	32/66	4/33
Castration	25/33	4/53
Hypophysectomy	2/8	0/8
Total	59/107 = 55%	8/94 = 8%
Androgen	12/26	2/24
Oestrogen	37/57	5/58
Anti-oestrogen	8/20	5/27
Total	57/103 = 55%	12/109 = 9%

in the body. Some observers claim that different samples of the same tumour almost always contain the same concentration of ER and conclude that there is only one cell population in respect to ER content (Leclerq et al., 1975). Other groups claim however, that ER levels may differ in metastases taken from different locations in the same patient (Braunsberg et al., 1973; Leung et al., 1975).

There are several possible explanations for the variation in ER level between specimens. It may be due to different degrees of differentiation between tumour sites, or to different proportions of non-epithelial connective tissue in each specimen (McGuire, 1975). Others suggest that the most likely reason is that human mammary cancer is multiclonal in origin and therefore each tumour may contain a genetic mixture of cells. Some of the clones may have a significant level of oestrogen receptors while others have none.

If the former cells predominate at a particular site, that particular tumour may show evidence of response to endocrine manipulation but if negative cells predominate, it will probably be hormonally autonomous. This has considerable relevance to the common observation that clinical response to endocrine therapy may vary from one site to another in the same patient. It bears also on tumour reactivation after temporary regression—further response will depend on the genetic characteristics of the surviving cells which have replaced the tumour.

We have seen that about 70% of human mammary cancers possess ER at a significant level but only 55% of these show significant clinical response to endocrine manipulation. Tumours possessing a particular receptor will undoubtedly be sensitive to that hormone but that does not necessarily mean either that the tumour is dependent on that hormone for growth, nor that a particular response is bound to follow stimulation of that receptor. A great deal of confusion results from the assumption by the clinician that clinical response to endocrine manipulation mirrors the biological hormonal sensitivity of a tumour (see Chapter 13).

The effect of administering oestrogen to a patient with mammary cancer will depend on its uptake by the tumour, and this will depend not only on the level of ER in the target organ but also on the concentration of the hormone in the vicinity of the tumour. Very high dosage of oestrogen may cause a local concentration at the tumour such that the receptors are saturated – something which does not occur physiologically (Terenius, 1974). This may lead to an effect on plasma membranes, capillary permeability or lysosomal activity, quite different from the usual physiological effects of oestrogen on RNA and protein synthesis.

Moreover it must be taken into account that oestrogen is probably only one of several hormones involved together in the regulation of human mammary cancer, and this may be another reason that the presence of significant levels of ER in the tumour is associated with response to androgens, progestogens or corticosteroids. In normal mammary tissue it seems that after oestrogen is taken up by the receptor, the oestrogen protein complex reacts with the progesterone, androgen and corticosteroid receptors inside the cell, or with receptors for polypeptides such as prolactin, growth hormone or insulin on the cell surface membrane. This may apply in breast cancer also.

It is of course possible that when the mammary cell undergoes malignant mutation it may lose some of these different receptor sites, but the fact remains that the mere presence of oestrogen receptor does not itself predict the certainty of response to endocrine manipulation. It is theoretically possible that the level of binding by the tumour of insulin, prolactin or growth hormone may be correlated with the likelihood of response (Holdaway et al., 1975).

Assays of progesterone receptors (Terenius, 1973) or androgen receptors (Engelsmann et al., 1974) may provide extra information. The latter group of investigators report the presence of androgen receptors in 18% of human mammary cancers, compared to a 41% incidence of oestrogen receptors in their series. It may be important in the treatment of breast cancer that the anti-oestrogen tamoxifen not only blocks oestrogen receptors but *in vitro* can block the androgen receptor in 35% of human mammary cancers (Lippman, 1976).

Breast cancers which are reported to be ER – have

an insignificant receptor level yet they have an 8-9% likelihood of clinical response to endocrine therapy. In addition, there is no correlation between the *absolute* level of ER in the tumour and the likelihood of clinical response (McGuire, 1975; Block et al., 1975). It has therefore been suggested that we should no longer regard breast cancer as being either hormonal dependent or independent "but rather as having varying degrees of dependence" (Leclerq et al., 1975). On this basis, ER-tumours need not necessarily be excluded from endocrine treatment, especially in view of the fact that there are other receptors and mechanisms by which endocrine manipulation may influence the growth of breast cancer.

ANTI-OESTROGENIC MECHANISMS

Any agent which reduces the response of a target tissue to oestrogen can be termed an anti-oestrogen. Steroidal agents with androgenic or progestogenic activity are sometimes included under this heading, but the term is more accurately restricted to those non-steroidal anti-oestrogens which, in addition to blocking the uptake of oestradiol, also exert a specific effect on oestrogen-sensitive tissue. This group of compounds not only has an affinity for oestrogen receptors but is also retained by the receptors.

The anti-oestrogens which have been especially studied for their ability to control the growth and spread of mammary cancer are clomiphene, nafoxidine and tamoxifen (Nolvadex®). Although the action of an anti-oestrogen in inhibiting the growth of mammary cancer could result from blocking the uptake of oestradiol by the ER in the tumour, there are other possible mechanisms. It may be taken up by oestrogen receptors in the hypothalamus or anterior pituitary tissue and thereby inhibit prolactin secretion or release, or it may act directly on the tumour by exerting an antimetabolic effect.

In the case of carcinogen-induced mammary cancer in rats, the first two of these effects have been demonstrated following the administration of anti-oestrogens such as clomiphene, nafoxidine and tamoxifen. The uptake of tritiated oestradiol by the tumour is reduced and the circulating prolactin level is also markedly reduced. The animals show inhibition of the tumour growth (Schultz et al., 1969; Terenius, 1971; Jordan and Koerner, 1975), and the degree of tumour inhibition is said to be correlated with the ER content of the tumour. However, if the rat is castrated first, the effect of anti-oestrogen is the same as that of oestrogen — it causes acceleration of tumour growth. The reason for this is not clear.

To some extent these observations are paralleled in the human. Advanced breast cancer, particularly in soft tissues and viscera, regresses in at least one-third of cases following anti-oestrogen therapy. Tumour regression may occur in premenopausal as well as in postmenopausal women (see Chapter 13). The uptake of tritiated oestradiol by human mammary cancer is reduced in vitro by clomiphene (Terenius, 1971), nafoxidine (Jensen et al., 1971) or tamoxifen (Hahnel et al., 1973; Jordan and Koerner, 1975). Clinical observations show conflicting evidence as to whether basal serum prolactin levels are reduced (L'Hermite et al., 1974; Willis, 1976; Griffiths, 1976). A close degree of correlation is shown between the likelihood of regression following tamoxifen therapy and the ER content of breast cancer (Band et al., 1976; Jordan, 1976).

Thus, the inhibitory effect of these anti-oestrogens on the growth of human mammary cancer may result from preventing replenishment of receptors in the tumour, and this explanation could apply equally to the postmenopausal as to the premenopausal woman. In the former, however, there may be in addition a metabolic effect similar to that ascribed to high dosage oestrogen therapy. This could involve an effect of cell membranes, capillary permeability or lysosomal activity. Nordenskjold et al. (1976) have examined serial aspiration biopsies of breast cancer in women during treatment either with tamoxifen or oestrogen. They report that using tritiated thymidine uptake as a marker, both treatments caused similar decrease in the proportion of cells labelled during regression. It is not clear whether the effect is due to delay in DNA synthesis or to actual death of the cells.

It is still possible that the inhibitory effect of anti-oestrogens on the growth of breast cancer could involve reduction in the circulating prolactin level by displacing oestradiol from the ER sites in the hypothalamus. Whereas the effect of oestradiol is to stimulate the pituitary release of prolactin but inhibit that of gonadotrophin, the effect of anti-oestrogen is to decrease prolactin release. Excessive stimulation of gonadotrophin-secreting cells in the pituitary gland may crowd out the prolactin secreting cells (Ben David et al., 1971).

MEASURING EFFECTIVENESS OF ADJUVANT THERAPY

Measuring the effectiveness of adjuvant therapy in patients with breast cancer presents unusual difficulties for three major reasons. First is the remarkable

variability in the course of the disease from patient to patient, which results from the biological balance between host and tumour factors (Stoll, 1976; Devitt, 1976). This makes the stratification of patients extremely difficult in the planning of clinical trials. Second is the minimal significance which can be attached to early recurrence-free rates, because these may represent short term inhibition of tumour growth and not a true prevention of metastases. Third is the relative unimportance of the 5 year survival rate which is used as a parameter in other types of cancer.

These difficulties are responsible for the contradictory results which have emanated from many of the prospective randomised trials which have been organised in the last 10 to 15 years. Although the prospective randomised trial has become something of a "sacred cow" in the evaluation of treatment in breast cancer, critics of such trials have cogently pointed out that "What is needed for interpreting the results of clinical investigations are objective criteria for evaluating treatments, knowledge of the important patient characteristics influencing prognosis, and quantitative models for predicting the outcome of treatment based upon knowledge of a given patient's characteristics" (Gehan and Freireich, 1976).

From an analysis of large patient groups in the U.S.A. and Canada, it has been shown by Mueller and Jeffries (1975) that after an initially high mortality in the first three years after diagnosis of breast cancer, women then die of the disease at a constant annual rate. About 8% of those at risk die year by year until ultimately at least 80% of all patients are shown to die with evidence of disease. From an analysis of 704 patients treated before 1950, Brinkley and Haybittle (1975) point out that at 21 years after diagnosis, only 18.5% of their patients are cured and even in the so-called "early cases" only 30% are alive at 21 years.

For these reasons, short-term survival rates and clinical recurrence rates have so far been found incapable of providing clear evidence of the degree of benefit from trials of adjuvant therapy in breast cancer.

Recurrence-Free and Survival Rates

There is no doubt that in a proportion of women with "early" breast cancer the recurrence-free interval shows considerable prolongation when the natural menopause intervenes after the primary treatment; the "dormant" interval in some cases extends to many years (Clemmesen, 1948; Hadfield and Holt, 1956; AMA Committee on Research, 1960). This is paralleled by observations in the four prospective randomised trials described below, that by carrying out ovarian ablation at the time of primary treatment, the first manifestation of recurrence can be considerably delayed.

There is no evidence to support the belief expressed by Burchenal (1976) and very widely assumed, that in the human "oophorectomy apparently works as well in clinically dectable metastases as on micrometastases". Certainly experimental observations in the rat mammary cancer model (see p. 78) suggest that a proportion of the tumours can be extinguished completely. The response to oophorectomy, androgen or anti-oestrogen treatment, is greatest when this is carried out early in the development of the tumour (Griswold and Green, 1970; De Sombre and Arbogast, 1974).

A prospective randomised trial of adjuvant X-ray castration in premenopausal and perimenopausal women (Cole, 1970) showed a significantly prolonged recurrence-free interval compared to a control series during the first 4 years (Table 2). There was however no significant increase in the 5 year survival rate in the castrated women. Another prospective randomised trial of adjuvant X-ray castration was reported by Nissen Meyer (1967) and this demonstrated not only an improved recurrence-free rate in the castrated group but also an improvement in the 4 year survival rate.

In 1969 Nevinny et al., reported a randomized prospective trial of adjuvant oophorectomy in premenopausal and perimenopausal women. Their figures showed "an apparent difference in the percentage of patients alive without disease, favouring the oophorectomy group" and the recurrence-free period was longer in the castrated group. In 1970, Ravdin et al., reported a randomised prospective trial of adjuvant oophorectomy, and showed that at 18 months the recurrence rate in the oophorectomy

Table 2. Randomized trial of ovarian ablation by X-rays at the time of mastectomy. Cumulative incidence of recurrence, metastasis or death up to 15 years in patients with positive axillary nodes. (After Cole, 1970.)

Years	*Ov. ablation*	*Control*
1	16.5%	35.1%
2	36.2%	51.1%
3	46.4%	56.5%
4	48.8%	59.5%
5	55.1%	61.1%
7	56.7%	61.8%
10	58.3%	65.6%
12	61.4%	66.4%
15	62.2%	71.0%
	127 cases	131 cases

Table 3. Randomised trial of oophorectomy at the time of mastectomy. Failure rate at intervals in premenopausal women with more than four positive axillary nodes. (After Ravdin et al., 1970.)

Months observation	*Treatment Failure Rate* *Oophorectomy*	*Control*
12	30%	42%
18	41%	58%
24	44%	62%
30	55%	62%
36	63%	67%

Table 4. Randomised trial of l-phenylalanine mustard (L-PAM) as adjuvant therapy after mastectomy. Failure rate in premenopausal and postmenopausal women with positive axillary nodes. (After Fisher et al., 1975.)

	Nodes positive	*Treatment Failure Rate* *L-PAM*	*Placebo*	
Premenopausal	1–3	0%	17%	Sig.
	4+	8%	42%	Sig.
Postmenopausal	1–3	3%	0%	Not sig.
	4+	18%	36%	Not sig.

group with four or more involved axillary nodes was "only two-thirds of that in the placebo group" (Table 3). The advantage was maintained up to 3 years after primary treatment but the 5 year survival rate was not improved.

There is evidence therefore that ovarian ablation can delay the onset of recurrence in a proportion of patients with microdissemination, for up to 4 years if not longer. What is more, the effect of ovarian ablation seems closely related to the results observed in the early NSABP trials of adjuvant cytotoxic chemotherapy (see Chapter 7). In 1968, Fisher reported the results of the NSABP trial of adjuvant thioTEPA given the day of mastectomy and on two successive days afterwards (Fisher et al., 1968). Significant difference between the thioTEPA group and the placebo group was found only in premenopausal women with four or more axillary nodes. Those receiving thioTEPA showed a recurrence rate approximately 40% less than the placebo group between the 18th and 36th months.

Subsequently the results were reported of the NSABP trial of adjuvant phenylalanine mustard (L-PAM) given in courses every 6 weeks for a period of 2 years after mastectomy (Fisher et al., 1975). Again there was a decreased recurrence rate in the L-PAM treated group involving only the premenopausal women (Table 4).

A very likely conclusion is that the decreased incidence of recurrence in premenopausal women in adjuvant trials involving alkylating agents is due to a "chemotherapeutic castration" (Stoll, 1963). Cytokinetic considerations make it extremely unlikely that a 3 day course of very moderate dosage of thioTEPA at the time of surgery could exert long term control of tumour growth by any other mechanism. Although amenorrhoea resulted in the majority of premenopausal women involved in these trials of thioTEPA, Fisher et al. (1975) chose to cast doubt on this mechanism being involved because no relationship could be shown between treatment failure and changes in menstrual activity. But it has clearly been shown by the writer that following irradiation of the ovaries, the presence of amenorrhoea is not necessary for regression of breast cancer to occur (Stoll, 1969). A *failing* ovarian secretion appears to be sufficient to cause the change in the tumour.

A recent preliminary report (Bonadonna et al., 1976) claims that a combination of cyclophosphamide, methotrexate and 5-fluorouracil used as adjuvant therapy has led to a decrease in the early recurrence rate in postmenopausal as well as in premenopausal women. At the date of writing however Bonadonna has reported privately that the premenopausal women are showing an increasingly greater advantage in freedom from recurrence. Persistent amenorrhoea occurred in all the premenopausal women given the CMF combination.

Biological markers of residual tumour

The results in the preceding section suggest that the effectiveness of adjuvant therapy in breast cancer is unlikely to be established accurately until we are able to use biological markers which are related to the mass of residual tumour in the body. Not only will this permit the results of treatment to be defined promptly and accurately, but it will also be possible to select the patients requiring adjuvant therapy.

At the present time it is customary to select for adjuvant therapy those patients whose axillary nodes are found to be positive at the time of mastectomy. But only two thirds of such patients are liable to show any effect on short term recurrence rate or survival rate by adjuvant therapy, because the other third will survive 5 years without such therapy. It is ethically desirable in any case that the presence of micrometastases or subclinical metastases should be demonstrated before embarking on a long course of

Table 5. Classification of tumour-associated biological markers which have been suggested in breast cancer. (After Coombes and Neville, 1977.)

1. Breast tissue products, e.g. casein, lactalbumen.
2. Oncofoetal antigens, e.g. carcinoembryonic antigen, alpha foetoprotein, ferritin.
3. Hormones, e.g. human serum chorionic gonadotrophin, calcitonin.
4. Enzymes, e.g. placental alkaline phosphatase, sialyl transferase.
5. Cell turnover products, e.g. polyamines, nucleosides.
6. Tumour specific antigens—specific to tumour cell.
7. Plasma proteins, e.g. pregnancy associated macroglobulin, beta macroglobulin, fucose-containing glycoprotein.
8. Urinary hydroxyproline excretion.

cytotoxic therapy which may involve the risk of immuno-suppression, myelosuppression and even possible carcinogenesis.

For the purpose of stratifying patients for a clinical trial which will assess the value of adjuvant systemic therapy, it is essential to be able to assess the presence of tumour in the body quantitatively. For this a biochemical or immunological method would be most valuable.

In the last few years we have accumulated a large number of tumour-associated markers which are thought to reflect, to a greater or lesser degree, the tumour burden in the patient with breast cancer (Table 5). In the table they are subdivided, perhaps somewhat arbitrarily, under the headings of breast tissue products, oncofoetal antigens, hormones, enzymes, cell turnover products, tumour specific antigens, plasma proteins and urinary metabolic products.

At present, none of the clinically explored tests is by itself capable of acting as a specific marker of the high risk patient who requires adjuvant treatment after primary surgery (Coombes and Neville, 1977). Levels of individual markers have been shown to be raised in varying proportions of patients with proven distant metastases, and some even in a small proportion of patients assessed postoperatively. It still remains to be proved, however, that these latter patients turn out to have a worse prognosis (Steward et al., 1974), and it is clear that the more facets of tumour metabolism measured, the more likely are we to establish a correlation with the presence of micrometastases after surgery. At this stage many institutions are measuring a spectrum of markers in each patient in order to correlate it with the tumour burden and the prognosis.

Table 6. Properties of the ideal tumour marker in the patient with breast cancer. (After Coombes and Neville, 1977.)

1. Measurement should be easy and inexpensive.
2. Specific to breast cancer and commonly associated with it.
3. A stoichometric relationship should exist between plasma level of the marker and the number of tumour cells in the body.
4. The plasma or urine level should become abnormal in the presence of micrometastases i.e. at a stage where no clinical or presently available diagnostic methods reveal their presence.
5. The plasma or urine level should not be subject to wide fluctuation.
6. If present in normal plasma, the factor should exist at a much lower concentration than that found in association with *any* stage of breast cancer.

When numbers of these multifactorial studies have been analysed, it will be possible to measure a group of selected markers in each patient at her first attendance. Those with all markers negative will be regarded as suitable for curative treatment. Those with evidence of residual tumour will proceed to adjuvant systemic therapy. The level of the markers will be watched and used for judging the dosage of the adjuvant drug and its duration of administration. After adjuvant therapy has been completed, assessment of markers will be used to watch for the first evidence of recurrence.

Coombes and Neville (1977) have defined the properties of the ideal marker in breast cancer (Table 6). Selecting carcinoembryonic antigen (CEA), serum human chorionic gonadotrophin (HCG) and the nucleoside dimethyl guanosine as parameters, Tormey et al. (1975) have reported the presence of an abnormal level of at least one of these markers in 97% of patients with metastatic breast cancer, and in 67% of post-operative patients found to have axillary nodes involved at operation.

Analysing their observations with 10 biological markers, Coombes and Neville (1977) have shown abnormality of at least one in 100% of patients with overt distant metastases; in 80% of those presenting with T4 tumours or Grade 3 histology or positive axillary nodes; but in 30% of patients whose clinical findings at operation suggested a good prognosis. Six of the markers were adequate to pick out *all* positive cases and two of them, CEA and Ferritin, picked out all those with evidence of overt distant metastases.

Whereas tumour markers show the presence of the tumour burden and may be able to quantitate it, tumour localising agents are intended to detect the

site and extent of tumour in patients with known primary or recurrent cancer. So far, these agents have shown their greatest accuracy in the detection of large clinically recognisable tumours but their sensitivity is being refined. They fall into three categories (Kaplan and Adelstyn, 1976);

- Tumour seeking isotopes, e.g. Gallium-67 and Indium-111
- Radiolabelled antibiotics, e.g. Bleomycin labelled with Cobalt-57, Gallium-57, Indium-111, or Technetium-99m, Tetracycline labelled with Technetium-99m.
- Radiolabelled antibodies to tumour-associated antigens such as CEA.

CONCLUSIONS

Animal mammary cancers showing the most complete response to castration, androgen or anti-oestrogen therapy are those treated early in their course, and the phenomenon of first order kinetics applies equally to endocrine as to cytotoxic therapy in this disease. However, all systemic adjuvant therapy aiming to control micrometastases persisting after the primary treatment of mammary cancer must face the problem that the disease in the human is almost certainly multiclonal. To be successful, the agents used will have to possess not only selectivity for breast cancer but also a very wide spectrum of activity; otherwise the death of the sensitive clones will be followed by their replacement by non-sensitive clones.

While endocrine therapy is selective for mammary cancer cells, cytotoxic therapy is anti-proliferative but not selective. The modest results achieved in the trials of adjuvant cytotoxic therapy to date suggest that the benefits achieved are due, at least in part, to an endocrine effect. If we are not to be disappointed in our future trials, there are strong reasons for the use of combined endocrine/cytotoxic regimes for this purpose. The argument applies with even greater force in those patients whose tumours show significant levels of oestrogen receptor protein.

The responsiveness of advanced breast cancer to the anti-oestrogen tamoxifen in several reported series, and the absence of significant side effects on long term administration (see Chapter 13) makes it highly suitable for such an adjuvant trial in high risk patients after primary surgery. A suggested flow chart for selection of treatment is shown (Table 7). The choice of combined endocrine/cytotoxic treatment is based on the presence of a significant oestrogen receptor assay, while the patients whose tumours are receptor negative will be referred for combined immune/cytotoxic therapy.

Table 7. The use of oestrogen receptor assay of the tumour as a guide to adjuvant therapy after primary treatment in breast cancer.

Operative finding	*Receptor assay*	*Adjuvant therapy*
Axillary nodes +	ER +	Anti-oestrogen/cytotoxic therapy
	ER –	Immuno/cytotoxic therapy
Axillary nodes –		WATCH

It is hoped that two emendations of the flow chart will be possible in the near furture. Firstly, there is evidence from several reports that even with oestrogen receptor negative tumours, patients respond to anti-oestrogen therapy in the remarkably high proportion of 15 to 20% of cases (McGuire, 1975). It may be relevant that tamoxifen can compete for the androgen receptor as well as for the oestrogen receptor of breast cancer, and this has been demonstrated in 35 of 100 breast cancers *in vitro* (Lippman, 1976). It may be that a negative oestrogen receptor assay is not adequate to exclude patients from a tamoxifen adjuvant trial, and that additional information from androgen receptor assays may be needed for a decision.

The second emendation of the flow chart which may soon be possible is in connection with the selection of high-risk patients. This is based at present on the presence of involved axillary nodes at the time of primary surgery. The next two or three years should see rapid development in multifactorial studies which will establish a spectrum of biological markers suitable for selecting patients for systemic therapy at the time of primary treatment. Not only will these tumour-associated markers identify the presence of persistent disease after primary treatment, but they will be useful for monitoring early recurrence and possibly for localizing it.

REFERENCES

AMA Committee on Research (1960). Androgens and estrogens in the treatment of disseminated mammary carcinoma. *J. Amer. Med. Assoc. 172,* 1271.

Band, P. R., Lerner, H., Israel, L. and Leung, B. (1976). In *Proceedings of Symposium on Hormonal Control of Breast Cancer,* ICI, Macclesfield, p. 35.

Baum, M. (1975). Effect of administered hormones on the immune reaction. In *Host Defence in Breast Cancer*, p. 130 (Ed. B. A. Stoll). London: Heinemann Medical.

Ben-David, M., Danon, A. and Sulman, F. G. (1971). Evidence of antagonism, between prolactin and gonadotrophin secretion. *J. Endoc. 51*, 719.

Berenbaum, M. C. (1975). Effect of cytotoxic drugs and ionising radiation on immune responses. In *Host Defence in Breast Cancer*, p. 147 (Ed. B. A. Stoll). London: Heinemann Medical.

Bonadonna, G., Brusamolino, E. and Valagussa, P. et al. (1976). Combination chemotherapy as an adjuvant treatment in operable breast cancer. *New Engl. J. Med. 294*, 405.

Bond, W. H. (1968). The influence of various treatments on survival rates in cancer of the breast. *The Treatment of Carcinoma of the Breast*, p. 24 (Ed. A. S. Jarrett). Amsterdam: Excerpta Medica.

Block, G. E., Jensen, E. V. and Polley, T. Z. (1975). Prediction of hormonal dependence of mammary cancer. *Ann. Surg. 182*, 342.

Brambilla, C., De Lena, M., Rossi, A. et al. (1976). Response and survival in advanced breast cancer after two non-cross-resistant combinations. *Brit. Med. J. 1*, 801.

Braunsberg, H., James, V. H. T., Irvine, W. T. et al. (1973). Prognostic significance of oestrogen uptake by human breast cancer tissue. *Lancet 1*, 163.

Brinkley, D. and Haybittle, J. L. (1975). The curability of breast cancer. *Lancet 2*, 95.

Bulbrook, R. D. (1976). Personal communication.

Burchenal, J. H. (1976). Adjuvant therapy-theory, practice and potential. *Cancer 37*, 46.

Clemmesen, J. (1948). Carcinoma of breast. Results from statistical research. *Brit. J. Radiol. 21*, 583.

Cole, M. (1970). Prophylactic compared with therapeutic X-ray artificial menopause. In *Second Tenovus Workshop on Breast Cancer*, p. 2 (Eds C. A. F. Joslin and E. N. Gleave). Cardiff: Tenovus.

Coombes, R. C. and Neville, A. M. (1977). Significance of tumour index substances in management of breast cancer. In *Secondary Spread in Breast Cancer*, (Ed. B. A. Stoll). London: Heineman Medical.

De Sombre, E. R. and Arbogast, L. Y. (1974). Effect of the anti-estrogen C1628 on the growth of rat mammary tumours. *Cancer Res. 34*, 1971.

Devitt, J. E. (1976). Clinical prediction of growth behaviour. In *Risk Factors in Breast Cancer*, p. 110 (Ed. B. A. Stoll). London: Heinemann Medical.

Engelsmann, E., Korsten, C. B., Persijn, J. P. and Cleton, F. J. (1974). Oestrogen and androgen receptors in human breast cancer. *Brit. J. Cancer, 30*, 177.

Feherty, P., Farrer-Brown, G. and Kellie, A. E. (1971). Oestradiol receptors in carcinoma and benign disease of the breast. *Brit. J. Cancer 25*, 697.

Fisher, B., Carbone, P., Economou, S. G., et al. (1975). L-PAM in the management of primary breast cancer. A report of early findings. *New Engl. J. Med. 292*, 117.

Fisher, B., Ravdin, R. G., Ausman, R. K., Slack, N. H., Moore, G. E., Noer, R. J. (1968). Surgical adjuvant chemotherapy in cancer of the breast. Results of a decade of co-operative investigations. *Ann. Surg. 168*, 337.

Gallager, H. S. and Martin, J. E. (1969). The study of mammary carcinoma by mammography and whole organ sectioning. *Cancer 23*, 855.

Gehan, E. A. and Freireich, E. J. (1974). Non randomized controls in cancer clinical trials. *New Engl. J. Med. 290*, 198.

Griffiths, K. (1976). In *Proceedings of Symposium on Hormonal Control of Breast Cancer*, ICI, Macclesfield, p. 61.

Griswold, D. P. and Green, C. H. (1970). Observations on the hormone sensitivity of DMBA induced mammary tumours in the rat. *Cancer Res. 30*, 819.

Gullino, P. M., Grantham, F. H., Losonezy, I. and Berghofer, B. (1974). Physiopathologic characteristics of hormone dependent tissue. *J. Nat. Cancer Inst. 49*, 1333.

Hadfield, G. J. and Holt, J. A. G. (1956). The physiological castration syndrome in breast cancer. *Brit. Med. J. 2*, 972.

Hahnel, R., Twaddle, E. and Ratajczak, T. (1973). The influence of synthetic anti-estrogen on the binding of tritiated estradiol-17β by cytosols of human uterus and human breast carcinoma. *J. Steroid Biochem. 4*, 687.

Hill, B. T. and Price, L. A. (1977). Concepts and prospects in adjuvant chemotherapy. In *Secondary Spread in Breast Cancer*, (Ed. B. A. Stoll). London: Heinemann Medical.

Holdaway, I. M., Friesen, H. and Worsley, I. (1975). Prolactin tumour binding. *Oncol. News 1*, 7.

Huseby, R. A. and Thomas, L. B. (1954). Histological and histochemical alterations in the normal breast tissues of patients with advanced breast cancer being treated with estrogenic hormones. *Cancer 7*, 54.

Jensen, E. V., Desombre, E. R. and Jungblut, P. W. (1967). Estrogen receptors in hormone responsive tissues and tumor. In *Endogenous Factors influencing Host-Tumour Balance*, (Eds R. W. Wissler, T. L. Dao and S. Wood). Illinois: Univ. Chicago Press.

Jensen, E. V. et al. (1971). In *Estrogen Target Tissues and Neoplasia*, p. 23 (Ed. T. L. Dao). Illinois: Univ. Chicago Press.

Jordan, V. C. (1976). In *Proceedings of Symposium on Hormonal Control of Breast Cancer*, ICI, Macclesfield, p. 11.

Jordan, V. C. and Koerner, S. (1975). Tamoxifen and the human carcinoma 8S oestrogen receptor. *Europ. J. Cancer*, 11, 205.

Kaplan, W. D. and Adelstein, S. J. (1976). The radionuclide identification of tumors. *Cancer 37*, Supplement, 487.

Korenman, S. G. and Dukes, B. A. (1970). Specific estrogen binding by the cytoplasm of human breast carcinoma. *J. Clin. Endoc. 30*, 639.

Leclerq, G., Heuson, J. C., Deboel, M. C. and Mattheiem, W. H. (1975). Oestrogen receptors in breast cancer; a changing concept. *Brit. Med. J. 1*, 185.

Leung, B. S., Moseley, H. S., Davenport, C. E. et al. (1975). In *Estrogen Receptors in Human Breast Cancer*, p. 127 (Ed. W. L. McGuire et al). New York: Raven Press.

L'Hermite, M., Robyn, C., Heuson, J. C. and Rozencweig, M. (1974). Breast cancer regression under oestrogen therapy. *Brit. Med. J. 1*, 390.

Lippman, M. (1976). In *Proceedings of Symposium on Hormonal Control of Breast Cancer*, ICI, Macclesfield, p. 25.

McGuire, W. L. (1975). Current status of estrogen receptors in human breast cancer. *Cancer, 36*, 638.

Mobbs, B. G. (1966). The uptake of tritiated estradiol by DMBA induced mammary tumors of the rat. *J. Endoc. 36*, 409.

Mueller C. B. and Jeffries, W. (1975). Cancer of the breast. Its outcome as measured by the rate of dying and causes of death. *Ann. Surg. 182*, 334.

Nevinny, H. B., Nevinny, D., Rosoff, C. B., Hall, T. C. and Muench, H. (1969). Prophylactic oophorectomy in breast cancer therapy—preliminary report. *Amer. J. Surg. 117*, 531.

Nissen Meyer, R. (1967). The role of prophylactic castration on the therapy of human mammary cancer. *Europ. J. Cancer 3,* 395.

Nordenskjold, B., Lowhagen, T. and Zajicek, J. (1976). In *Proceedings of Symposium on Hormonal Control of Breast Cancer,* ICI, Macclesfield, p. 43.

Qualheim, R. E. and Gall, E. A. (1967). Breast carcinoma with multiple sites of origin. *Cancer 10,* 460.

Ravdin, R. G., Lewison, E. F., Slack, N. H. et al. (1970). Results of a clinical trial concerning the worth of prophylactic oophorectomy for breast carcinoma. *Surg. Gynec. Obstet. 131,* 1055.

Schabel, F. M. (1975). Concepts for systemic treatment of micrometastases. *Cancer 35,* 15.

Schmahl, D. (1974). Carcinogenic hazards from drugs. In *Advances in Tumour prevention, detection and characterisation,* Vol. 2, p. 34 (Ed. C. Maltoni et al). Amsterdam: Excerpta Medica.

Schultz, K. D., Haselmeier, B. and Holzel, F. (1969). *Acta Endoc. Supp. 138,* 236.

Sieber, S. M. and Adamson, R. H. (1975). Toxicity of antineoplastic agents in man. Chromosomal aberrations, antifertility effects, congenital malformations and carcinogenic potential. *Advances in Cancer Research 22,* 57.

Spaeren, U., Olsnes, S., Brennhovd, I. et al. (1973). Content of estrogen receptors in human breast cancers. *Europ. J. Cancer 9,* 353.

Steward, A. M., Nixon, D., Zamcheck, N. and Aisenberg, A. (1974). CEA in breast cancer patients. Serum levels and disease progress. *Cancer 33,* 1246.

Stoll, B. A. (1963). Thio TEPA and breast cancer. *Brit. Med. J. 1,* 54.

Stoll, B. A. (1969). In *Hormonal Management in Breast Cancer,* (Ed. B. A. Stoll). London: Pitman Medical and J. B. Lippincott.

Stoll, B. A. (1972). In *Endocrine Therapy in Malignant Disease,* p. 128 (Ed. B. A. Stoll). London: W. B. Saunders.

Stoll, B. A. (1976). Effect of age on growth pattern. In *Risk Factors in Breast Cancer,* p. 129 (Ed. B. A. Stoll). London: Heinemann Medical.

Terenius, L. (1971). Anti-estrogen and breast cancer. *Europ. J. Cancer 7,* 57.

Terenius, L. (1973). Estrogen and proestogen binders in human and rat mammary carcinoma. *Europ. J. Cancer 9,* 291.

Terenius, L. (1974). Anti-oestrogens and their role in mammary cancer. In *Mammary Cancer and Neuro-endocrine therapy,* p. 82 (Ed. B. A. Stoll). London: Butterworth.

Tormey, D. C., Waalkes, T. P., Ahmann, D. et al. (1975). Biological markers in breast carcinoma (1). Incidence of abnormalities in CEA, HCG, three polyamines and three minor nucleosides. *Cancer 35,* 1095.

Willis, K., London, D. R. and Butt, W. R. (1976). In *Proceedings of Symposium on Hormonal Control of Breast Cancer,* ICI, Macclesfield, p. 59.

SECTION 2

Treatment for Palliation

Chapter

9

ARTHUR J. DONOVAN

Sequential Therapy of Advanced Disease

INTRODUCTION

The majority of individuals in whom a diagnosis of mammary cancer is established will require palliative therapy and ultimately will die of the disease. The primary therapy of "operable" mammary cancer may have little effect on the final outcome (Mueller, and Jeffries, 1975); while 5 year survival may exceed 50% (Berg and Robbins, 1966), the crude 15 year survival has been reported as 17% (Brinkley and Haybittle, 1968). Thus, most cases of mammary cancer will require several forms of therapy sometimes extending over a period of years.

The physician responsible for the care of the patient with mammary cancer is presented at each stage of the disease with a bewildering variety of therapy from which to choose. It has been noted in previous chapters that the primary treatment of "operable" mammary cancer is highly controversial. In this section discussion is confined to the patient with advanced disease. In such cases some form of sequential therapy is almost universally used, but the sequence to be described represents the personal choice of the writer. In a field of uncertainty and imprecision such as this, no apology is offered for such prejudice. Unless otherwise indicated, statements regarding results are based on the writer's published experience (Johnson et al., 1970; Sievers and Donovan, 1973).

BASIS OF SEQUENTIAL THERAPY

The group of patients to be considered include those with advanced local disease or overt remote metastases at the time of initial diagnosis. Also included are patients with either local or remote recrudescence of disease appearing after surgical treatment of "operable" disease. Such cases of advanced mammary cancer will need several forms of therapy, but in the writer's philosophy, the term "sequential" therapy means more than just this.

Sequential therapy denotes stepwise progression from simple to more complex forms of therapy, and

avoidance (when reasonable), of the simultaneous use of multiple methods of therapy. Sequential therapy embodies also a concept of moderation in the intensity of the methods used. The justification for such moderation is an acknowledgement of the fact that progression of the disease is inevitable, and that the dominant goal of treatment is palliation which is "relief of symptoms without hope of cure" (Dorland, 1944).

Therefore, when a form of therapy is selected for trial, one does not progress to another form of therapy until adequate time has been allowed to show that the therapy in use will not achieve palliation. If, however, control of disease is observed, therapy is continued until further progression occurs.

The basis for selection of a particular sequence of therapy is empirical, that is, arbitrary and based on experience. Intense efforts to develop objective predictive criteria to apply in selection of therapy have not achieved proven success. The current status of tests of prediction has been summarized by Bulbrook (1974) as follows:

> The overall results of the last 20 years' work are depressing. As far as metastatic breast cancer is concerned, there is not a single predictive test that is so firmly established that its use is mandatory. In the strictest scientific sense, there is no definitive proof of the efficacy of the published methods of prediction and, for this reason, it is perfectly ethical to select particular treatments for patients by the standard clinical methods (precedent or instinct).
>
> Even when there is evidence that selection of patients for a particular treatment by means of predictive measurements will lead to a substantial increase in benefit, this is almost certainly accomplished by denying treatment to a small proportion of potential responders. The question of prediction and selection then becomes a subjective one, and every clinician has to make up his own mind about the level of response he requires in his responsive patients and the degree of misclassification he will accept, in the light of the severity of the disease and the burden of the proposed treatment.

As already stated, the goal of therapy in advanced mammary cancer is palliation. It is unfortunate that a confusing tendency has arisen to equate palliation with objective regression of measurable tumor. While it is true that effective palliation is more likely when objective regression of disease occurs, the duration of control and the quality of life must also be critical considerations.

Intensive therapy associated with major morbidity may sometime achieve objective regression. If, however, its duration is only a few weeks and the disease is again recrudescent by the time morbidity from therapy has abated, one must question whether palliation has indeed been achieved. The mere objective regression of tumor is not the goal of palliative therapy and must not be confused with improved quality of life. Injection of morphine sulfate for relief of bone pain may be extraordinarily effective palliation.

PRETREATMENT EVALUATION

The selection of a particular sequence of treatment is based mainly upon a pretreatment evaluation of the extent of the disease and of the estrogen status of the patient. The response of tumor to prior therapy and the site and rate of progression of the disease will also influence the decision.

(1) Extent of disease

When advanced mammary cancer is diagnosed, a decision must be made as to how assiduously one should try to establish the full extent of the disease. It is widely believed that early dissemination occurs in most, if not all, cases of mammary cancer, but that the foci of disseminated disease may remain covert for many years. Thus, many patients with obviously inoperable or recrudescent disease on the chest wall may not show clinical evidence of remote metastases. On the other hand, some patients with remote metastases may not show evidence of chest wall, mammary or regional node tumor, while other patients will show evidence of both remote and local disease.

One important aim of pretreatment evaluation in advanced mammary cancer is to distinguish patients with apparently limited disease from those with clinical evidence of widespread metastases. Selection of therapy is considerably affected if the disease appears clinically to be localized—be it to the mammary region, nodes or a solitary metastatic deposit.

Physical examination will reveal the extent of overt disease in the breasts, on the chest wall and in the axillary and supraclavicular nodal areas. When feasible, tissue should be removed for histological examination to verify the presence of malignant tissue and a portion of tissue should be analysed for estrogen binding, if such studies are available. Hepatomegaly, pleural effusion or ascites may also be detectable on physical examination while areas of tenderness over the spine and pelvis should be sought.

A radiogram of the chest is mandatory. If available, a scintiscan of the skeletal system is preferred to a standard radiographic skeletal survey, as it may identify metastatic disease not discernible on standard radiograms (Silberstein et al., 1973). In most

institutions the difference in cost between a scintiscan and a skeletal survey is not great, and the greater accuracy of the scintiscan will help to determine whether the disease is limited in extent.

The incidence of both false positive and false negative results with the scintiscan must be recognized and a standard radiogram should therefore be obtained of areas noted as suspect in the scintigram. If the radiogram does not confirm the presence of osseous metastases and local symptoms are not present, the area is observed. Conversely, if symptoms suggest metastasis but the scintigram is indeterminate, a standard radiogram may show a metastatic focus which was not noted on the scintigram.

Additionally, a radiographic record of bone metastases is desirable for the purpose of serial observations. Repeat radiograms are more easily obtained than repeat scintigrams; the behavior of the tumor in response to therapy is recorded more accurately by radiography than by scintiscan.

The level of alkaline phosphatase in the serum should be assessed, and if elevated, the isoenzymes are determined in order to ascertain whether the osseous or hepatic fraction is responsible. The serum calcium should also be determined.

Some might suggest that a more assiduous search for metastases should be carried out and that this might include scintigrams of liver and brain. We have not adopted such a policy because we direct therapy towards overt and, in particular, symptomatic metastases. Obviously, if a diagnosis of hepatic metastases is suspected because of hepatomegaly or a persistently elevated alkaline phosphatase level, a scintiscan of the liver will be obtained. If signs or symptoms suggesting cerebral metastases are noted, further studies will be indicated. If available, computerized transaxial tomography (EMI scan) should be carried out, but alternatively, brain scintiscan or arteriography are indicated.

(2) **Estrogen status**

Approximately one-third of cases of mammary cancer are "hormone dependent". This dependency is reflected in the objective regression of tumor that may occur following oophorectomy (Beatson, 1896). Such regression is seen most commonly in premenopausal or "estrogen-rich" women. Conversely, postmenopausal or "estrogen-poor" women may show tumor regression following administration of estrogenic steroids (Biden, 1943). This paradox has not been explained but the dichotomy in response necessitates a judgement as to the estrogen status of the patient before instituting hormone therapy.

Estimation of estrogen status is fairly obvious in the menstruating woman or in the women beyond the seventh decade. The difficulty in defining estrogen status is related mainly to the early postmenopausal patient. Unfortunately, analysis of urinary excretion of estrogenic steroids is not particularly helpful in resolving the issue. The occurrence of "hot flashes" following cessation of menstruation may suggest the persistence of active ovarian function. Studies of vaginal smears in the early postmenopausal patient generally reveal good to moderate estrogen effect.

An arbitrary policy has been pursued by us in defining estrogen status. Cases are divided into "estrogen rich" and "estrogen poor" by the empiric criteria shown in Table 1. In this arbitrary classification it should be noted that women under age 50 in whom an artificial menopause has been induced even many years previously, are listed as estrogen rich. This reflects the fact that such patients tend to respond to hormonal manipulation more in the fashion of menstruating women than of estrogen poor women.

This arbitrary classification does not claim to identify the case that is hormone dependent. It merely serves to identify the patient who will be subjected either to endocrine ablation (estrogen rich) or to additive therapy with estrogenic steroids (estrogen poor). However, a revolution in the identification of the hormone dependent tumor may currently be in process. Techniques for determination of the affinity of mammary cancer for estrogenic steroids have been developed (Jensen and Jacobsen, 1962). Early results suggest that when estrogen

Table 1 Classification of estrogen status in women with advanced mammary cancer

Estrogen rich	*Estrogen poor*
Menstruating	
< 3 years following natural cessation of menstruation	> 3 years following natural cessation of menstruation
< 50 years of age following surgically* or radiologically induced menopause	> Age 50 following surgically* or radiologically induced menopause

* Verification of oophorectomy at time of hysterectomy by pathology report is mandatory.

binding by the mammary cancer is present, the rate of objective regression following ablative hormonal therapy is high, approaching two-thirds of cases (Block et al., 1975).

(3) Other modifying factors

The sequence of treatment in advanced breast cancer is affected also by the history of the tumor's response to prior hormonal therapy. A patient who has responded favorably to one form of sex hormone therapy tends to respond favorably to other forms. The converse is also true.

Modification of sequential therapy may also result from our knowledge that a specific therapy is less efficacious for disease at a particular site, that response to one therapy modifies the selection of subsequent therapy, or that a particular mode of behaviour by the tumor suggests the need for a particular form of therapy. These modifications will be discussed more fully later (p. 96).

THERAPEUTIC SEQUENCE

The basic sequence of therapy employed in treatment of advanced mammary cancer is summarized in Figure 1. The progression from one step to another is determined by a documented failure to respond favorably, or by further progression of the disease after a period of favorable response.

Assuming that the determination of estrogen binding becomes established as a useful predictive criterion of hormone dependency, this sequence will become modified. At the least, the ablative hormonal sequence will be followed in cases with positive estrogen binding while in cases with negative estrogen binding, ablative hormonal therapy will be bypassed in favor of chemotherapy.

Radiation therapy is the first choice for apparently localized disease, regardless of the age of the patient or her estrogen status. In general, cases with widespread disease at the time of initiation of therapy, or cases with localized disease which is not controlled by radiation therapy, should receive systemic therapy, i.e. additive or ablative hormonal therapy or chemotherapy.

In the patient whose tumor exists in an estrogen rich environment, primary reliance for systemic therapy is on endocrine ablation performed sequentially, i.e. oophorectomy, followed by adrenalectomy or hypophysectomy. Primary reliance for systemic therapy in the estrogen poor patient is on additive hormonal therapy by estrogenic steroids. Chemo-

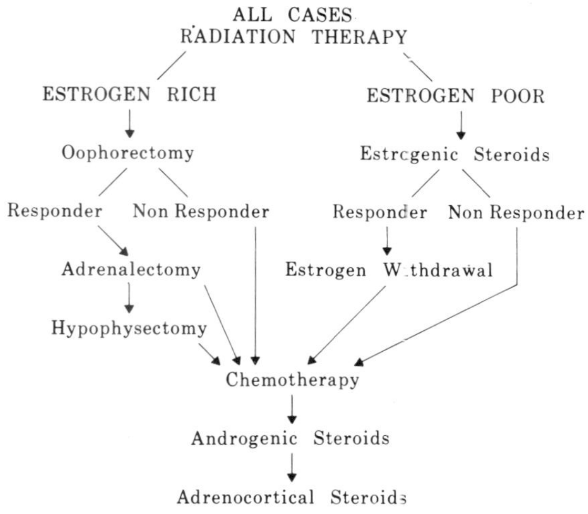

Figure 1 Basic sequence of therapy in women with advanced mammary cancer.

therapy is employed in cases of failure from additive or ablative hormonal therapy, irrespective of estrogen status. Androgenic steroids are occasionally used as a near-final resort and following failure of chemotherapy. The final therapy employed is usually by adrenocortical steroids.

RESPONSE TO THERAPY

(1) Recording the response

The objective response of measurable tumor to therapy must be documented. If accessible, deposits of tumor are measured by caliper and the results recorded on a line drawing. Visual estimates of size of tumor deposits are notoriously unreliable. With chest wall or mammary disease, serial photographs are especially helpful while sequential imaging of the lungs, bone or liver will assess the behaviour of tumor at these sites.

The frequency and extent of follow-up examinations is a matter of practical importance because the costs of repeated diagnostic studies can be very heavy. The aphorism of the late Gertrude Stein may be relevant: "A difference to be a difference must make a difference". If one or more metastatic foci have been identified, these foci are rescrutinized by the appropriate study after 6 weeks of therapy. For example, if the only metastatic disease identified was an osteolytic lesion in the lumbar spine, a single film of the lumbar spine is obtained. If symptoms suggestive of disease at a new site develops, then the appropriate study is performed. The only routine

investigations are chest radiograms and bone scintigrams at the completion of three months of therapy and before any change in therapy.

The evidence for objective response of osseous metastases is of various types. Osteolytic lesions may recalcify with a rim of dense calcification and appear as areas of increased calcification. On the other hand, the progress of osteoblastic metastases may be difficult to evaluate. Following the institution of systemic therapy, foci of increased calcification may be noted on radiography of areas in which metastatic disease was not previously identified. These foci may be in areas suspected of metastases on the scintigram but not confirmed by radiograms. Recognition of this phenomenon is most important because of the danger of assuming that such areas of increased calcification represent newly developing osteoblastic metastases.

(2) **Evaluating the response**

Responses are categorized as either favorable or unfavorable; the two categories include both objective and subjective components.

A favorable therapeutic response includes those cases with objective regression of disease. (Objective regression is defined as a 50% decrease in the size of a measurable tumor without new deposits of tumor appearing.) Also included as a favourable response are those patients in whom the disease was progressive at the initiation of therapy but in whom a period of stability followed therapy. Although such a period of stability may represent a spontaneous event, it constitutes satisfactory palliation. The goal of therapy is the establishment of a situation in which the patient may enjoy a meaningful quality of life.

In either instance, there must be subjective improvement to justify designation of favorable therapeutic response. Precise categorization of subjective response is most difficult, although it has been recently attempted (Patterson, 1975). Taken into consideration are the ability to continue work, the potential for meaningful social activity and the degree of dependence on pharmacological agents for the relief of pain.

Those patients in whom there is objective progression of disease at three months after initiation of therapy, and in whom increase in symptoms has occurred at that time are considered as having an unfavorable therapeutic response.

(3) **Duration of therapy**

How long should a specific course of therapy be pursued? If a favorable therapeutic response has been observed, the therapy in use is continued until further progression is noted. In the case of ablative treatment or additive sex hormone therapy, a minimum period of observation/trial of three months is desirable. Evidence of objective regression may be delayed for this period. On the other hand, if a favorable response occurs with cytotoxic chemotherapy it is almost always apparent within 6 weeks. If the disease continues to progress after 6 weeks of such therapy, further trial is not worthwhile.

Rampant progression of disease may ensue following institution of a course of therapy. In this instance the period of trial of three months must be abandoned and another therapeutic option exercised.

A mixed response to therapy presents particular problems. Disease at one site may show objective regression, while at the same time disease has appeared or progressed at another site. For example, mammary or regional nodal disease may have regressed with chemotherapy but a painful osseous metastasis may have become apparent. In this instance chemotherapy can be continued, and radiation therapy should be employed for the newly manifest osseous disease.

STEPS IN SEQUENTIAL THERAPY

The steps in the therapeutic sequence shown in Figure 1 are discussed in detail in following chapters. They are referred to here in a cursory fashion, mainly in order to illustrate the writer's personal philosophy.

Radiation therapy

In cases of localized disease, radiation therapy will, in a predictable fashion, result in the highest incidence of favorable response of any therapy available. Approximately three-fourths of cases will experience favorable response. This applies both to disease in the breast itself and to metastases in regional lymph nodes, soft tissue, bone or central nervous system. Unless unusual circumstances exist, patients with localized disease should be offered the opportunity of a beneficial response from radiation therapy before proceeding to systemic therapy.

Oophorectomy

Ovarian ablation is the first systemic therapy to be employed in the estrogen rich patient. Surgical ablation of the ovaries is preferred. Approximately one-third of estrogen rich cases of mammary cancer

will show objective tumor regression following oophorectomy. Because of the sharp decrease in favorable response to oophorectomy after the menopause (Treves and Finkbeiner, 1958), the writer does not advise oophorectomy in women who are more than three years postmenopausal.

Adrenalectomy and Hypophysectomy

At the University of South Alabama prior favorable biological response in the estrogen rich patient to oophorectomy has remained the primary indication for adrenalectomy and approximately 40% of such cases will respond favorably (MacDonald, 1962). Because of the low response rate, the writer has not recommended adrenalectomy either in estrogen poor cases or in estrogen rich cases without evidence of favorable biological response to previous oophorectomy. The likelihood of favorable response must be high enough to balance the morbidity following adrenalectomy.

The indications for ablation of pituitary function are similar to those for adrenalectomy and the incidence of regression is comparable to that achieved with adrenalectomy. Patients in whom disease is again progressive following a favorable response to adrenalectomy may be subjected to trans-sphenoidal cryohypophysectomy (Conway and Collins, 1969).

Estrogenic steroids

Estrogenic steroids are the initial choice of systemic therapy for estrogen poor patients with advanced mammary cancer. Cases with dominant osseous disease are an exception because of the low incidence of favorable response of osseous disease to therapy with estrogenic steroids (Stoll, 1950). However, soft tissue and pulmonary metastases respond well to therapy with estrogens, 34% of cases experiencing objective regression, and an additional 23% stability of disease (Sievers and Donovan, 1973).

The phenomenon of *withdrawal regression* requires emphasis (Kaufman and Esher, 1961). When a patient has experienced a favorable response to additive therapy with sex hormones and subsequent progression of disease occurs, all hormonal therapy should be discontinued. Withdrawal regression will occur in at least one-third of cases. An exception to this advice would be a case with rampant progression of disease. If withdrawal regression occurs and further progression subsequently occurs, a second trial of therapy with the same sex hormone is worthwhile.

Cytotoxic chemotherapy

In general chemotherapy is employed after demonstrable failure of control by additive or ablative hormonal therapy. In contrast to additive or ablative hormonal therapy in which failure to respond to one form of therapy reduces sharply the likelihood of subsequent response to another form of hormone therapy, the likelihood of favorable response to chemotherapy is not related to the prior response to hormone therapy. If single agent chemotherapy is chosen, a series of chemotherapeutic programs will usually be employed.

Androgenic steroids

Because of its masculinizing effects and a lower rate of favorable response than with other additive or ablative sex hormonal therapy, androgen is not selected as the initial systemic therapy in any patient. In estrogen rich patients endocrine ablation is preferred; in estrogen poor cases therapy with estrogenic steroids is preferred. The incidence of favorable response to androgen therapy is so low in cases which have failed to respond to either ablative or additive hormonal therapy, that chemotherapy should be employed before a trial of androgenic steroids. Androgens are employed as a last resort for systemic therapy prior to the use of adrenocortical steroids.

Adrenocortical steroids

Adrenocortical steroids are extremely valuable in the treatment of certain specific manifestations of advanced mammary cancer including cerebral metastases, hypercalcemia and "lymphangitic" pulmonary metastases. Tumor regression may occur with soft tissue and osseous disease but the incidence of regression is the lowest of any of the more common forms of therapy. With the above first mentioned exceptions, administration of adrenocortical steroids alone cannot be justified until the potential benefit of other therapeutic modalities has been exhausted.

EXCEPTIONS TO THERAPEUTIC SEQUENCE

The usual therapeutic sequence may be modified for three reasons—because of the location of the tumor, because of its rapid rate of progression or because of its response to prior therapy. In addition, employment of some types of combined therapy may be based on personal experience. Included among these exceptions are the following:

Osseous metastases—estrogen poor case

The less favorable response of osseous metastases to therapy with estrogenic steroids was noted in the discussion of estrogen therapy. As a consequence, the estrogen poor case with predominantly widespread osseous metastases is submitted to cytotoxic chemotherapy rather than to additive hormonal therapy.

Cerebral metastases

Intracranial metastases respond very poorly to hormonal manipulation. The usual chemotherapeutic agents employed in the treatment of advanced mammary cancer do not cross the blood brain barrier and thus are not effective in the treatment of intracranial metastases. However, adrenocortical steroids are believed to abort the reactive edema surrounding cerebral metastases and the resultant remission of neurological findings is often dramatic. Initial control of the clinical manifestations of intracranial metastases having been achieved, the physician can proceed with total cerebral radiation.

Hypercalcemia

Hypercalcemia associated with metastatic mammary cancer can develop spontaneously or may be induced by additive sex hormone therapy. When either spontaneous or induced hypercalcemia develops, other therapies are bypassed and treatment with adrenocortical steroids is instituted. Control of hypercalcemia will occur in over 70% of cases but if not achieved, mithramycin is administered. With stabilization of the level of calcium, the physician can proceed with other appropriate systemic therapy such as ablative hormonal therapy or chemotherapy. Effective palliation persisting for 12-24 months is not uncommon.

"Lymphangitic" pulmonary metastases

"Lymphangitic" pulmonary metastases may in fact be a manifestation of embolization of tumor cells (Case Records, 1972). The prognosis is ominous (Goldsmith et al., 1967) and the course of disease, unless arrested promptly, follows a rapidly fatal course with fulminant respiratory insufficiency. Administration of a pharmacological dose of adrenocortical steroids may induce a dramatic response with prompt improvement in pulmonary function although the mechanism of its action is unknown.

The physician can then initiate immediate additional treatment for which my choice is cytotoxic chemotherapy. In general, the response to chemotherapy, if it occurs, is more rapid in onset than that observed following initiation of sex hormonal therapy. If progression is arrested, or objective regression occurs, further therapy can be instituted. In this instance, aggressive therapy with a combination of modalities—adrenocortical steroids, chemotherapy and endocrine ablation is warranted because of the otherwise dismal prognosis.

Hepatic metastases

Hepatic metastases are not suitable for radiation therapy and respond very poorly to additive or ablative hormonal therapy. Therefore, if hepatic metastases are the dominant manifestation of disease, other therapies are omitted and the patient is submitted to cytotoxic chemotherapy.

Pleural metastases

Intrapleural instillation of a chemotherapeutic agent has a special role in the treatment of pleural effusion and for this purpose there appears to be little to choose between nitrogen mustard and 5-Fluorouracil. The treatment by cytotoxic agents is combined with other therapy when the pleural effusion is not the only evidence of advanced mammary cancer. If disease is present in the mammary area radiation therapy is indicated, or appropriate sequential systemic therapy is employed if the disease is disseminated or if further radiation therapy to the mammary area is not feasible.

Radiation therapy combined with systemic therapy

In a variety of instances radiation therapy may be desirable for a localized focus of disease with simultaneous systemic therapy for diffuse disease. The pre-eminent example is the patient with one or two foci of painful osseous metastasis in the presence of widespread disease. Radiation therapy can be directed to the specific pain-producing site while systemic therapy is initiated or continued. Response to systemic therapy is evaluated by the response observed in sites other than those subjected to radiation.

The potential benefits of both radiation therapy and oophorectomy may be required for treatment of active disease in the mammary area with or without regional nodes and distant metastases. This is illustrated in *inflammatory cancer of the breast* in the estrogen rich patient. Oophorectomy is performed first and the breast is observed for evidence of

biological response–decrease in skin redness and softening of the tumor mass. As soon as it is observed, radiation therapy is instituted. If regression does not occur or progression is relentless, radiation therapy is instituted after about 4 weeks.

This evidence of biological response to oophorectomy is sought because it will be a basis for a decision to proceed to adrenalectomy when further progression of the tumor occurs. It is possible that evidence of estrogen binding in a tumor specimen may eliminate the need for this period of observation.

Extirpative surgery

Excisional surgery may have an occasional role in the sequential therapy of advanced mammary cancer. Either a primary tumor or a metastasis in the opposite breast may coexist with advanced regional nodal disease or remote metastases. A palliative resection of the tumor in the breast may be advisable but cases with locally advanced disease in the breast in which the resection would transect tumor, or in which the line of resection would be marginal, should be excluded.

RESULTS OF SEQUENTIAL THERAPY

We have previously reported the duration of survival in 195 consecutive cases of advanced mammary cancer with mammary, soft tissue, nodal or pulmonary disease who received sequential therapy according to the principles that have been outlined (Sievers and Donovan, 1973). These results are summarized in Table 2 as an example of results that may be anticipated with sequential therapy.

In this chapter a simple and stepwise sequence of therapy has been outlined for treatment of advanced mammary cancer. Reports from more aggressive approaches such as combination of oophorectomy, adrenalectomy and 5-Fluorouracil (Wilson et al., 1971) or combination chemotherapy (Cooper, 1969) are impressive, but it remains to be proven that they result in a greater prolongation of life of meaningful quality than that achieved by the summation of responses to sequential therapy.

Data which will bear valid statistical scrutiny in comparing various approaches to the treatment of advanced breast cancer are extraordinarily rare. The vagaries in the behaviour of mammary cancer are limitless. Disease at different sites may respond differently to a particular form of therapy, and there are never two instances in which the course of the disease is identical. Periods of dormancy are frequent and may persist for protracted periods. Progressive disease may, after a period of aggressive growth, remain stable for a variable period of time and host resistance undoubtedly plays a role in these vagaries of behavior.

All of these factors may explain the widely different results that are reported for the same therapy. The physician should beware of extravagant claims of therapeutic efficacy based on a small number of cases followed for a short period of time. Although statistical methods can be applied and may reveal "significance", the number of uncontrolled variables are such as to question the justification for applying statistical methods.

Without treatment, a small percentage of patients with advanced mammary cancer will survive for many years. Perhaps those with advanced disease who survive for several years with treatment are those with biologically less aggressive tumors. The higher incidence of favorable response to palliative therapy in patients with a longer "free interval" supports such a concept. However, when dramatic regression of progressive disease occurs following institution of therapy, and tumor remains in regression for 2-3 years, it is indeed difficult not to conclude that life has been prolonged.

Data on total duration of survival, with different therapeutic regimens which can be compared, is almost non-existent. Criteria for evaluation of response vary widely. Reports indicating the incidence of objective regression with specific therapies abound but too often such reports contain only sparse information on total duration of survival. Survival data concerning a particular mode of therapy are often presented without indicating the total duration of survival with *all* therapies employed during the course of the disease.

Table 2 Results of sequential therapy in personal series

Survival	*All cases (195)*	*Favorable response *(115)*	*Progression †(80)*
	(%)	(%)	(%)
6 months	63	80	38
12 months	45	61	21
18 months	27	42	5
36 months	11	18	0

* Documented favorable response to any therapy employed; 57 cases alive at time of report.
† No documented favorable response to any therapy.

CONCLUSION

The care of the patient with advanced mammary cancer demands a particular relationship between the physician and patient. The inevitable outcome is obvious, but only rarely will even the intelligent patient admit that therapy will not control the disease. This denial can contribute importantly to the quality of life that will be enjoyed by the patient. That the physician must not destroy this illusion is a profound conviction of the writer, and the attitude of the physician therefore becomes a most important agent in palliation.

An additional factor concerns the degree to which attention is focused on the patient's disease. The patient who experiences a favorable response to oophorectomy or whose disease is in remission following radiation therapy can be seen at prolonged intervals. On the other hand, the patient receiving weekly chemotherapy or requiring maintenance therapy following adrenalectomy has constant attention focused on her morbid state, and this causes extra anxiety.

Sequential therapy can be compared to guerilla warfare, in contrast to a frontal assault. All forms of weapons are employed and with sequential therapy there is nearly always an additional therapeutic option that can be utilized. By jealous rationing of therapeutic modalities the day is postponed when the physician is required to inform the patient that further therapy is not available. The latter necessity can be a devastating experience for the patient whose disease is still progressive but not yet terminal.

In summary, with sequential therapy the physician jealously guards the therapies available and rations them to the patient at what is deemed to be the appropriate time. The potential of the more simple single agent therapy to achieve beneficial results is emphasized—radiation therapy for localized disease, oophorectomy rather than combined oophorectomy and adrenalectomy, single agent chemotherapy rather than agressive combination chemotherapy. The more aggressive therapies and combination of therapies are reserved for use in special instances and for cases that have failed to be controlled with simpler methods.

REFERENCES

Beatson, G. T. (1896). On the treatment of inoperable cases of carcinoma of the mamma: suggestions for a new method of treatment with illustrative cases. *Lancet ii*, 104.

Berg, J. W. and Robbins, G. F. (1966). Factors influencing short and long term survival of breast cancer patients. *Surgery, Gynecology & Obstetrics 122*, 1311.

Biden, W. M. (1943). Stilboestrol for breast cancer. *British Medical Journal ii*, 57.

Block, G. E., Jensen, E. V. and Polley, T. Z. (1975). The prediction of hormone dependency of mammary cancer. *Annals of Surgery 182*, 342.

Brinkley, D. and Haybittle, J. L. (1968). A 15-year follow-up study of patients treated for cancer of the breast. *British Journal of Radiology 41*, 215.

Bulbrook, R. D. (1974). Tests of prediction. *The Treatment of Breast Cancer*, p. 177 (Ed. S. H. Atkins). Baltimore: University Park Press.

Case Records of the Massachusetts General Hospital (1972). *New England Journal of Medicine 287*, 604.

Conway, L. W. and Collins, W. F. (1969). Results of trans-sphenoidal cryohypophysectomy for carcinoma of the breast. *New England Journal of Medicine 281*, 1.

Cooper, R. (1969). Combination chemotherapy in hormone resistant breast cancer. *Proc. American Association Cancer Research 10*, 15.

Dorland's Illustrated Medical Dictionary (1944). W. B. Saunders Co.

Goldsmith, H. S., Bailey, H. D., Callahan, E. L. and Beattie, E. J. (1967). Pulmonary lymphangitic metastases from breast carcinoma. *Archives of Surgery 94*, 483.

Jensen, E. V. and Jacobson, H. I. (1962). Basic guides to the mechanism of oestrogen action. *Recent Prog. Horm. Res. 18*, 387.

Johnston, M. J., Lipsett, J. A. and Donovan, A. J. (1970). Osseous metastasis in mammary cancer; response to therapy. *Archives of Surgery 101*, 578.

Kaufman, R. J. and Escher, G. C. (1961). Rebound regression in advanced mammary carcinoma. *Surgery, Gynecology & Obstetrics 113*, 635.

MacDonald, I. (1962). Endocrine ablation in disseminated mammary carcinoma. *Surgery, Gynecology & Obstetrics 115*, 215.

Mueller, C. B. and Jeffries, W. (1975). Cancer of the breast. *Annals of Surgery 182*, 334.

Patterson, W. B. (1975). The quality of survival in response to treatment. *Journal American Medical Association 233*, 280.

Sievers, D. and Donovan, A. J. (1973). Palliative treatment of mammary cancer. *Archives of Surgery 107*, 43.

Silberstein, E. B., Saenger, E. L., Tofe, A. J. and Park, H. M. (1973). Imaging of bone metastases with Sn-EHDP-^{99m}Te(Diphosphonate), ^{18}F and skeletal radiography: comparison of sensitivity. *Radiology 107*, 551.

Stoll, B. A. (1950). Hormone therapy in relation to radiotherapy in the treatment of advanced carcinoma of the breast. *Proc. Roy. Soc. Med. 43*, 875.

Treves, N. and Finkbeiner, J. A. (1958). An evaluation of therapeutic surgical castration in the treatment of metastatic, recurrent and primary inoperable mammary carcinoma in women. *Cancer 11*, 421.

Wilson, R. E., Piro, A. J., Aliapoulious, M. A. and Moore, F. D. (1971). Treatment of metastatic breast cancer with a combination of adrenalectomy and 5-fluorouracil. *Cancer 28*, 962.

Chapter

10

FLORENCE C. H. CHU

Radiotherapy for Symptomatic Relief

A majority of patients with breast cancer will eventually require treatment for advanced or disseminated disease. These patients are usually managed by hormonal manipulation or chemotherapy, with simultaneous or sequential use of irradiation to relieve localized symptoms. Palliative radiation treatment not only improves patients' quality of survival, but in certain instances, treatment of metastatic lesions involving a vital organ may actually prolong the patient's life. For these reasons radiotherapy should be utilized fully in the management of advanced cancer.

A few general rules are to be observed in the palliative treatment of cancer:

- The purpose of palliation is to make the patient's remaining life more comfortable and more tolerable. Palliative therapy should not be too aggressive, resulting in complications whose symptoms may be even worse than those from the cancer itself.
- Good palliative therapy aims to deliver an effective radiation dose within the shortest possible time. Prolonged treatment in patients with a relatively short life span is not justified.
- Even though treatment is palliative, patients still deserve the best possible technique. Every effort should be made to give the maximum dose to the tumor-bearing volume and to spare the surrounding normal tissues. Megavoltage photon beam or high energy electron beam sources should be utilized whenever feasible. Careful treatment planning and accurate beam direction is essential.
- For patients with widespread disease, ablative or additive hormonal treatment or chemotherapy can be instituted, without precluding the use of irradiation to one or more sites.

Since breast cancer may metastasize to any part of the body, radiation treatment of various sites of metastases will be discussed separately.

SKIN METASTASES

Local skin recurrence after initial mastectomy is a very common problem in the management of patients with breast carcinoma. Skin recurrence may be of the nodular or the "inflammatory" forms. Nodular recur-

rence may be solitary or multiple, occurring most frequently in the skin and subcutaneous tissues in or near the mastectomy scar. Small nodules are usually asymptomatic, but the larger ones cause pain, itching and ulceration. In the most advanced cases, confluent nodules may encircle the chest to form "cancer en cuirasse".

The "inflammatory" type of recurrence is relatively uncommon. The lesions appear as a diffuse reddening of the skin, associated with slight induration and an increase in the local temperature. Diagnosis must be confirmed by skin biopsy which shows cancer cell invasion of the skin lymphatics. Patients with this form of skin lesions have a grave prognosis and usually die of widespread metastases within a short period of time.

The radiotherapeutic management of skin recurrence depends on the extent of the disease. If there is no clinical evidence of distant metastases and the local recurrence is of limited extent, one may aim for permanent eradication or long term control. If the disease is locally extensive or if distant metastases are present, only palliative therapy can be offered.

When planning the treatment of recurrent skin disease, one should take into consideration not only the delivery of an adequate radiation dose to the tumor bearing volume, but also how to minimize the dose to the underlying normal tissues, particularly the lung. Electron beam therapy is advocated for chest wall irradiation because of the unique physical characteristics of electrons which permit excellent dose distribution with relatively simple methods (Chu et al., 1967; Chu, 1968).

The chief advantages of high energy electron beam include: controllable depth of penetration of radiation by varying the energy of electrons; abrupt termination of radiation at a specific depth; minimal differential energy absorption in bone; and easy beam shaping with the use of tissue equivalent compensators. Electron beams can be applied directly to the chest to deliver a homogeneous dose to the skin and subcutaneous tissue without unnecessary irradiation to the underlying lung. On the other hand, when megavoltage X-ray or telecobalt therapy is used for chest wall treatment, tangential field arrangements are required because these beams are highly penetrating.

For patients with limited local recurrence without evidence of distant metastases, intensive treatment is indicated. The radiation field should cover the site of recurrence with a wide margin in order to include other occult lesions which may exist in the neighboring skin. In most cases the whole anterior chest wall on the affected side is treated, even though the recurrent nodule may appear solitary. The radiation dose recommended is about 5,000 rads tumor dose in 5 weeks. A supplementary local dose of 500 to 1,000 rads in 1 week may be given to bulky lesions if necessary for residual disease.

The results of radiotherapy of 215 patients with recurrent disease limited to the chest wall and/or regional lymph nodes were evaluated by Chu et al. (1976). Complete control of the local disease was achieved in 67% of cases for a mean duration of 32 months and a median duration of 22 months. Another 24% showed partial control for mean and median durations of 11 months and 8 months respectively. The total response rate therefore was 91%. The survival data showed that 44 patients (21%) survived 5 years, and 10 (5%) survived 10 years following radiotherapy of recurrent disease. There were seven patients, or 3%, who were free of cancer at 5 to 15 years. Intensive radiotherapy, therefore, was worthwhile in patients with a limited extent of local disease.

Most patients with skin recurrence however, have extensive local involvement or evidence of generalized dissemination and only palliative therapy can be offered to these cases. The radiation dose most frequently used is about 3,500-4,000 rads delivered in a period of 3-4 weeks. Effective control of the symptomatic lesions can be achieved in the majority of patients treated (Chu et al., 1957; Chu et al., 1967).

In the 1967 study, Chu et al. evaluated the local response of inoperable, recurrent and metastatic breast lesions to electron beam therapy. There were 630 cases of chest wall recurrences treated and most of these had advanced disease. Many represented difficult clinical problems such as recurrence in previously irradiated areas, failure after ablative or additive hormonal treatment, chemotherapeutic failures and combinations of these. Evaluation of response showed complete contro of local disease in 464 cases, or 74%, for a mean duration of 13 months. Partial control was achieved in 64 cases, or 10%, for a mean duration of 5 months. The total response rate

Table 1 Local control of chest wall recurrences by electron beam therapy (Chu et al., 1967)

	Number of areas treated	*(%)*	*Mean duration (months)*
Complete control	464	74 } 84	13
Partial control	64	10 }	5
Failure	102	16	
Total	630	100	

was 84% (Table 1) and included the disappearance of painful lesions and healing of ulcers after irradiation.

LYMPH NODE METASTASES

The most frequent sites of lymph node metastases from breast cancer are the axilla and the supraclavicular regions. These lymph nodes if untreated tend to grow, become fixed, and ulcerate. They may produce the brachial plexus syndrome, either by pressure or by direct tumor invasion.

Internal mammary lymph node metastasis usually manifests as a parasternal nodule, growing through the intercostal space. Most patients who develop internal mammary nodal recurrence are those with an inner quadrant or central primary tumor, who did not have internal mammary lymph node dissection or postoperative therapy directed to this chain. The nodule is usually asymptomatic at the beginning, but, when a large size is reached, there may be pain and ulceration. In late cases, there may be destruction of the sternum and involvement of the mediastinal and other intrathoracic structures.

Supraclavicular and axillary lymph nodes are treated either by megavoltage photon or high energy electron beams, with equally good tumor control, dose for dose. Small parasternal masses from internal mammary lymph node involvement are best treated with electron beams. Large parasternal masses, particularly those associated with mediastinal involvement, may require megavoltage photon therapy. They show excellent response to radiotherapy.

If a patient with regional lymph node recurrence has no evidence of distant metastases an attempt should be made to eradicate the disease. A tumor dose of 5,000 rads in 5 weeks should be delivered. If a residual mass persists, a supplementary dose of about 500 to 1,000 rads in 1 week may be given through a reduced field. As in the treatment of limited skin recurrence, these patients may live without evidence of disease for a long period of time (Chu et al., 1976). Most patients, however, already have distant dissemination and the treatment is for palliation. The dose given is about 3,500-4,000 rads, delivered in a period of 3-4 weeks.

Table 2 Local control of lymph node metastases by electron beam therapy (Chu et al., 1967)

	Number of areas treated	*(%)*	*Mean duration (months)*
Complete control	212	71 } 79	16
Partial control	24	9 }	9
Failure	61	21	—
Total	297	100	

In an evaluation of 297 lymph node areas treated by radiation therapy (Chu, 1967), 71% were shown to be completely controlled for a mean duration of 16 months and 8% were partially controlled for a mean duration of 9 months. The total response rate was 79% (Table 2).

BONE METASTASES

The majority of patients with widespread metastatic breast carcinoma often have painful and disabling bone lesions. Although disseminated osseous metastases must be treated by systemic therapy, irradiation to localized symptomatic areas offers the highest expectation of pain relief and of recalcification of bone destruction. Radiotherapy is also indicated in the treatment of osteolytic lesions in a weight bearing bone, to prevent pathological fracture.

Our current dose schedule for bone metastases is to deliver a tumor dose of 400 rads daily for five treatments, or a total dose of 2,000 rads in 5 to 7 days, utilizing megavoltage X-ray or cobalt therapy. In order to avoid untoward local or systemic reactions in the treatment of large volumes such as the whole pelvis, or in the case of deeply seated bones such as the lumbar spine, a more protracted course of therapy, 2,400 rads in 2 weeks is given. These regimes offer prompt pain relief in 80%-90% of patients. This is followed in a few weeks by signs of recalcification in the areas of bone destruction.

LUNG METASTASES

Pulmonary metastases are seldom treated by radiotherapy because effective dose of irradiation, particularly to a large lung volume, may produce symptomatic pneumonitis followed later by fibrosis. Occasionally, patients with severe respiratory symptoms due to relatively localized pulmonary lesions may warrant palliative radiotherapy. The most important indications for treating such patients include hemoptysis and the symptoms and signs of bronchial obstruction. Less important indications include a rapidly growing tumor, persistent cough, chest pain and dyspnea. Doses in the range of 3,000-3,500 rads in 3 to 4 weeks may be given to relatively small areas and in most instances produce satisfactory palliation.

Bronchial obstruction with Atelectasis

Metastatic lesions may occur in the bronchus causing obstruction of the lumen and atelectasis of the lung. The clinical picture resembles bronchogenic carcinoma. Bronchoscopy and biopsy are required to rule out primary bronchogenic carcinoma and to establish the diagnosis of metastatic breast cancer. These lesions should be treated with relatively small fields accurately aimed at the involved bronchus. A tumor dose of 3,000 rads delivered over a period of 2 weeks usually relieves the obstruction, resulting in reaeration of the lung.

PLEURAL EFFUSION

Malignant pleural effusion proved by cytology, is best treated with thoracentesis, followed by instillation of colloidal ^{32}P or an appropriate chemotherapeutic agent (see Chapter 17). In our experience, external irradiation to the hemithorax appears to be helpful in treating patients with bloody pleural effusion, uncontrolled by ^{32}P or chemotherapy. A tumor dose of 2,000 to 2,500 rads in 2 to 3 weeks to the hemithorax usually stops the bleeding and slows down reaccumulation of fluid.

MEDIASTINAL METASTASES

Metastases to the mediastinal lymph nodes may cause chest pain, cough, shortness of breath, compression of the esophagus or superior vena caval syndrome. Metastatic lesions may also occur intrinsically in the walls of the esophagus, obstructing the lumen. Doses in the range of 3,500-4,000 rads in 3-4 weeks are effective in achieving good palliative results.

Superior vena caval obstruction constitutes one of the genuine emergency situations for prompt radiotherapy. Prolonged obstruction may result in organized thrombosis, which cannot be reversed by radiotherapy or anticoagulants. The diagnosis of superior vena caval syndrome is usually made by the clinical manifestation of venous engorgement in the neck and upper chest, shortness of breath, puffiness of the face, and the demonstration of filling defects by the use of an upper extremity venogram. Our current radiotherapy regimen is to give 400 rads tumor dose daily for 3 days, followed by 200 rads daily dose for a total dose of about 3,600 rads in 3 weeks. The initial high doses of radiotherapy are given to achieve rapid shrinkage of the tumor and rapid decompression of the obstruction.

CARDIAC AND PERICARDIAL METASTASES

A difficult problem is metastatic involvement of the heart and its pericardium, producing distressing symptoms and threatening life. The correct diagnosis is frequently missed and as a result, the patients are often not given proper treatment.

Actually, cardiac metastasis is not uncommon in patients with advanced cancer. DeLoach et al. (1953) found cardiac involvement in 14% of all cancer cases at autopsy while Bisel et al. (1953) reported a frequency of 21%. Carcinoma of the lung, carcinoma of the breast and malignant melanoma are the most frequent tumors involving the heart and, in the series by Bisel et al. (1953), cardiac metastases were found in 33% of patients who died of breast cancer. The most commonly involved area is the pericardium, although metastatic tumors to the heart may involve any part of that organ, including the endocardium and myocardium.

The clinical diagnosis of cardiac metastases may be difficult due to the lack of characteristic symptoms and signs. However, when a cancer patient with no previous history of heart disease suddenly develops arrhythmia, congestive heart failure or pericarditis, not responding to the usual conservative treatment, cardiac metastases should be strongly suspected. Diagnostic procedures such as an electrocardiogram, echogram, angiocardiogram and pericardiocentesis should be utilized to establish the diagnosis.

A review of our experience in the treatment of 38 patients with cardiac and pericardial metastases from various primary cancers with radiotherapy has been reported (Cham et al., 1975). It was found that approximately 60% of patients responded to radiotherapy and 11 of 16 breast carcinoma patients showed improvement of symptoms and signs for periods ranging from 2 to 36 months. The mean duration of remission was 6 months and the median was 4 months. Radiotherapy of the heart may not only relieve the distressing symptoms, it may also avert a life threatening situation.

For the treatment of malignant pericardial effusion, external beam therapy may be combined with intracavitary instillation of ^{32}P. Martini et al. (1976) described a method of intrapericardial catheterization and instillation of ^{32}P which provides prompt relief of symptoms of malignant pericardial effusion.

BRAIN METASTASES

Brain metastasis is associated with devastating physical, emotional and nursing problems and radio-

therapy is invaluable in its treatment. Relief of symptoms of neurological dysfunction by irradiation is most gratifying to the physician, the patient and the family. Some patients may even resume work and have a useful life for several months, or even years.

The most frequent symptoms and signs of intracranial metastases are headache, motor weakness and mental changes, and when brain involvement is suspected a neurological consultation should be obtained immediately. The diagnostic approach used at Memorial Hospital has been described by Posner (1974) and is based firstly on history and physical examination, secondly on electroencephalogram and brain scan, and finally, on contrast studies such as arteriogram or pneumoencephalogram. More recently the computerized transaxial tomogram (CTT) is being explored to see if small lesions in the brain may be detected by this method. In most cases electroencephalogram and brain scan are adequate in demonstrating lesions in the brain.

Since cerebral metastases are usually multiple, the radiotherapy field should cover the entire brain. Over the years the time dose schedule for brain irradiation has undergone a series of changes. In the 1950's when orthovoltage X-rays were used, treatment was started cautiously with small daily doses in the order of 50 rads and these were gradually increased to 300 rads per day. The planned dose was in the range of 3,000 rads delivered in a period of 3 weeks (Chao et al., 1954; Chu et al., 1961; Nisce et al., 1971).

With the availability of megavoltage therapy and corticosteroids it became possible to deliver a higher dose within a shorter period of time and Hindo et al. (1971) even advocate 1,000 rads in a single treatment. However, in our experience (Young et al., 1974) a rapid course of radiotherapy (1,500 rads in 2 treatments over a period of 3 days) appeared to produce shorter remission duration and higher complication rates than a slow course of therapy. Our current dose schedule is therefore 3,000 rads, delivered in 10 fractions, over a period of 2 weeks. All patients receive corticosteroids, which are capable of decreasing cerebral symptoms and signs, as well as minimizing radiation side effects.

The results of radiotherapy of brain metastases reported in the literature (Chao et al., 1954; Chu et al., 1961; Deeley et al., 1968; Order et al., 1968; Horton et al., 1971; Young et al., 1974) have shown that approximately 60% of cases treated improved for a mean duration of several months. Patients with breast carcinoma did somewhat better than those with bronchogenic carcinoma, melanoma or other types of cancer. It is generally agreed that not only is radiotherapy effective in prolonging life, but the quality of survival is improved as well.

SPINAL CORD COMPRESSION

Compression of the spinal cord caused by extradural metastatic cancer is not uncommon in patients with breast cancer and it is of paramount importance that this condition is recognized early and treatment is instituted promptly. Extradural tumor masses which cause spinal cord compression usually occur in the presence of vertebral metastases. Spinal cord compression should be suspected in patients with breast cancer who have progressive back pain associated with appropriate neurological symptoms. A myelogram is essential to define the exact level of compression and to identify other occult extradural lesions.

Spinal cord compression is an emergency situation and in most Centers, spinal deroofing with no attempt at resection is regarded as the first step necessary to avoid the development of paraplegia (see Chapter 11). Subsequent radiation therapy is usually combined with corticosteroids. The regimen currently in use at Memorial Hospital is to give initial high doses, i.e. 400 rads for the first three doses, followed by daily doses of 200 rads to a total dose of about 3,000 to 3,500 rads. The high initial dose treatment is used to accomplish quick radiation decompression by shrinkage of the tumor mass (Rubin, 1969; Rubin et al., 1969).

The results of treatment depends on many factors, one of which is the duration of symptoms prior to therapy. The patients with paraplegia for many days will do less well than the patients with minimal neurological deficits and whose symptoms are treated almost immediately after appearance. In most reports (Mones et al., 1966; Bansal et al., 1967; Kahn et al., 1967; Millburn et al., 1968; Rubin et al., 1969; Raichle and Posner, 1971; Posner, 1971) between 40% and 50% of patients with varying degrees of spinal compression become ambulatory after a course of radiotherapy. Decompression laminectomy is the treatment indicated in patients who suddenly develop spinal cord compression, or whose neurological deficits continue to worsen while receiving radiotherapy.

CHOROID METASTASIS

Breast carcinoma is the most frequent cancer involving the eye, particularly the choroid. There is simultaneous or sequential bilateral involvement in about 25% of cases. The principal symptom is blurred vision, but other less common symptoms include scotoma, pain and photophobia. Most lesions are situated on the temporal side of the choroid and produce elevation, wrinkling or mottling of the

retina. In more advanced cases there is detachment of the retina.

The clinician should suspect choroid metastasis when a patient with a history of breast carcinoma suddenly complains of blurred vision. Ophthalmologic consultation should be obtained immediately and if a diagnosis of choroid metastasis is confirmed, radiotherapy should be instituted without delay. It can produce dramatic and gratifying results.

Orenstein et al. (1972) reviewed the literature and also reported their own seven cases of choroid metastases treated by megavoltage X-ray therapy through a small lateral field. A high response rate with complete or partial restoration of vision was observed in the majority of patients treated. Thatcher et al. (1975) reviewed 42 cases of choroid metastases and reported similar results for radiotherapy.

At the Memorial Hospital, Chu (1976) has analyzed the results of radiotherapy in 44 cases of choroidal metastases. Most were treated with high energy electron beam irradiation and in this series, 89% of choroidal metastases were from breast carcinoma. The dose given was usually 3,000 to 4,000 rads in 3 to 4 weeks. There was a response rate of 64% for a median duration of 6 months and those patients who failed to respond to radiation therapy had either an inadequate dose of radiation (less than 2,500 rads in 2 to 3 weeks) or advanced lesions with massive detachment of the retina. Those patients who received 3,500 to 4,000 rads in 3 to 4 weeks showed a higher rate of response than those who received lower doses.

ORBITAL METASTASES

Metastases to the extraocular orbit may be similarly palliated. For example, retrobulbar metastases may cause proptosis, decrease in visual acuity, diplopia, pain and sometimes bone destruction. A dose of 3,000 to 4,000 rads in 3 to 4 weeks to the retrobulbar region may reduce the symptoms and signs.

Recently Huh et al. (1974) reported a series of 70 cases of extraocular orbital metastases treated by irradiation at Memorial Hospital. Carcinoma of the breast and lymphoma were the most common types. Radiotherapy was effective in producing worthwhile palliation and of the 79 lesions treated, 39% showed marked improvement for an average duration of 17 months. In addition, 33% showed slight improvement for a duration of 7 months, and only 28% failed to respond.

ABDOMEN AND PELVIS

Localized symptomatic tumor mass or masses in the abdomen or pelvis may be palliated by radiotherapy. Shrinkage of the tumor by irradiation not only relieves the pain, but also may prevent or reverse an impending intestinal obstruction.

Diffuse abdominal carcinomatosis with ascites is sometimes treated by a combination of total abdominal external irradiation plus the instillation of colloidal ^{32}P. Such treatment is, however, poorly tolerated by patients and not more than 3,000 rads can usually be delivered over a period of approximately 4 weeks. Proper shielding of the kidneys, so that they do not receive in excess of 2,000 rads, is imperative in order to minimize the risk of subsequent radiation nephritis.

LIVER METASTASES

The liver is another organ which does not tolerate irradiation well. The threshold dose for radiation hepatitis is about 3,000 rads in 3 weeks, and liver metastases are usually managed by hormonal or chemotherapeutic agents. Radiotherapy is seldom used except for relief of severe pain, and then the dose should be about 2,500 rads delivered in 3 weeks.

Patients with obstructive jaundice secondary to enlarged lymph nodes at the porta hepatis, can be effectively treated by external radiation to a tumor dose of 3,500 rads in 3 to 4 weeks, with disappearance of jaundice and relief of symptoms.

URETERAL METASTASES WITH HYDRONEPHROSIS

Ureteral metastasis is an uncommon manifestation of breast cancer involvement. The lesions occur in the periureteral tissue, causing encasement and constriction of the ureter and hydronephrosis. Patients with this complication usually show urinary symptoms and signs of frequency, polyuria, oliguria, or anuria with elevation of BUN. The characteristic radiographic findings have been described by Grabstald and Sherman (1969) and consist of fusiform narrowings of the ureter with marginal waviness or beading.

Grabstald and Kaufman (1969) reported a series of 24 cases of metastatic breast cancer causing ureteral obstruction seen at the Memorial Hospital. They discussed the clinical syndrome and methods of management. Treatment was essentially individualized and included systemic antitumor therapy, radio-

therapy, nephrostomy, ureteral catheters and dialysis. The authors emphasized that recognition of the hydronephrosis and institution of appropriate therapy have relieved the symptoms and prolonged the lives of several patients. Two patients survived for 31 and 37 months and seven of 24 patients survived for more than 1 year by virtue of recognition and management of hydronephrosis. Radiotherapy was the primary treatment in five patients and of these one survived 17 months.

Radiotherapy should be utilized more often in the treatment of ureteral metastases because of its effectiveness in relieving obstruction. The technique consists of parallel opposing fields irradiating the segment of the ureteral narrowing. There is a high frequency of bilateral involvement and in such cases both ureters are treated. Sometimes ureteral metastases are also associated with bulky disease in the pelvis. Both ureters and the pelvis can be irradiated through U-shaped portals. A tumor dose of about 3,500 rads, delivered in a period of 3-4 weeks, will usually relieve the obstruction and avoid the necessity of surgical intervention, such as nephrostomy.

SUMMARY

Metastatic breast cancer may involve any part of the body and the severity of symptoms produced by these secondary deposits depends on the location and size of the lesions. The treatment of disseminated breast cancer requires a multidisciplinary approach utilizing ablative or additive hormonal manipulation, chemotherapy and irradiation.

The technique of radiotherapy and its results at various sites of metastasis have been discussed. Irradiation is highly effective in palliation if the proper dosages and techniques are skilfully employed. Not only are distressing symptoms relieved in the great majority of patients treated, but also life may be prolonged in situations involving vital organs.

REFERENCES

Bansal, S., Brady, L. W., Olsen, A., Faust, D. S., Osterholm, J. and Kazem, I. (1967). The treatment of metastatic spinal cord tumors. *Journal of the American Medical Association 202,* 686.

Bisel, H. F., Wroblewski, F. and LaDue, J. S. (1953). Incidence and clinical manifestations of cardiac metastases. *JAMA 153,* 712.

Cham, W. C., Freiman, A. H., Carsteins, P. H. B. and Chu, F. C. H. (1975). Radiation therapy of cardiac and pericardial metastases. *Radiology 114,* 701.

Chao, J. H., Phillips, R. and Nickson, J. J. (1954). Roentgen-ray therapy of cerebral metastases. *Cancer 7,* 682.

Chu, F. C. H. (1968). The role of electron beam therapy in the treatment of breast cancer. *Frontiers of Radiation Therapy Oncology 2,* 224. New York: Karger, Basel.

Chu, F. C. H. (1975). Radiation therapy of recurrent breast cancer. In *Strahlentherapie der Mammakarzinome.* Switzerland: Springer-Verlag.

Chu, F. C. H. (1976). Radiation therapy of choroid metastases of the eye. In preparation.

Chu, F. C. H. and Hilaris, B. S. (1961). Value of radiation therapy in the management of intracranial metastases. *Cancer 14,* 577.

Chu, F. C. H., Lin, F. J., Kim, J. H., Huh, S. H. and Garmatis, C. J. (1976). Locally recurrent carcinoma of the breast—Results of radiation therapy. *Cancer, in press.*

Chu, F. C. H., Nisce, L. Z., Baker, A. S., Sattar, A. and Laughlin, J. S. (1967). Electron-beam therapy of cancer of the breast. *Radiology 89,* 216.

Chu, F. C. H., Sved, D. W., Escher, G. C., Nickson, J. J. and Phillips, R. F. (1957). Management of advanced breast carcinoma with special reference to combined radiation and hormone therapy. *American Journal of Roentgenology 77,* 438.

Deeley, T. J. and Edwards, J. M. R. (1968). Radiotherapy in the management of cerebral secondaries from bronchogenic carcinoma. *Lancet 1,* 1209.

DeLoach, J. F. and Haynes, J. W. (1953). Secondary tumors of the heart and pericardium. *A.M.A. Arch. Internal Medicine 91,* 224.

Grabstald, H. and Sherman, R. S. (1969). Radiographic diagnosis of ureteral involvement by metastatic breast cancer. *Radiology 92,* 1184.

Grabstald, H. and Kaufman, R. (1969). Hydronephrosis secondary to ureteral obstruction by metastatic breast cancer. *Journal of Urology 102,* 576.

Hindo, W. A., DeTrana, F. A. III, Lee, M. S. and Hendrickson, F. R. (1970). Large dose increment irradiation in treatment of cerebral metastases. *Cancer 26,* 138.

Horton, J., Baxter, D. H. and Olson, K. B. (1971). The management of metastases to the brain by irradiation and corticosteroids. *American Journal of Roentgenology 3,* 334.

Huh, S. H., Nisce, L. Z., Simpson, L. D. and Chu, F. C. H. (1974). The value of radiation therapy in the treatment of orbital metastasis. *American Journal of Roentgenology 120,* 589.

Kahn, F. R., Glicksman, A. S., Chu, F. C. H. and Nickson, J. J. (1967). Treatment by radiotherapy of spinal cord compression due to extradural metastases. *Radiology 89,* 495.

Martini, N., Freiman, A. H., Watson, R. C. and Hilaris, B. S. (1976). Malignant pericardial effusion. *American Journal of Roentgenology* (submitted for publication).

Millburn, L., Hibbs, G. G. and Hendrickson, F. R. (1968). Treatment of spinal cord compression from metastatic carcinoma—Review of the literature and presentation of a new method of treatment. *Cancer 21,* 447.

Mones, R. T., Dozier, D. and Berrett, A. (1966). Analysis of medical treatment of malignant extradural spinal cord tumors. *Cancer 19,* 1842.

Nisce, L. Z., Hilaris, B. S. and Chu, F. C. H. (1971). A review of experience with irradiation of brain metastases *American Journal of Roentgenology 111,* 329.

Order, S. E., Hellman, S., Von Essen, C. F. and Kligerman, M. M. (1968). Improvement in quality of survival following whole-brain irradiation for brain metastasis. *Radiology 91,* 149.

Orenstein, M. M., Anderson, D. P. and Stein, J. J. (1972). Choroid metastasis. *Cancer 29,* 1101.

Posner, J. B. (1971). Spinal cord compression: a neurological emergency. *Clinical Bulletin 1,* 65.

Posner, J. B. (1971). Diagnosis and treatment of metastases to the brain. *Clinical Bulletin 4,* 47.

Raichle, M. E. and Posner, J. B. (1971). Role of surgery in the treatment of spinal cord compression by metastatic neoplasm. *Cancer 27,* 558.

Rubin, P. (1969). Extradural spinal cord compression by tumor. Part I: experimental production and treatment trials. *Radiology 93,* 1243.

Rubin, P., Mayer, E. and Poulter, C. (1969). Extradural spinal compression by tumor. Part II: high daily dose experience without laminectomy. *Radiology 93,* 1248.

Thatcher, N. and Thomas, P. R. M. (1975). Choroidal metastases from breast carcinoma: a survey of 42 patients and the use of radiation therapy. *Clin. Radiol. 26,* 549.

Young, D. F., Posner, J. B., Chu, F. C. H. and Nisce, L. Z. (1974). Rapid-course radiation therapy of cerebral metastases: results and complications. *Cancer 34,* 1069.

Chapter

11

T. H. ACKLAND

Surgery for Symptomatic Relief

In this section it is intended to discuss the role of surgery in providing symptomatic relief in breast cancer, and discussion is under the following headings:

- Excision of localized tumour.
- Surgical relief of lymphoedema.
- Repair of post-radiation damage.
- Surgical methods of pain relief.
- Management of malignant paraplegia and bone deposits.

EXCISION OF LOCALIZED TUMOUR

Before a decision is made to treat advanced or recurrent breast cancer with either radiotherapy, hormonal manipulation or chemotherapy, consideration should be given to the possibility of surgical excision for the purpose of palliation. This applies chiefly to the local lesion or to nodal metastases, but occasionally a solitary visceral deposit may call for similar management. Several specific circumstances require mention.

(1) When there is local recurrence of tumour after inadequate surgery such as lump excision, radical dissection may offer a hope of cure and more than mere palliation, provided that the local recurrence is sufficiently restricted in area and without deep attachment.

(2) An apparently incurable carcinoma which is ulcerated or about to become so, is often best managed by a palliative simple mastectomy. Removing an offensive lesion of this type is particularly useful if it is a slowly growing tumour occurring in an elderly patient. After the simple mastectomy the patient may survive several years without metastases or local recurrence, before succumbing to another disease.

However, it must be stressed that excision must never be attempted if the growth is fixed deeply to the chest wall, or if there is surrounding "peau d'orange" or inflammatory carcinomatous infiltration. Under such circumstances, surgical interference may precipitate widespread ulcerated dissemination

over the chest wall, and this is perhaps the most distressing of all the many manifestations of breast cancer.

(3) Recurrence of carcinoma in the axilla is rarely seen after a carefully performed radical mastectomy of either the Halsted or Patey type, but is certainly common after simple mastectomy. If the metastatic nodes are mobile, a radical axillary dissection is the treatment of choice, and is more likely to offer some prospect of cure than is radiotherapy.

(4) After mastectomy, several nodules of recurrent disease may appear on the chest wall, grouped closely together, and if they lie within a circle of not more than 5 cm in diameter, they can be treated by means of a full thickness chest wall resection. This is especially indicated if the nodules are subcutaneous and suggest a localized implantation in or near the scar, rather than diffuse permeation recurrence at the periphery of the operated area.

The full thickness resection of skin, ribs and pleura should be a circular one and well clear of the nodules, after which closure of the chest wall is effected by a fascia lata graft, with skin flap rotation ensuring that the fascia lata is covered by normal skin and subcutaneous tissue. The area from which the skin flap has been advanced is then covered by a split skin graft. The writer has sometimes performed this operation with no more than a hope of palliation, yet after the passage of many years, no further local or distant metastases have developed.

(5) It is very rare for carcinoma of the breast to produce a solitary visceral metastasis in spite of occasions when clinical investigation suggests that no other deposits are present. An apparently single metastasis in lung, liver or brain is almost always associated with lesions elsewhere; there is therefore not the scope for resections such as partial hepatectomy which may well be the proper management for a metastasis for carcinoma of the colon.

Nevertheless, the writer recently removed an enormous and apparently solitary omental metastasis from a patient treated by mastectomy for carcinoma of the breast many years previously. This mass was on the point of producing a large bowel obstruction, and its removal was clearly desirable. Although it is very likely that further tumour will develop in the abdomen, the process may possibly be delayed by the cyclical combination chemotherapy now being given.

RELIEF OF LYMPHOEDEMA

Causation and prevention

A serious degree of arm lymphoedema is a complication of radical mastectomy in approximately 12% of patients. The major aetiological factor is known now to be impairment of lymph flow brought about by obstruction of the main lymphatic trunks in the axilla, and lymphangiography invariably reveals both tortuosity of lymph trunks and dermal backflow. Clearance rates of subcutaneously injected radioiodinated human serum albumin, measured before and after radical mastectomy, reveal a 40% flow reduction after the operation, with higher figures occurring in cases treated with post-operative radiotherapy (Britton and Nelson, 1962; Ju et al., 1954).

It is now known that a radical axillary gland dissection necessarily involves resection of the main lymphatic collecting channels which usually lie anterior and medial to the axillary vein; but if post-operative conditions are favourable, regeneration of lymph channels follows within 4 to 6 weeks. Careful lymphangiographic studies by Goffrini et al. (1962) and Bobbio et al. (1962) have shown that lymphoedema develops only if such regeneration is impaired and if collateral channels accompanying the cephalic vein fail to become established. The factors which are most often responsible for preventing this normal sequence are sloughing, wound infection with fluid collections, and radiotherapy.

Treatment

When arm swelling is only moderate in degree and the patient's chief complaint is an unsightly appearance, management should be conservative. This is fully discussed in Chapter 21. Operative treatment is indicated when gross oedema produces a heavy arm which is not only useless, but also a severe and continual burden. The first attempt to improve lymph flow from a swollen limb was made by Handley in 1909, when he introduced the operation of lymphangioplasty by inserting multiple silk threads, passed subcutaneously along the length of the limb to the chest wall, where the proximal ends were buried. Although unsuccessful, later variations on this method were attempted, including the use of strips of fascia (Lexer, 1919) and nylon threads (Zieman, 1951). But none of these methods was useful, the most common sequence being infection, followed by the extrusion of the implanted foreign material.

Kondoleon in 1912, introduced an operation which seemed more reasonable; he attempted to achieve anastomosis of superficial to deep lymphatic channels by excising long strips of deep fascia. Results were poor, probably because regeneration of deep fascia quickly occurs. Sistrunk (1927) added wide sleeve resection of subcutaneous fat to the

radical excision of deep fascia, but this too, met with very limited success.

The use of tubed pedicle skin flaps containing normal lymphatics, and passing from the upper arm to the chest wall to bypass the axilla, has been advocated (Mowlein, 1958; Smith and Conway, 1962). Although some reduction in tissue tension is achieved, the effect of gravity on lymph flow prevents a satisfactory result. The whole upper arm from axilla to elbow has been sutured to the trunk by Standard (1942), but although this does achieve significant lymph drainage, it is, of course, at the price of abolishing all shoulder movement.

The excisional operation of Charles (1912) had an entirely different objective, which was to eliminate completely all lymphoedematous tissues. McCormack (1954) has claimed some success for this procedure, excising all tissues of the forearm and dorsum of the hand, down to muscles, and covering with thick split skin grafts. However, most surgeons who have used this operation have found that joint stiffness, finger swelling, and skin graft changes lead to poor end-results.

More recently, Goldsmith et al. (1967) have used omental transposition, mobilizing omentum upon gastroepiploic vessels and passing it subcutaneously into the swollen arm as far as the elbow. Not surprisingly, viability problems with the graft have made this an unsatisfactory procedure.

The first operation to be both sound in concept and successful in practice was that described by Thompson (1967, 1969). The principle of this operation is to excise deep fascia and oedematous fat, and to bury into a deep muscular crevice, a long flap of dermis denuded of its epidermis and attached to skin along one edge. In this way a permanent communication is created capable of directing lymph flow into the deep compartment of the limb where it can drain proximally along deep muscle planes.

It leads to the establishment of anastomoses between superficial lymphatic vessels and either deep lymph trunks or muscle venules. Satisfactory clinical results have been reported by Larson et al. (1966) in the United States and by Fontaine and Fontaine in Germany (1969). Tests of lymphatic function, using subcutaneously injected radio-iodinated human serum albumin pre-operatively and one year post-operatively, demonstrate a doubling of proximal lymph flow after the operation.

It now seems possible that recent developments in micro-surgical techniques may lead to the above described operations being abandoned in favour of the creation of artificial lymphovenous anastomoses. Since it is known that lymphatico-venous communications occur both normally and pathologically, attempts have been made to create artificial lymphovenous anastomoses to drain the excess lymph in cases of lymphoedema. Chiefly for technical reasons the initial attempts involved the anastomosis of transected lymph nodes to veins (Firica et al., 1969; Politowski and Bortowski, 1969; Rivero et al., 1967), but these anastomoses were usually sealed by fibrous tissue after three months.

The micro-vascular work of Yamada (1969), and more recently that of O'Brien et al. (1976) have both been successful in achieving direct anastomosis of lymph *vessels* to veins in experimental animals. In this work, O'Brien has found a persisting patency rate of 66% using both re-exploration and lymphangiography to check the results. O'Brien and his co-workers have, as yet, only a limited clinical series (eight cases at the time of writing of this paper). Through small incisions at the elbow level and in the upper arm, up to eight anastomoses have been made. Significant early reduction in limb volume has been claimed, but long term evaluation is awaited. If a lymphoedematous arm is not improved by this technique, recourse may still be had to Thompson's operation.

Lymphangiosarcoma

Lymphangiosarcoma apparently arising from the endothelial lining cells of lymphatics is recognized as being a complication of post-mastectomy lymphoedema. It was first described by Stewart and Treves (1948) and subsequent reports by various authors have brought the total number of recorded cases to approximately 100. Although some pathologists such as Salm (1963) have suggested that these arm lesions are metastases from the original breast carcinoma, the generally accepted opinion is that they are a distinct tumour.

The duration of the oedema before the development of sarcoma has varied from 6 to 24 years in the cases recorded, with a mean of 9 years. Purplish red macules and nodules appear in the skin of the oedematous arm and unless one is aware of the condition, it may be confused with simple ecchymoses or recurrent carcinoma of the breast. Ulceration usually follows and widespread metastases soon develop.

Most cases have been treated in the past by interscapulo-thoracic amputation, but with few exceptions this have been unsuccessful in preventing a fatal outcome. Conservative management, perhaps associated with radiotherapy, is to be preferred as there is some evidence that the tumour is at least moderately radiosensitive (Rawson and Frank, 1953).

Hermann and Ariel (1967) have reported 5 year survival in a patient treated by intra-arterial injection of radioactive yttrium.

REPAIR OF POST-RADIATION DAMAGE

Post-irradiational brachial plexus damage

With increasing understanding of the limiting factors for megavoltage therapy (see Chapter 5) serious brachial plexus damage in radiotherapy will probably become rare in the future. Nevertheless, we still have no precise knowledge as to the maximum dose of irradiation which can be tolerated by the nerve trunks, and there is a need for experimental work on this subject. The writer has had the opportunity of seeing more than twenty of these cases, in all of which the history closely follows the following pattern.

For 1 or 2 years following surgery and post-operative radiation therapy nothing amiss is noted. There then occurs paraesthesia followed occasionally by severe pain radiating down the arm and fingers. In the most severe cases this is followed by paresis, which often begins in the thumb and index finger and tends to extend slowly, in some cases to the point of total abolition of all movements of the elbow, wrist and hand. In most cases, pain slowly subsides or even disappears, but paralysis remains together with varying degrees of loss of sensation.

The pathological basis of this condition has not yet been clarified. The most likely explanation is that there occurs a slowly developing endarteritis of small vessels supplying the brachial plexus; but it is possible that irradiation may cause direct but delayed neuronal damage. A further explanation which has been advanced is that the brachial plexus becomes constricted by advancing fibrosis of the axillary sheath. There may well be a combination of all these processes and it is uncertain whether any treatment apart from prophylaxis is possible. The writer has explored the brachial plexus above the clavicle in several of these cases, without finding any evidence of constricting fibrosis; not surprisingly, severe healing problems follow the making of an incision through heavily irradiated skin.

More recently, O'Brien (1975), believing that fibrosis around the plexus is in fact the cause, had used a long incision extending from the scalene muscles to the upper arm, with excision of the middle third of the clavicle, in order to "free" the whole length of the brachial plexus. Then, anticipating inevitable healing problems, this wound is not sutured, but closed by a free full-thickness skin graft employing vessel suture by microvascular techniques. Results of this operation are not yet available. The writer has on one occasion carried out fore-quarter amputation to rid a patient of the burden of a totally useless, heavy, oedematous and insensitive upper limb.

Radionecrotic ulceration or necrosis

Heavy doses of radiation to the cervico-axillary lymphatic chain may on rare occasions lead to the development of infraclavicular radionecrotic ulceration. With sequestrating first or second rib in its base, this ulcer not only shows no tendency to heal, but has the axillary artery and vein lying immediately subjacent to its lateral end. When arterial pulsations are visible in the ulcer's base, the danger of sudden and fatal secondary haemorrhage is great, and interscapulo-thoracic amputation should be carried out. The writer has carried out this operation for three such cases, in one after a secondary haemorrhage had actually occurred.

The technique of fore-quarter amputation for infraclavicular ulceration requires modification of the standard procedure. The anterior incision, instead of passing from the junction of the inner and medial thirds of the clavicle straight across the anterior axillary fold, must curve well medially, avoiding the ulcer by at least 5 cm, while the posterior incision may utilize a convexity of healthy deltoid skin, which fits conveniently into the anterior concavity.

Radionecrotic destruction of the head of the humerus, associated with severe pain and limitation of movement of the shoulder joint, has been seen in the past as a rare complication of radiotherapy. No treatment other than excision of the humeral head is effective. Pain is relieved although this is at the cost of a flail arm with poor shoulder control.

Osteosarcoma is a complication sometimes added to the humeral head necrosis and should be suspected before the radiological appearance becomes typical. If biopsy confirms the diagnosis, interscapulo-thoracic amputation is required, although, as in the case of osteosarcoma elsewhere, pulmonary metastases may later become evident.

SURGICAL METHODS OF PAIN RELIEF

When advanced breast cancer is associated with severe pain, the local treatment of choice should always be

radiotherapy, provided that the lesion or lesions under consideration are sufficiently localized to allow it. An advanced primary growth may show fungation, chest wall attachment or associated enlarged fixed axillary glands, but surprisingly, pain is rarely a severe problem. On the other hand, pain is a common accompaniment of osseous metastases. If lesions are too widely disseminated to permit the use of radiotherapy, some form of systemic therapy, such as the administration of exogenous hormones, ablative endocrine surgery, or chemotherapy will usually be employed, in addition to the administration of pain relieving, or tranquillizing, drugs. For these reasons it does not often happen that the pain of advanced breast cancer calls for a neurosurgical procedure aimed at the interruption of pain conducting pathways.

The most likely situation calling for neurosurgical pain relief is severe pain arising from tumour infiltration of the brachial plexus, when the patient has already had local irradiation to a cancericidal dose and it cannot therefore be repeated. Such circumstances are, however, rare in the writer's experience. Another possible indication for neurosurgical operative intervention is post-irradiational damage to the brachial plexus, especially if tumour recurrence in the brachial plexus is also suspected.

Patients with chronic pain arising from some non-cancerous cause, such as causalgia after a limb amputation, may have a normal life expectation and the problem of relieving their pain adequately is a difficult one. On the other hand, those with advanced breast cancer have a limited life expectation and in this group, satisfactory techniques should be able to provide complete abolition of pain until death.

The techniques available for the interruption of pain conducting fibres are chemical nerve blocking and posterior rhizotomy, cordotomy and tractotomy, thalamotomy and leucotomy.

Chemical nerve blocking and posterior rhizotomy

Chemical nerve blocking as the sole procedure is seldom indicated in advanced breast cancer. Nevertheless it should be regarded as an alternative to tractotomy or posterior rhizotomy under three circumstances:

- When a patient, with intractable pain localized to specific nerve roots or trunks, will not live longer than 2 months;
- when pain is both localized and bilateral;
- when pain is increasing with the likelihood that other segments will be involved in a short time.

Cole (1965) has used the method extensively, and for subarachnoid and epidural blocks, prefers to use 5% phenol and glycerin, having found this material to be associated with less risk than alcohol. With careful posturing, sclerosis of posterior roots only will be achieved, with muscle power little affected.

Since Abbe (1896) reported the first sensory rhizotomy for chronic pain, there have been varying reappraisals of the procedure. Strangely, although the efficacy of trigeminal or glossopharyangeal section is beyond question, posterior spinal root section carries a somewhat uncertain prognosis for pain relief. Since function will be severely affected, an extremity should be denervated only if it is already without function, as may be the case when the brachial plexus is infiltrated by a malignancy, and perhaps in addition damaged by radiotherapy. The patient should be in good enough condition to tolerate a laminectomy, should have a moderate life expectancy, and should have pain distribution involving a limited number of nerve roots.

Suitable patients should, of course, be those in whom analgesics or mild narcotics have become ineffective and it is generally accepted that at least three contiguous sensory nerve roots should be divided. Preliminary diagnostic xylocaine nerve root blocking is often carried out, but the wide experience of Onofrio and Campa (1972) at the Mayo Clinic leads them to conclude that diagnostic blocking is not a reliable predictor of the results to be expected from section of the same roots.

The neural mechanism of pain transmission is not fully understood, in spite of the standard anatomical teaching that pain fibres enter the spinal cord and ascend a few segments in the posterior columns before crossing the midline to form the antero-lateral tract. Thus, although after appropriate posterior root section for pain the corresponding area of the arm may be quite anaesthetic, pain may persist at least to some degree. The reason for this is unknown, and it has been suggested that pain may be transmitted by the anterior spinal roots. This is, however, very unlikely and attempts by White and Sweet (1955a) to relieve residual pain by additional motor root section has not succeeded. On the other hand, they report that residual pain can often be relieved by interrupting secondary neurones in the spinothalamic tract.

Recent reports still speak favourably of posterior rhizotomy. Barrach and Leavens (1973), reviewing a series of 70 multiple dorsal rhizotomies, performed at the M.D. Anderson Hospital for the relief of pain secondary to malignancy, report total relief in 40 cases and good relief in 18 patients. They consider that the operation is "safe" and effective.

Cordotomy and tractotomy

Open transection of the spinal pain pathway, the anterolateral column, was first carried out by Martin in 1912, on the basis of Spiller's observations in 1905. More recently, however, the open operation has been replaced in centres where the necessary facilities and experience are available, by percutaneous cordotomy as described by Mullam et al. (1963), or by the Rosomoff et al. (1965) modification of the procedure. A spinal needle is inserted intrathecally between C1 and C2 below the mastoid process under local anaesthesia, and after the dentate ligament has been visualized radiologically by the injection of radio-opaque material, an insulated electrode is introduced through the needle with its bare sharpened end penetrating the anterolateral tract to a depth of 2 mm. A 5 x 4 mm lesion is produced by a radiofrequency current of 1 to 3 W lasting 2 to 5 seconds in a number of applications, and in all for approximately 30 seconds. During and between the coagulations, motor power is tested and the analgesic level on the opposite side checked by pinprick.

The percutaneous approach offers two advantages over cordotomy; a general anaesthetic and recuperation from a major surgical procedure is avoided, and more important, the extent of the lesion produced may be carefully monitored. Lipton (1973) has reported an impressive series of 450 percutaneous cordotomies with a very small mortality and morbidity, and comments that "although the technique looks difficult, it is not so, as performed at the Walton Hospital, Liverpool".

However, in breast cancer, cordotomy is indicated less frequently than rhizotomy because surgical division of pain conducting fibres is most likely to be required for supraclavicular metastases with brachial plexus infiltration. Since pain fibres after entering the cord ascend for a varying number of segments before crossing the midline to form the anteroclateral tract, the highest possible contralateral cordotomy cannot be guaranteed to be successful in treating such a case. Indeed, for practical purposes it may be said that this operation should rarely be advised for the control of pain arising from a lesion above the level of nipple.

From a theoretical point of view, spinothalamic tractotomy in the medulla, pons or midbrain has anatomical advantages which should guarantee success in the relief of pain. However, these operations find little favour with neurosurgeons since the surgical approach to these regions is no easy task and is associated with an excessive mortality, quite apart from a high incidence of paraesthesias.

Thalamotomy and leucotomy

Concurrent with the development of stereotaxic procedures in the treatment of Parkinsonism, has been the endeavour to find suitable points in the thalamus for interrupting pathways for the perception of pain. Hécaen et al. (1949) provided one of the earliest reports; lesions made in the dorso-medial nuclei in six cases relieved pain to some extent, but only temporarily. Later reports by Riechert (1960) and Brodal (1969) reached the general conclusion that the results of thalamotomy are disappointing; some three-quarters of patients derive considerable immediate benefit, but pain soon returns in about one-half. It is very unlikely that pain arising from advanced breast cancer will be treated successfully by this method.

Similarly, bifrontal leucotomy has very little, if any, applicability to pain relief in breast cancer. Not only does this operation offer uncertain relief from pain, but more important, the price paid in sacrifice of personality qualities, and the severe mental deterioration that may follow, justify the procedure only in very special circumstances. Indeed, White and Sweet (1955b) state that leucotomy "should never be performed in any condition where there is at least an even chance of pain relief by rhizotomy or cordotomy". Although it could be maintained that in some conditions the conservatively leucotomized individual, with all his limitations, is preferable to the chronic morphine addict, this would rarely, if ever, apply to a patient with recurrent breast cancer, where life expectation is of necessity limited.

MANAGEMENT OF MALIGNANT PARAPLEGIA AND BONE DEPOSITS

When deposits of malignant tissue in vertebrae or in the vertebral canal begin to exert pressure on the spinal cord, a surgical emergency has arisen. This is so, even although the symptoms and signs of neurological deficit may be minimal. Only too often in the past, valuable time has been allowed to elapse until pressure has brought about irreversible paraplegia, partly by direct pressure on neuronal structures, and partly by causing ischaemia.

Although irreversible damage may not be brought about for hours or days, it may occur within minutes following a fracture. There is no place for the use of cytotoxic or hormonal systemic therapy or even irradiation as the initial measures under these circumstances. The patient should be admitted to hospital

immediately, myelography should be carried out and laminectomy should follow

The aim of operation should be a wide deroofing to relieve, as thoroughly as possible, the pressure from bone or tumour. No attempt should be made to remove the tumour completely, and this in any case is most unlikely to prove possible. If posteriorly situated tumour is evident, it may be removed gently from the dural surface. The theca should not be retracted, and if tumour is present only anteriorly, no attempt should be made either to remove it or even to biopsy a portion. Localized radiotherapy should follow as soon as possible, assisted perhaps by cytotoxic drugs or hormonal manipulation if indicated.

The management of metastatic deposits of breast carcinoma in bone calls for some comment. If metastases are widespread and pain is multifocal, treatment should be primarily systemic, employing either hormonal administration, surgical endocrine ablation or the use of cytotoxic agents. When, however, only one or two sites seem to be involved by metastases, it should be remembered that no form of therapy is as effective as radiotherapy, in its ability to control the pain of localized bone metastases. Even if metastases are very widespread, it may be very helpful to select one particular painful region (perhaps one side of the bony pelvis) for irradiation. There is approximately a 90% prospect of achieving pain relief, and associated with this there is likely to occur some degree of healing with sclerosis.

When an osteolytic deposit in a long bone is found, treatment by radiotherapy is urgent even if it appears that there is no immediate likelihood of pathological fracture. In the case of a non weight-bearing bone such as the humerus, preliminary internal fixation may not be necessary if a reasonable bridge of intact bone spans the metastasis, and in such cases, there is an excellent chance of healing with sclerosis following. If, however, a fracture has actually occurred or is impending, some suitable form of internal fixation must be achieved before irradiation is given. In the case of weight bearing sites such as the shaft or neck of the femur, this will be indicated more often, because of the greater risk of fracture occurring (see Chapter 15).

It was once believed that secondary radiation from the presence of a metal nail or plate might contribute to tumour destruction, but it is now recognized that the effect of this secondary radiation is to cause damage to Haversian systems and localized bone necrosis. For this reason megavoltage therapy should always be employed in these cases, this quality of beam being associated with a minimal risk of this danger.

REFERENCES

Abbe, R. (1896). Intra-dural section of the spinal nerves for neuralgia. *Boston Med. Surg. J. 135*, 329.

Barrach, J. M. and Leavens, M. E. (1973). Dorsal rhizotomy for the relief of intractable pain of malignant tumour origin. *J. Neurosurg. 38*, 755.

Bobbio, P., Perracchia, G. and Pellegrino, F. (1962). La Circolazione linfatica nell'edema del bracchio secondario ad intervento di mastectomia radicale. *L'Ateneo Parmense. 33*, (Suppl 3), 110.

Britton, R. C. and Nelson, P. A. (1962). Causes and treatment of postmastectomy lymphedema of the arm: report of 114 cases. *J.A.M.A. 180*, 95.

Brodal, A. (1969). *Neurological Anatomy in Relation to Clinical Medicine* (2nd Ed.). London: Oxford University Press.

Charles, R. H. (1912). Elephantiasis scroti. In *A System of Treatment* (A. Latham and T.C. English) (Vol. 3). London: Churchill, 1912.

Cole, R. (1965). The problem of pain in persistent cancer. *Med. J. Aust. 1*, 682.

Firica, A., Ray, A. and Murat, J. (1969). Les anastomoses lympho-veineuses, étude experimentale. *Lyon Chirurgical 65*, 384.

Fontaine, R. and Fontaine, J. L. (1969). Die operative therapie des lymphedema. *Arch. Chir. 325*, 89.

Goffrini, P., Bobbio, P., Perracchia, G. and Pellegrino, F. (1962). Modalita di repristino della circolazione linfatica dell'arto superiore e dell'ascella dopo l'intervento di mastectomia radicale. *L'Ateneo Parmense 33*, (Suppl. 3), 60.

Goldsmith, H. S., Santos, R. de los and Beattie, E. J. (1967). Relief of chronic lymphedema by omental transposition. *Ann. Surg. 166*, 573.

Handley, W. S. (1909). A prospective cure for elephantiasis. *Lancet 1*, 31.

Hécaen, H., Talairach, J., David, M. and Dell, M. B. (1949). *Rev. Neurol. 81*, 917.

Herrmann, J. B. and Ariel, I. M. (1967). Therapy of lymphangiosarcoma of the chronically oedematous limb. *Am. J. Roentgenol. 99*, 393.

Hogeman, K. E. (1955). Artificial subcutaneous channels in draining lymphoedema. *Acta Chir. Scand. 110*, 154.

Ju, D. M. C., Blakemore, A. and Stevenson, T. W. (1954). A lymphatic function test: Clin. Congress Am. Coll. of Surgeons, *Surgical Forum*, 607.

Kondoleon, F. (1912). Die operative Behandlung der Elephantiastischen Oedema *Munch. Med. Wschr. 59*, 1823.

Larson, D. L., Coers, C. R., Doyle, J. E., Rapperport, A. S., Kloehn, R. and Lewis, S. R. (1966). Lymphedema of the lower extremity. *Plast. Reconstr. Surg. 38*, 293.

Lexer, E. (1919). Vereins und Kongressgerichte Naturwissenschafte medizinische Gesellschaft Zu Jena. *Munchen Med. Wschr. 66,* 1274.

Lipton, S. (1973). Pain control and the management of advanced malignant disease. *Proc. Roy. Soc. Med. 66,* 607.

Mowlein, R. (1958). Lymphatic oedema: an evaluation of surgery in its treatment. *Amer. J. Surg. 95,* 216.

Mullam, S., Harper, P. V. and Hekmatpanah, J. et al. (1963). Percutaneous interruption of spinal pain tracts by means of a strontium-90 needle. *J. Neurosurg. 20,* 931.

McCormack, R. M. (1954). The surgical treatment of postmastectomy lymphedema. *Plast. Reconstr. Surg. 14,* 62.

O'Brien, B. M., Gilbert, A., Vorrath, J. M., Sykes, P. J. and Baxter, T. J. (1976). *Lymphatico-Venous Anastomosis by Microvascular Technique.* Not yet published.

O'Brien, B. M. (1975). Personal communication.

Onofrio, B. M. and Campa, H. K. (1972). Evaluation of rhizotomy: review of 12 years experience. *J. Neurosurg. 36,* 751.

Politowski, M. and Bortowski, S. (1969). Treatment of lymphoedema of the limbs by lymphatico-venous fistula. *Surgery 66 (4),* 639.

Rawson, A. J. and Frank, J. L. (1953). Treatment by irradiation of lymphangiosarcoma in post-mastectomy lymphedema. *Cancer 6,* 269.

Riechert, T. (1960). Die chirurgische behandlung der zentralen schmerzzustände. *Acta Neurochirurg. 8,* 136.

Rivero, O. R., Calnan, J. S., Reis, N. D. and Mercurius Taylor, L. (1967). Experimental peripheral lymphovenous communications. *Brit. Jnl. Plast. Surg. 20,* 124.

Rosomoff, H. L., Brown, C. J. and Sheptak, P. (1965). Percutaneous radio-frequency cervical cordotomy technique. *J. Neurosurg. 23,* 639.

Salm, R. (1963). The nature of the so-called postmastectomy lymphangiosarcoma. *J. Path. Bact. 85,* 445.

Sistrunk, W. E. (1927). Kondoleon operation for elephantiasis. *Ann. Surg. 85,* 185.

Smith, J. W. and Conway, H. (1962). Selection of appropriate procedures in lymphoedema: introduction of the hinged pedicle. *Plast. Reconstr. Surg. 30,* 10.

Spiller, W. G. (1905). The occasional clinical resemblance between caries of the vertebrae and lumbo-thoracic syringomyelia and the location within the spinal cord of the fibres for the sensations of pain and temperature. *Univ. Pennsylvania Med. Bull. 18,* 147.

Standard, S. (1942). Lymphedema of the arm following radical mastectomy for carcinoma of the breast: new operation for its control. *Ann. Surg. 116,* 816.

Stewart, F. W. and Treves, N. (1948). Lymphangiosarcoma in post mastectomy lymphedema. *Cancer 1,* 64.

Thompson, N. (1967). The surgical treatment of chronic lymphedema of the extremities. *Surg. Clin. N. Amer. 47,* 445.

Thompson, N. (1969). The surgical treatment of advanced postmastectomy lymphoedema of the upper limb. *Scand. J. Plast. Reconstr. Surg. 3,* 54.

Walter, C. (1918). Note sur une nouvelle methode de traitement de l'elephantiasis des membres. *Bull. Acad. Nat. Med. (Paris) 79,* 195.

White, J. C. and Sweet, W. H. (1955). In *Pain,* (a) p. 176, (b) p. 289. Springfield, U.S.A.: Charles C. Thomas.

Yamada, V. (1969). The study on lymphatic venous anastomosis in lymphoedema. *Nagoya Jnl. Med. Sci. 32,* 1.

Zieman, S. A. (1951). Reestablishing lymph drainage for lymphedema of the extremities. *J. Internat. Coll. Surg. 15,* 328.

Chapter

12

DOUGLASS C. TORMEY and JAMES P. NEIFELD

Chemotherapeutic Approaches to Disseminated Disease

INTRODUCTION

The chemotherapeutic approach to clinically disseminated carcinoma of the breast has undergone marked changes in recent years. The traditional approach to management of patients with metastatic cancer has been single agent chemotherapy only after exhausting potentially useful hormonal manipulation. Recently, combination chemotherapy has been shown to be more effective than single agents for inducing objective tumor regression. As a result combination chemotherapy is being increasingly considered as the first therapeutic modality for disseminated disease either alone or in combination with hormonal approaches. Since the survival of responding patients is generally greater than that of those who do not respond, considerable emphasis has been placed upon developing more effective remission inducing regimens.

This chapter will examine the effectiveness of single agent and combination chemotherapy, with special emphasis on response rates and durations, length of survival, and the influence of pre-therapeutic variables upon response. Toxicity and selected inter-relationships between chemotherapy and hormonal therapy will also be discussed. We shall attempt to survey these topics separately, utilizing the data from randomized prospective trials wherever possible.

Since corticosteroids are a frequent component of combination chemotherapy, these drugs, when incorporated into combinations, will be considered as chemotherapeutic agents. Throughout this review "intermittent" therapy refers to an interval of 2 or more weeks between drug courses and "continuous" therapy refers to an interval of less than 2 weeks between drug doses. The use of the term "response" or "remission" generally implies at least a 50% reduction in measurable tumor, although this is not always stated by the authors.

Before discussing the current "state of the art" it is germane to first consider the comparability of the results across reported trials. Different trials vary in their eligibility criteria, drug doses and their modification criteria, toxicity and response criteria and in their definitions of remission duration. In addition

not all trials report the data across prognostic variables. It is for these reasons that the general conclusions reached below must be tempered with caution. This is especially true when the conclusion is based on a single trial.

WHAT IS THE RELATIVE EFFECTIVENESS OF COMBINATION CHEMOTHERAPY AND SINGLE AGENT CHEMOTHERAPY?

Many cytotoxic agents have been utilized in the management of disseminated carcinoma of the breast. The cumulative data in Table 1 suggests that the most effective and commonly used single agents appear to be cyclophosphamide (CYT), thiotepa (TSPA), methotrexate (MTX), 5-fluorouracil (5-FU), adriamycin (ADR), and vincristine (VCR). Other agents have been investigated in smaller numbers of patients with varying degrees of efficacy. The highest response rates among these agents have been reported with ADR. The cumulative data with this drug was recently summarized by Tormey (1975) and in patients not exposed to previous chemotherapy the response rate was 43%. This drug has also been found to be effective in 28% of patients who have failed previous chemotherapy.

There have been few clinical studies directly comparing various single agents. Those studies that have been performed have not found a statistical advantage between the fluorinated pyrimidines 5-FU and 5-Fluorodeoxyuracil riboside (5-FUDR) and CYT or MTX (Talley et al., 1965; Eastern Cooperative Oncology Group, 1967). Response durations with most single agents appear to range from 4 to 6 months; however, several investigators have reported response durations as long as 9 to 14 months. Complete responses are uncommon with single

Table 1 Cumulative single agent response rates in advanced breast carcinoma*

Drug	*No. of patients evaluable*	*No. of patients responding*	*% response*
Antimetabolites			
5-Fluorouracil (5-FU)	1,236	324	26
Methotrexate (MTX)	356	120	34
Cytosine arabinoside	64	6	9
6-Mercaptopurine (6-MP)	44	6	14
Hydroxyurea	16	2	12
Alkylating agents			
Cyclophosphamide (CYT)	529	182	34
Thio-tepa (TSPA)	162	48	30
Nitrogen mustard	92	32	35
Phenylalanine mustard (L-PAM)	86	20	23
Chlorambucil (CLB)	54	11	20
Anti-tumor antibiotics			
Adriamycin (ADR)	221	81	37
Mitomycin C (MITO C)	60	23	38
Others (actinomycin D, mithramycin, streptonigrin, bleomycin, daunomycin)	99	13	13
Mitotic inhibitors			
Vincristine (VCR)	226	47	21
Vinblastine (VLB)	95	19	20
Random synthetics			
CCNU†	155	18	12
BCNU†	76	16	21
MCCNU†	33	2	6
Hexamethylmelamine (HMM)	39	11	28
Imidazole Carboxamide	29	2	7
Dibromodulcitol (DBD)	22	6	27
Procarbazine	21	1	5

* Modified from Broder and Tormey (1974)
† Abbreviations: CCNU = 1-(2-chloroethyl)-3-cyclohexyl-1-nitrosourea; BCNU = 1,3-bis(2-chloroethyl)-1-nitrorourea; MCCNU = 1-(2-chlorethyl)-3-(4-methylcyclohexyl)-1-nitrosourea.

agents, occurring in 5% of patients with L-PAM (Taylor et al., 1973), 4% of patients on ADR (Tormey, 1975), and 1-2% of patients on 5-FU (Ansfield, F. J., personal communication). Survival in responding patients has been shown to be increased when compared to non-responders. Responders have been reported to survive from 9 to 15 months and non-responders from 4 to 5 months (Talley et al., 1965; Eastern Cooperative Oncology Group, 1967).

Among the various idealized prerequisites for combination chemotherapy the most often quoted ones include: the agents should be effective when used as single agents against the disease; the agents should have differing biochemical mechanisms of action; cell-cycle specificities should be different; and the toxicities of the various agents should overlap as little as possible. These criteria were reasonably well met in the early studies of combination chemotherapy reported by Greenspan (1966, 1967).

The modern era of combination chemotherapy was formally introduced in 1969 by Cooper who reported that 53 of 60 patients treated with a five-drug regimen (CYT, MTX, 5-FU, VCR and Prednisone) obtained complete remission with a mean response duration of 10 months; survival data was not reported. Other investigators have not been able to reproduce these results, but using this and similar regimens objective tumor regressions appear to occur in approximately 50-60% of patients with no previous chemotherapy.

Available data with two, three, four, and five drug combinations from randomized (Tables 2 through 5) and nonrandomized trials indicates the remission rate for previously untreated patients has ranged from 153/375 (41%) with two drug combinations to 478/912 (52%) with three drug, 277/463 (60%) with four drug, and to 340/616 (55%) with five drug regimens. The cumulative response rates from the data in Table 1 with the single agents used in these combinations, and the response rate data with the combinations summarized above are plotted in Figure 1 as a function of the number of drugs used.

There appears to be a trend toward higher response rates with the combinations but the curve

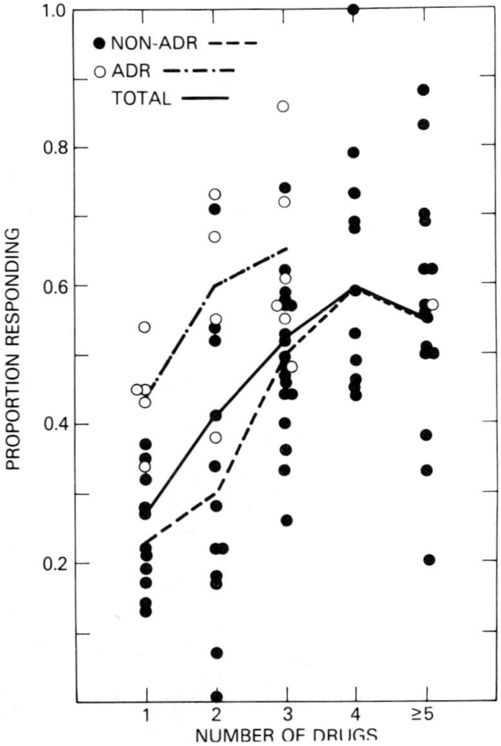

Figure 1. Response rates to single and combination chemotherapy regimens. The data is extracted from Tables 1-5 and the references in the bibliography marked with an asterisk (*). The figure includes only those patients not previously exposed to chemotherapy. The lines indicate the mean for each subset of data.

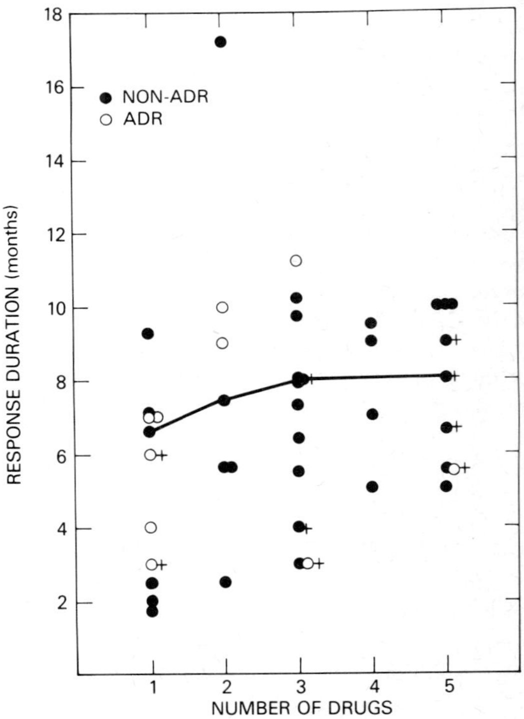

Figure 2. Response durations to the single and combination chemotherapy regimens utilized in Figure 1. Response duration data was not available for the majority of the trials. Symbols followed by a + indicate the median is not yet reached. The line indicates the median for each subset and does not include the points indicated by a +.

tends to level off at 3-4 drug combinations. It also appears that the ADR containing combinations may be slightly superior to those not containing this drug. This latter trend will be further explored below. There is less information available concerning response durations but again there appears to be a leveling off at 7-8 months with three to five drug combinations (Figure 2). In contradistinction to the response rate data there is no indication that the introduction of ADR has yet altered the response duration.

There have been few randomized studies directly comparing combinations to single agents (Table 2). Hoogstraten and George (1974) compared an intermittent CYT, MTX, 5-FU, VCR, and Prednisone (PRED) schedule against the same drugs given weekly and against ADR. The response rates were similar, but the combinations were associated with longer response durations; survival data has not yet been reported. Taylor et al. (1975) in the Eastern Co-operative Oncology Group (ECOG) compared a regimen of CYT, MTX, and 5-FU to 1-phenylalanine mustard (L-PAM). The combination regimen was significantly better than the single agents in inducing complete (15% vs. 5%) and partial (38% vs. 15%) responses. Both response duration and survival were also improved in the group receiving the combination regimen. Nemoto et al. (1975) have compared CYT, 5-FU, and PRED to ADR and to adrenalectomy (ADX); preliminary results show a slightly increased response rate and survival in patients who receive the combination as primary therapy.

Several studies have compared combinations to the same agents given sequentially. Baker et al. (1974) reported a study comparing CYT, 5-FU, and VCR to sequential 5-FU, CYT, then VCR. In the sequential arm each drug was used until progressive disease occurred at which time the next drug was begun. There was no reported difference in overall response rates, durations, or survival. It should be noted, however, that there is data available to suggest that the combination used may be less than optimal (vide infra). Smalley (1973) has reported the preliminary results of a trial comparing 5-FU, MTX, CYT, VCR, and PRED given in combination or sequentially. Patients receiving the combination had a 38% response rate while only 9% of the patients who were in the sequential arm experienced objective responses to 5-FU. The reason for these low response rates is not apparent in their report. The median survival in this study was significantly greater in the patients treated with the combination.

The data from these randomized trials suggests that the response rate and survival of patients treated with intensive combination chemotherapy is increased when compared to patients treated with single agents. The institution of still more effective combination regimens should theoretically augment this difference by placing more patients in the more favorable response category.

WHICH ARE THE CRITICAL DRUGS IN THE CYT, MTX, 5-FU, VCR, PRED COMBINATION?

The sudden development of a regimen employing five drugs simultaneously created immediate concerns regarding whether or not all five drugs were necessary. If any of the agents could be deleted the toxicity could theoretically be reduced and a hopefully effective drug regimen provided for relapsing patients. Many trials have been initiated to dissect the five drug combination, but the data currently available enables only cautious statements regarding an optimal minimal drug combination. As comparability of patient groups and definitions is more likely within randomized trials, these will be considered in more detail than the non-random studies.

Several tentative conclusions may be reached from a consideration of the available randomized trials outlined in Table 3. Brunner et al. (1975) found a lower response rate when VCR was substituted for PRED in a CYT, MTX, PRED combination. Tucker et al. (1975) reported a decreased response rate with CYT, 5-FU and VCR compared to CYT and 5-FU. Finally, Ahmann et al. (1975) have observed a decreased response rate and survival when VCR was added to a CYT, 5-FU, PRED combination. Thus, there is no evidence at present from randomized trials to suggest that VCR provides increased effectiveness in the combination regimens derived from CYT, MTX, 5-FU, VCR and PRED.

There is less data concerning CYT since most investigators have included this drug in their combinations. Brunner et al. (1975) found no difference in the two drug combinations of CYT and MTX versus chlorambucil (CLB) and MTX. In the sequential trials by Brunner et al. (1975), three drug combinations of CYT + MTX and either VCR or PRED appeared superior to the two drug combinations. This is perhaps a critical trend since Tucker et al. (1975) reported no difference between CYT + 5-FU and 5-FU + VCR, and the Acute Leukemia Group B (Leone and Rege, 1973) data suggests the superiority of the full five drug regimen over a combination of 5-FU, VCR and PRED. When this data base is coupled with the VCR data (vide supra) it is difficult

Table 2 Randomized combination vs. single agent chemotherapy trials

Reference		*Regimen*	*Resp./total†*	*CR†*	*% Resp.*	*Resp. duration*	*Survival*
Smalley (1973)*	1.	CYT 100 mg/m^2/d p.o. MTX 20 mg/m^2/wk p.o. 5-FU 400 mg/m^2/wk i.v. VCR 1 mg/m^2/wk i.v. PRED 45 mg/d p.o., then tapering course	14/37		38		9 +
	2.	q 28 d courses CYT 400 mg/m^2 i.v. d 1,8 5-FU 400 mg/m^2 i.v. d 1,8 VCR 1 mg/m^2 i.v. d 1,8 PRED 80 mg d 1-8 p.o.	7/35		20		9 +
	3.	5-FU 600 mg/m^2/wk i.v. then MTX 20 mg/m^2 2x/wk p.o. then CYT 100 mg/m^2/d p.o. then VCR 1 mg/m^2/wk i.v. then PRED 45 mg/d taper	3/34		9		4.5
Baker et al. (1974)	1.	q 28 d courses CYT 4 mg/kg i.v. d 1-5 5-FU 7.5 mg/kg i.v. d 1-5 VCR 0.015 mg/kg i.v. d 1,8	20/46	2	44	6.4	11.25
	2.	5-FU 15 mg/kg i.v. d 1-5 q 28 d	9/30	0			
		then CYT 8.0 mg/kg d 1-5 q 28 d	10/25	0			
		then VCR 0.02 mg/kg/wk i.v.	0/12	0			
		Total patients	16/30	0	53		13.9
Taylor et al. (1974)	1.	q 28 d courses CYT 100 mg/m^2 d 1-14 p.o. MTX 40 mg/m^2 d 1,8 i.v. 5-FU 600 mg/m^2 d 1,8 i.v.	49/93	14	53	8	12
	2.	PAM 6 mg/m^{2}d 1-5, p.o. q 6 wk	18/91	5	20	4	9
Hoogstraten and George (1974)*	1.	CYT 60 mg/m^2/d p.o. MTX 15 mg/m^2/wk i.v. 5-FU 300 mg/m^2/wk i.v. VCR 0.625 mg/m^2/wk i.v. PRED 30 mg/m^2/d, then tapering course	53/92	14	57	10	
	2.	q 28 d courses CYT 120 mg/m^2 i.v. d 1-5 MTX 4 mg/m^2 i.v. d 1-5 5-FU 180 mg/m^2 i.v. d 1-5 VCR 0.625 mg/m^2 i.v. d 1,5 PRED 40 mg/m^2 d 1-5	42/82	7	51	10	
	3.	q 3 wk courses ADR 60 mg/m^2 i.v.	38/66	3	57	4	
Nemoto et al. (1975)*	1.	q 35 day courses CTX 4 mg/kg/d i.v., d 1-5 5-FU 8 mg/kg/d i.v., d 1-5 PRED 30 mg/d d 1-4, then tapering course	24/46		52		9
	2.	ADR 75 mg/m^2 i.v. q 21 d	12/32		38		7
	3.	ADX	13/38		34		5

* Data updated from reference via personal communication from authors or in Broder and Tormey (1974).
† = number; Resp. = responders; CR = complete response. Resp. duration and survival are expressed in months. A blank indicates no data is available. ADX = adrenalectomy.

Table 3 Randomized trials of combination chemotherapy regimens not containing ADR

Reference		*Regimen*	*Resp./total†*	*CR†*	*% Resp.*	*Resp. duration*	*Survival*
Leone and Rege (1973)*		1. CYT 2 mg/kg/d p.o. VCR 0.025 mg/kg/wk i.v. MTX 0.75 mg/kg/wk i.v. 5-FU 12 mg/kg/wk i.v. PRED 0.75 mg/kg/d x 21, then taper	41/82	7	50	5-6	12
		2. VCR, 5-FU, PRED as above	30/82	6	36	5-6	8
Ahmann et al. (1975)		1. q 35 day courses CYT 4 mg/kg i.v. d 1-5 5-FU 8 mg/kg i.v. d 1-5 PRED 30 mg p.o. d 1-14, then taper to 10 mg/d	29/49		59	10.2	30
		2. CYT, 5-FU, PRED as above VCR 1.4 mg/m² i.v. d 1,5	19/41		46	9.5	18
Brunner et al. (1975)	A	1. CYT 2 mg/kg/d MTX 0.12 mg/kg 3 x/wk	4/23	1	22	5.6	12.7
		2. CLB 0.14 mg/kg/d MTX 0.12 mg/kg 3 x/wk	7/39	2	18	5.6	12.7
	B	1. CYT + MTX + VCR 0.025 mg/kg/wk	15/46	3	33	7.9	18.5
		2. CYT + MTX + PRED 1 mg/kg/d x 14, then tapering course	23/49	3	47	7.3	15.4
	C	1. CYT + MTX + PRED	8/18	1	44		
		2. CYT + VCR + PRED + MTX 0.4 mg/kg/wk + 5-FU 10 mg/kg/wk	44/91	6	48	3.0	16.0
Edelstyn et all (1975)	I.	1. CYT 500 mg d 1 MTX 50 mg d 1 5-FU 500 mg d 1 VCR 2 mg d 1	20/41		49		
		2. CYT 300 mg d 1,5 MTX 20 mg d 1,4 5-FU 500 mg d 1-5 VCR 1 mg d 2,5	23/39		59		
	II.	1. CYT 300 mg d 1,5 MTX 20 mg d 1,4 5-FU 500 mg d 1-5 VCR 1 mg d 2,5	27/51		53		
		2. CYT 500 mg d 1,8 MTX 50 mg d 8 5-FU 750 mg d 1 VCR 1 mg d 1,8	34/49		69		
Ramirez et al. (1975)		1. CYT 2 mg/kg/d p.o. MTX 0.5 mg/kg/wk 5-FU 10 mg/kg/wk VCR 0.02 mg/kg/wk	23/52		44		
		2. CYT + MTX + 5-FU + VCR + PRED 45 mg/d d 1-14, then tapering course	30/48		62		
Rossi et al. (1975)		1. L-PAM 4 mg/m² d 1-5 p.o. 5-FU 300 mg/m² d 1-5 i.v. PRED 30 mg/m² d 1-5 p.o.	6/15		40	3	
		2. L-PAM + 5-FU i.v.	4/18		22	2.5	
		3. L-PAM + 5-FU p.o.	1/14		7		
Tucker et al. (1975)		1. CYT 150 mg i.v. d 1,4 VCR 1 mg i.v. d 2,4 5-FU 300 mg/m² i.v. d 1-4			26		
		2. CYT + 5-FU			52		
		3. VCR + 5-FU			54		

* Data updated from reference via personal communication from authors or in Broder and Tormey (1974).
†= number; Resp.= responders; CR=complete response. Resp. duration and survival are expressed in months. A blank indicates no data is available.

to discard an important role for CYT in the more effective combinations.

The situation with PRED, MTX and 5-FU is equally complex. The Central Oncology Group (Ramirez et al., 1975) evaluated the five drug regimen with and without PRED. No significant differences were observed in response rates or durations after correction for prognostic variables. In view of the accumulating VCR data (vide supra), the Eastern Cooperative Oncology Group initiated a trial chaired by Band and Tormey comparing CYT, MTX and 5-FU with and without PRED. With over 50 cases analyzed in each regimen there is no demonstrable difference at the present time. This sequence of trials suggests that a combination of CYT, MTX and 5-FU is as effective as the five drug program, however, no trial has directly compared a CYT, MTX and 5-FU combination to the five drug combination.

Another trial by Brunner et al. (1975) found no difference by deleting 5-FU and VCR from the five drug regimen, thus it is possible that CYT + MTX + PRED and CYT + MTX + 5-FU are equivalent regimens. Although never compared to the above regimens the CYT + 5-FU + PRED regimen of Ahmann et al. (1975) appears to provide response rates equivalent to these other three drug programs and may be equivalent to them. The tentative conclusions which could therefore be suggested from the available randomized trials are: (1) regimens of CYT + MTX + PRED, or CYT + MTX + 5-FU and possibly CYT + 5-FU + PRED, appear to be as effective as the CYT + MTX + 5-FU + VCR + PRED regimens; (2) VCR does not appear to provide significant therapeutic benefit in these programs; (3) 5-FU or PRED appear to be equally effective when combined with CYT and MTX; and (4) MTX or 5-FU may be equivalent when combined with CYT and PRED.

WHAT HAS BEEN THE IMPACT OF ADR IN COMBINATION THERAPY?

The discovery of the marked efficacy of ADR as a single agent led to its utilization in combination regimens. ADR containing regimens have been reported to be associated with response rates from 55% to 86% in patients not previously exposed to chemotherapy. In patients receiving prior chemotherapy other than the study drugs, combination of ADR with VCR (Bonnadonna et al., 1975), dibromodulcitol (Tormey et al., 1975a), or BCNU and CYT (Presant and Kolhouse, 1975) have led to responses in 5/28 (18%), 20/50 (40%), and 4/9 (44%) patients, respectively.

Randomized trials in patients not exposed to prior chemotherapy suggest that an alkylator is an important component of the more active ADR combinations (Table 4). The studies of Ahmann et al. (1975b) and Eagen et al. (1975) show no difference between CYT + 5-FU + PRED and either ADR + MTX + VCR or ADR + MTX. Similarly, the Milan Group (Brambilla et al., 1974; DeLena et al., 1975; Bonnadonna et al., 1975) found an equal efficacy of CYT + MTX + 5-FU and ADR + VCR ± PRED. However, we have observed a superiority for a combination of CYT + ADR + 5-FU over CYT + MTX + 5-FU (Bull et al., 1975). These results suggest that alkylator containing ADR combinations mark an improvement over those regimens not containing ADR or incorporating it without an alkylator. Trials now in progress will help to further delineate the role of CYT, other alkylating agents, and 5-FU in these combinations.

Despite the higher remission rates there is as yet no substantial indication that the introduction of ADR has improved the remission duration. Similarly, although the population as a whole is placed into the more favorable response categories the data is too early to assess the impact of this feature upon survival.

ARE HORMONAL AND CHEMOTHERAPEUTIC APPROACHES COMPATIBLE?

The possibility that previous hormone response or lack of response could influence the response to subsequent chemotherapy has been examined retrospectively. Henderson et al. (1975) evaluated 63 patients and was unable to predict a response to chemotherapy based upon the response to endocrine therapy. This study confirmed previous reports of such a lack of predictive ability (Nemoto and Dao, 1971).

Another approach to this question concerns the value of hormonal and chemotherapeutic approaches administered simultaneously (Table 5). Falkson (1972) has reported a group of 75 randomized premenopausal patients treated either by oophorectomy alone or oophorectomy plus CYT. Two year survival figures were identical (60%); however, survival at five years was 33% in the oophorectomy plus CYT group and only 18% in the oophorectomy alone group. Patients who received CYT in addition to oophorectomy were further analyzed by whether the CYT was or was not initiated within two months

Table 4 Randomized trials of Adriamycin-containing combinations

Reference	*Regimen*	*Resp./total†*	*CR†*	*% Resp.*	*Resp. duration*	*Survival*
Ahmann et al. (1975a)	1. q 4 weeks ADR 60 mg/m² d 1 i.v. MTX 15 mg/m² d 1, 4 i.v.	9/24		38		
	2. q 35 days CYT 150 mg/m² d 1-5, i.v. 5-FU 300 mg/m² d 1-5 i.v. PRED 30 mg/m² d 1-14, then tapering course	7/12		58		
	3. CYT, 5-FU, PRED as above VCR 1.4 mg/m² d 1,5 i.v.	6/10		60		
Brambilla et al. (1974)	1. q 21 d courses ADR 75 mg/m² i.v. d 1 VCR 1.4 mg/m² i.v. d 1,8	10/15	1	67		
	2. ADR + VCR as above PRED 100 mg/m² i.m. d 1-5	12/21	2	57		
Bull et al. (1975)*	1. q 28 d courses CYT 100 mg/m² d 1-14 p.o. MTX 40 mg/m² d 1,8 i.v. 5-FU 600 mg/m² d 1,8 i.v.	25/40	2	62	9.7	
	2. q 28 d courses CYT 100 mg/m² d 1-14 p.o. ADR 30 mg/m² d 1,8 i.v. 5-FU 500 mg/m² d 1,8 i.v.	32/37	7	86	11.2	
De Lena et al. (1975) and Bonadonna et al. (1975)	1. q 21 d courses ADR 75 mg/m² d 1 VCR 1.4 mg/m² d 1,8	27/52	4	52		
	2. q 28 d courses CYT 100 mg/m² d 1-14 MTX 40 mg/m² d 1,8 5-FU 600 mg/m² d 1,8	28/53	6	53	6	
Eagen et al. (1975)	1. q 35 days CYT 150 mg/m² d 1-5 i.v. 5-FU 300 mg/m² d 1-5 i.v. PRED 30 mg/d x 14, then tapering course	8/14		57		
	2. CYT, 5-FU, PRED as above Calusterone 200 mg/d p.o.	6/12		50		
	3. q 35 days ADR 40 mg/m² d 2 i.v. VCR 1.4 mg/m² d 1,5 i.v. MTX 10 mg/m² d 1,5 i.v.	11/23		48		
Smalley and Bornstein (1975)*	1. q 21 d courses CYT 500 mg/m² i.v. ADR 50 mg/m² i.v. 5-FU 500 mg/m² i.v.	17/31		55		
	2. q 28 d courses CYT 100 mg/m² i.v. VCR 1 mg i.v. d 1,8 MTX 30 mg/m² p.o. d 1,8 5-FU 400 mg/m² i.v. d 1,8 PRED 20 mg/d d 1-7 p.o.	11/33		33		

* Date updated from reference via personal communication from authors or in Broder and Tormey (1974).
† = number; Resp. = responders; CR = complete response. Resp. duration and survival are expressed in months. A blank indicates no data is available.

of the development of metastases. Three and five year survivals were 78% and 58% if the CYT was begun within two months, but only 46% and 16% it it was not. Nemoto et al. (1975) have compared adrenalectomy to single agent and combination chemotherapy (ADR vs. 5-FU, CYT, PRED) in a randomized trial with a cross-over after treatment failure; preliminary results revealed no difference in rate of response or response duration in small groups of patients (Table 2). Unfortunately, estrogen receptor analyses were not used to enter patients into these studies as the value of this test was not yet available.

Additive hormonal therapy has also been combined with single agent chemotherapy in several studies with disappointing results (Table 5). Cole et al. (1973) added Nandrolone decanoate to CYT and compared the response rates obtained to both agents used singly; there was no advantage to the combination. Goldenberg et al. (1975) reported a randomized study comparing testolactone plus 5-FU to each agent used singly; again, no advantage was seen in the group given the combination.

Estrogen therapy has also been combined with single agent chemotherapy. Nowakowski et al. (1971) in a nonrandom trial combined ethinyl estradiol with CYT in 49 postmenopausal patients with 21 objective responses and a mean response duration of 15.4 months. Firat et al. (1968) combined diethylstilbestrol (DES) with CYT and compared this to DES alone. Using greater than 50% tumor regression as a criteria for objective response, 5 of 18 responded to DES alone and 4 of 14 to DES plus CYT. Kiang and Kennedy (1975) reported a slight response advantage to DES + CYT compared to DES, but a survival disadvantage. Taylor et al. (1975) added physiologic doses of conjugated estrogens to weekly intravenous 5-FU; no difference in response rate or survival was noted compared to 5-FU alone.

Table 5. Randomized Chemotherapy + Hormonal Therapy Trials

Reference		*Regimen*	*No. Evaluated*	** Resp*	*% Response*	*Survival*	
Firat et al. (1968)	A.	1. DES	18	5	28		
		2. DES+ CYT	14	4	29		
	B.	1. Oophorectomy	7	2	29		
		2. Oophorectomy + CYT	5	3	60		
Falkson (1972)		1. Oophorectomy	75 total			2 yr = 60%;	5 yr = 18%
		2. Oophorectomy + CYT				= 60%;	= 33%
Cole et al. (1973)		1. CTX 150 mg/d	30	7	23	Resp = 21	
		2. Nandrolone 50 mg q3w	26	0	0	Non-Resp = 12	
		3. CTX + Nandrolone	22	1	5		
Goldenberg et al. (1975)		1. Testolactone 1 g/d	40	8	20		
		2. 5-FU 500 mg/d	35	2	6		
		3. Testolactone + 5-FU	36	5	14		
Stott et al. (1973)		1. CTX, VCR, MTX, 5-FU, PRED	10	5	50		
		2. CTX, VCR, MTX, 5-FU, Medroxyprogesterone acetate	16	11	69		
Kiang and Kennedy (1975)		1. DES 15 mg/d	21	5	24	2 yr = 52%	
		2. DES 15 mg/d + CTX 200 mg/d	23	8	35	= 25%	
Taylor et al. (1975)		1. 5-FU 15 mg/kg/wk Premarin 2.5 mg/d PO	28		17	16	
		2. 5-FU 15 mg/kg/wk	32			16	
Goldenberg et al. (1973)		1. CLB 0.2 mg/kg/d	82	8	10	12	*Resp Only* 24
		2. CLB 0.2 mg/kg/d PRED 15 mg/d	87	10	21	7	14
		3. HCT 30 mg/d T_3 0.050 mg/d	85	10	12	11	18

* = Number; Resp = responders; CR = complete response. Resp duration and survival are expressed in months.
A blank indicates no data is available.

The substitution of medroxyprogesterone acetate for PRED in a CYT, MTX, 5-FU, VCR, PRED regimen by Stott et al. (1973) increased the response rate from 5/10 to 11/16. Finally, Eagen et al. (1975) reported no benefit by adding Calusterone to a CYT, 5-FU, PRED regimen (Table 4).

All of the above studies have in common the disadvantage of not using hormone receptor data as a criterion for evaluating the treatments used. Optimal doses of cytostatic agents do not appear to have been utilized in all the studies and patient cooperation in at least one study (Taylor et al., 1975) was reported as poor. The suggestion of an additive effect of the combination of ablative hormone and chemotherapy is currently under more vigorous test by several groups. Similarly, the evaluation of combination chemotherapy plus additive hormone therapy is now under investigation.

WHAT IS THE EFFECT OF PRE-THERAPEUTIC VARIABLES UPON THE RESPONSE RATE?

It is difficult to compare single agent to combination regimens with regard to various pre-therapeutic variables because very little data is available. The effect of menopausal status upon single agent response rates has been evaluated in several reports (Table 6).

There appears to be no difference in response to CYT depending on the menopausal status, but 5-FU appears most effective in patients within one year of the menopause; ADR, however, appears most effective in patients greater than ten years post-menopausal. There is as yet no clear pattern for the various combination regimens although there is a trend for higher response rates with ADR + VCR in patients greater than ten years post-menopausal (Table 7).

It appears that patients with a disease free interval longer than two years have a decreased response rate to either CYT or 5-FU, but the response rate to ADR alone appears to be greater in this group of patients. It is of interest, therefore, that in the combination regimens which have looked at this question, ADR plus VCR ± PRED (Table 7) shows a decreased response rate in patients with longer disease free intervals, and CYT, 5-FU, PRED plus/minus VCR appears to have a greater response rate with increased disease free intervals. The reason for this dichotomy in the trends is not clear.

The site of dominant disease appears to be an important variable regarding response. Once again, varying response definitions make analysis of reported response rates difficult. It appears that both ADR and CYT are most effective against dominant soft tissue disease, relatively less so against visceral disease, and even less effective against osseous disease.

Table 6. The Influence of Pretherapeutic Variables on Response to Single Agent Chemotherapy*

Drug	*% Response by Dominant Disease Site* Soft Tissue	Osseous	Visceral	*% Response by Years Post-Menopausal* 0-1	1-5	5-10	10+	*% Response by DFI* 0-2	2+
CYT	42	24	28	38	26	18	32	35	22
5-FU	29	28	18	33	18	19	17	24	9
ADR	60	10	42	20	33	28	43	29	41

* Modified from Broder and Tormey. DFI = time from mastectomy to first disease recurrence.

Table 7. The Influence of Menopausal Status and DFI on the Response Rate to Combination Chemotherapy

Reference	Drug Regimen	*% Response by years Post-Menopausal* Pre	0-1	1-5	5+	10+	*% Response by DFI* 0-1	1+	5+
DeLena et al. (1973)	CYT, MTX, 5-FU, VCR	21		43	28	41			
Brambilla et al. (1973)	ADR, VCR, ± PRED		57	55	69		68	60	43
DeLena et al. (1975)	ADR, VCR		50	38	67	80	65	43	
	CTX, MTX, 5-FU		85	63	40	57	72	50	67
Ahmann et al. (1975)	CTX, 5-FU, PRED ± VCR		56	52	9	38	33	46	60
Bull et al. (1975)*	CTX, ADR, 5-FU	80	100	100	80	80	75	93	100
	CTX, MTX, 5-FU	73		0	67	67	60	65	67

* Data updated from reference via personal communication from authors or in Broder and Tormey (1974).
DFI = time from mastectomy to first disease recurrence.

5-FU, however, appears equally effective against soft tissue and osseous disease but less effective against visceral disease. As can be seen from Table 8 the response rates even with similar combination regimens vary greatly. Averaging these results demonstrates that about 70% of patients with dominant soft tissue disease, 50% of patients with dominant visceral disease, and 35% of patients with dominant osseous disease have undergone objective regressions. The wide response rates preclude any comparative analysis of the varying combinations.

In general, it appears that combination chemotherapy does not markedly change the differential single agent response rates obtained across different pretherapeutic variables. Instead, there appears to be an increase of the response rate observed in all the categories which have been examined.

HOW DISABLING IS THE TOXICITY OF COMBINATION REGIMENS?

The toxicity encountered with the various combinations which have been utilized depends on the drugs used and their dosages, schedule of administration, and experience of the oncologist. General information concerning the types of side-effects to be expected with each agent can be found in various reviews (Greenwald, 1973; Bergevin, 1972). Only the more commonly potentially disabling toxicities will be noted here.

An important and potentially lethal complication of ADR is congestive heart failure; this complication is related to the total dose of ADR administered. Current recommendations are not to exceed a cumulative dosage of 500 to 550 mg/m^2 (Lefrak et al., 1975), and in patients with prior cardiac radiation or in combination with alkylating agents the total dose should probably be still less.

Neurologic toxicity is common in patients receiving VCR. In experienced hands it is rarely severe, usually consisting of parethesias and numbness which are not always reversible.

Cystitis is a potentially severe complication of CYT. The incidence can probably be decreased by adequate hydration before and immediately after drug administration. If not, the drug can be replaced by another alkylating agent.

Gastrointestinal toxicity is present in 25% to 75% of patients receiving combinations; nausea and vomiting are the most common manifestations although diarrhea also occurs in some patients. Stomatitis and/or mucositis is fairly common in MTX and ADR regimens, but is also reversible.

Table 8. The Influence of Dominant Disease Upon the Response Rate to Combination Chemotherapy

		% Response by Dominant Disease Site		
Reference	*Drug Regimen*	*Soft Tissue*	*Osseous*	*Visceral*
Deemarsky & Chernomordikova (1970)	CYT or TSPA, 5-FU	100	85	50
Freckman et al. (1964)	CLB + PRED	44	29	31
Brunner et al. (1975)	CYT + MTX; CLB + MTX	67	43	54
	CYT, MTX, VCR	75	50	42
	CYT, MTX, PRED	100	48	69
	CYT, MTX, 5-FU, VCR, PRED	83	63	81
Cooper (1969)	CYT, MTX, 5-FU, PRED, VCR	100	88	87
Ansfield et al. (1971)	CYT, MTX, 5-FU, VCR, PRED	80	29	70
Davis et al. (1974)	CYT, MTX, 5-FU, VCR, PRED		3	46
Kaufman et al. (1973)	CYT, MTX, 5-FU, VCR, PRED	79	56	50
Leone & Rege (1973)*	CYT, MTX, 5-FU, VCR, PRED	55	15	37
Jones et al. (1975)	CYT + ADR	80	84	72
Ahmann et al. (1975)	CYT, 5-FU, PRED, ± VCR	43	33	44
Canellos et al. (1974)	CYT, MTX, 5-FU, PRED	60	15	48
DeLena et al. (1973)	CYT, MTX, 5-FU, VCR	49	5	33
Brambilla et al. (1973)	ADR, VCR, ± PRED	75	25	47
DeLena et al. (1975)	ADR + VCR	60	33	22
	CYT, MTX, 5-FU	60	25	47
Creech et al. (1975)	CYT, MTX, 5-FU	56	0	46
Bull et al. (1975)*	CYT, MTX, 5-FU	80	70	56
	CYT, ADR, 5-FU	100	91	80
DeJager et al. (1975)	CYT, ADR, 5-FU	61	23	50
Blumenschein et al. (1974)	CYT, ADR, 5-FU	100	10	40

* Data updated from reference in Broder and Tormey (1974).

The most common complications, which may be life-threatening, are granulocytopenia and thrombocytopenia. Unfortunately, even careful hematologic monitoring may not always prevent these complications. Depending on the regimen utilized, from 10% to 80% of patients may have peripheral granulocyte counts less than 1000 and/or platelet counts less than 100,000. The nadir and duration of the depressed counts is dependent upon the drugs and schedules used. The current more effective intermittent regimens tend to have nadirs 10-15 days after the last I.V. drug with full recovery occurring in another 5-10 days.

The prevention of hematologic complications can usually be accomplished by careful monitoring of peripheral platelet and white blood cell counts. We monitor these parameters weekly and utilize both the nadir during the preceding cycle and the counts on the day of drug administration to determine the appropriate drug dosage. If moderately severe granulocytopenia or thrombocytopenia occur during any cycle of intermittent therapy, drug dosage should usually be diminished for the next cycle; if this is not done, further potentiation of hematologic toxicity, which may be fatal, could occur.

The mortality of combination regimens ranges from 0% to 10%, depending upon the patient population, agents and dosages administered, and experience of the oncologist. Drug-related deaths are usually due to sepsis related to severe granulocytopenia or, rarely, hemorrhage from severe (less than 20,000) thrombocytopenia. Accordingly, it is occasionally helpful to have white blood cell and platelet support facilities available.

Compared to single agent therapy one can only rely upon the impressions of experience at the present time. In general the severity of complications seen with intensive single agent therapy is qualitatively similar to that with intensive combination regimens. However, since the combinations involve more drugs, there exists the potential for a wider spectrum of interacting complications. It is this facet that makes the "experience factor" more critical with combination therapy than with single agents. If a particular toxicity occurs, such as severe mucositis or an hepatic enzyme change, it becomes important to know which of the drugs in the combination are implicated so that appropriate changes are made in the regimen.

SOME FUTURE CONSIDERATIONS

Steady progress is occurring in the palliative therapy of disseminated carcinoma of the breast. New applications of current therapeutic tools and the development of new agents appear to have improved response rates. Although these improvements appear to be leading to improved population survivals, there is as yet no clear evidence that the response durations obtained with 3-5 drug regimens are improved with higher response rates, e.g. CYT, ADR, and 5-FU as compared to CYT, MTX, and 5-FU.

One approach to improving overall survival is to develop techniques that allow treatment of the disease at what are now called subclinical tumor burdens. It has been demonstrated that many patients with disseminated carcinoma of the breast secrete non-specific tumor markers in abnormal amounts. Tormey et al. (1975b) have demonstrated that using a matrix analysis with carcinoembryonic antigen, human chorionic gonadotropin, and N^2, N^2-dimethylguanosine over 90% of patients with metastatic breast cancer have one or more elevations. It is theoretically possible that utilizing these and other markers after "curative" breast cancer surgery will identify patients with disseminated disease before it is clinically evident. Wang et al. (1975) have found a higher recurrence rate in patients with postoperative CEA elevations. The development of more highly specific and sensitive tumour markers may further refine this technique and enable patients to be treated with smaller tumor burdens when systemic therapy should be more effective and hopefully curative.

Analysis of the fail rates in remission duration in metastatic disease may offer a further insight into the manipulation of chemotherapeutic regimens. Appropriate life-table plots of available data from the trials of Bull et al. (1975) and Jones et al. (1975) demonstrate a change in the slope at 6-7 months; the negative slope doubles for each chemotherapeutic regimen at that time. One interpretation of these curves is that they are the summation of curves from two different populations of cells; those that are initially sensitive and those that are initially resistant to the agents employed. According to this hypothesis the resistant population becomes dominant at 6-7 months. It may be possible to alter this break in the curve by the addition of a second combination of drugs, a combination which has different mechanisms of action than the first. The second regimen could be employed before the break in the curve or in alternating cycles with the first regimen.

Another major interpretation of these curves could be that there is cumulative limiting host toxicity to the agents employed such that the dose of drugs delivered falls below the therapeutic level after three to four months of therapy; such an observation is not uncommon in the clinic and has been suggested by the data of DeLena et al. (1975). If this is the case

the incorporation of drugs that enhance host tolerance to the cytotoxic agents could improve the response durations. Finally, it is conceivable that continued perturbation of the tumor by cytotoxic agents on a rigid schedule could alter the kinetics of the tumor such that the cells are no longer in a sensitive portion of the cell cycle during drug delivery, a form of so-called kinetic resistance. This hypothesis would suggest that the therapeutic drug concentration during the time the cells are in a sensitive portion of their cell cycle is relatively low. An analysis of tumor kinetics under conditions of continued drug perturbation would be necessary to evaluate this hypothesis and, if appropriate, serve as a guide to an improved scheduling of therapy.

Combined modality therapy, as well as new chemotherapeutic drugs, may also improve response rates and survival. Tumor "debulking", with irradiation or surgery, should theoretically increase the proportion of cells that are chemotherapeutically-approachable by increasing the relative size of the proliferating pool. Immunotherapy and hormonotherapy in combination with chemotherapy might also improve response rates and help to consolidate responses. The further development of these approaches and new ones yet to be formulated should continue to provide further improvements in the therapy of this disease.

REFERENCES

Ahmann, D. L., Hahn, R. G. and Bisel, H. F. (1974). A Phase II evaluation of ifosfamide (NSC-109724) treatment of disseminated breast cancer. *Proceedings of the American Society of Clinical Oncology, 15,* 182.

Ahmann, D. L., Eagan, R. T., Bisel, H. F., Hahn, R. G., O'Connell, M. J. and Edmonson, J. H. (1975a). Evaluation of combination therapy with adriamycin (NSC-123127) and methotrexate (NSC-740) in patients with disseminated breast cancer. *Cancer Chemotherapy Reports Part 3, 6,* 335.

Ahmann, D. L., Bisel, H. F., Hahn, R. G., Eagan, R. T., Edmonson, J. H., Steinfeld, J. L., Tormey, D. C. and Taylor, W. F. (1975b). An analysis of a multiple-drug program in the treatment of patients with advanced breast cancer utilizing 5-fluorouracil, cyclophosphamide, and prednisone with or without vincristine. *Cancer, 36,* 1925.

Baker, L. M., Vaughn, C. B., Al-Sarraf, M., Reed, M. L. and Vaitkevicius, V. K. (1974). Evaluation of combination vs. sequential cytotoxic chemotherapy in the treatment of advanced breast cancer. *Cancer 33,* 513.

Bergevin, P. R., Tormey, D. C. and Blom, J. (1972). Guide to the use of cancer chemotherapeutic agents. *Modern Treatment 9,* 185.

Blumenschein, G. R., Cardenas, J. O., Freireich, E. J. and Gottlieb, J. A. (1974). FAC chemotherapy for breast cancer. *Proceedings of the American Society of Clinical Oncology 15,* 193.

Bonadonna, G., Beretta, G., Tancini, G., Brambilla, C., Bajetta, E., DePalo, G. M., DeLena, M., Bellani, F. F., Gasparini, M., Valagussa, P. and Veronesi, U. (1975). Adriamycin (NSC-123127) studies at the Institute Nazionale Tumori, Milan. *Cancer Chemotherapy Reports Part 3 6,* 231.

Brambilla, C., DeLena, M. and Bonadonna, G. (1974). Combination chemotherapy with adriamycin (NSC-123127) in metastatic mammary carcinoma. *Cancer Chemotherapy Reports 58,* 251.

Broder, L. E. and Tormey, D. C. (1974). Combination chemotherapy of carcinoma of the breast. *Cancer Treatment Reviews 1,* 183.

Brunner, K. W., Sonntag, R. W., Martz, G., Senn, H. J., Obrecht, P. and Alberto, P. (1975). A controlled study in the use of combined drug therapy for metastatic breast cancer. *Cancer 36,* 1208.

Bull, J., Tormey, D., Falkson, G., Blom, J., Perlin, E. and Carbone, P. (1975). A comparison of cyclophosphamide, adriamycin, and 5-fluorouracil versus cyclophosphamide, methotrexate, and 5-fluorouracil in metastatic breast cancer. *Proceedings of the American Society of Clinical Oncology 16,* 246.

Canellos, G. P., DeVita, V. T., Gold, G. L., Chabner, B. A., Schein, P. S. and Young, R. C. (1974). Cyclical combination chemotherapy for advanced breast carcinoma. *British Medical Journal 1,* 218.

Cole, M. P., Todd, I. D. H. and Wilkinson, P. M. (1973). Cyclophosphamide and nandrolone decanoate in the treatment of advanced carcinoma of the breast—results of a comparative controlled trial of the agents used singly and in combination. *British Journal of Cancer 27,* 396.

Cooper, R. J. (1969). Combination chemotherapy in hormone resistant breast cancer. *Proceedings of the American Association for Cancer Research 10,* 15.

*Corder, M. P., Stone, W. H., Justice, G. R., Herbst, K. H. and Flannery, E. P. (1975). Combination chemotherapy with or without leucovorin in the treatment of poor risk breast cancer patients. *Proceedings of the American Association for Cancer Research, 16,* 202.

Creech, R. H., Catalano, R. B., Mastrangelo, M. J. and Engstrom, P. F. (1975). An effective low-dose intermittent cyclophosphamide, methotrexate, and 5-fluorouracil treatment regimen for metastatic breast cancer. *Cancer 35,* 1101.

Davis, H. L., Ramirez, G., Ellerby, R. A. and Ansfield, F. J. (1974). Five-drug therapy in advanced breast cancer: Factors influencing toxicity and response. *Cancer 34,* 239.

Deemarsky, L. Y. and Chernomordikova, M. F. (1970). Combination chemotherapy in the management of breast cancer metastases. *Cancer 26,* 771.

DeJager, R., Kaufman, R., Ochoa, M. and Krakoff, I. H. (1975). Chemotherapy of advanced breast cancer with a combination of cytoxan, adriamycin, and 5-FU (CAF). *Proceedings of the American Society of Clinical Oncology 16,* 273.

DeLena, M., DePalo, G. M., Bonadonna, G., Beretta, G. and Bajetta, E. (1973). Terapia del carcinoma mammariv metastatizzato con ciclofosfamide, methotrexate, vincristina e fluorouracile. *Tumori 59,* 11.

DeLena, M., Brambilla, C., Morabito, A. and Bonadonna, G. (1975). Adriamycin plus vincristine compared to and combined with cyclophosphamide, methotrexate, and 5-fluorouracil for advanced breast cancer. *Cancer 35,* 1108.

Eagen, R. T., Ahmann, D. L., Edmonson, J. H., Hahn, R. G. and Bisel, H. F. (1975). Controlled evaluation of the combination of adriamycin (NSC-123127), vincristine (NSC-67574), and methotrexate (NSC-740) in patients with disseminated breast cancer. *Cancer Chemotherapy Reports (Part 3) 6,* 339.

Eastern Cooperative Group in Solid Tumor Chemotherapy (1967). Comparison of antimetabolites in the treatment of breast and colon cancer. *Journal of the American Medical Association 200,* 100.

*Edelstyn, G. A. and MacRae, K. D. (1973). Cyclical combination chemotherapy in advanced breast cancer. *British Journal of Cancer, 28,* 459.

Edelstyn, G. A., Bates, T. D., Brinkley, D., MacRae, K. D., Spittle, R. F. and Wheeler, T. (1975). Comparison of 5-day, 1-day, and 2-day cyclical combination chemotherapy in advanced breast cancer. *Lancet ii,* 209.

Falkson, G. (1972). An annotation on the treatment of disseminated breast cancer in premenopausal women. *South African Journal of Surgery 10,* 41.

Firat, D. and Olshin, S. (1968). Treatment of metastatic carcinoma of the female breast with combination of hormones and other chemotherapy. *Cancer Chemotherapy Reports 52,* 743.

Freckman, H. A., Fry, H. L., Mendez, F. L. and Maurer, E. R. (1964). Chlorambucil-prednisolone therapy for disseminated breast carcinoma. *Journal of the American Medical Association 189,* 23.

*Foley, J. F., Lemon, H. M. and Miller, D. (1970). Low dosage methotrexate (NSC-740) and cyclophosphamide (NSC-26271) for solid tumors. *Cancer Chemotherapy Reports 54,* 41.

Goldenberg, I. S. (1973). Secondary chemotherapy of advanced breast cancer. *Cancer 31,* 660.

Goldenberg, I. S., Sedransk, N., Volk, H., Segaloff, A., Kelley, R. M. and Haines, C. R. (1975). Combined androgen and anti-metabolite therapy of advanced female breast cancer: A report of the Cooperative Breast Cancer Group. *Cancer 36,* 308.

Greenspan, E. M. (1966). Combination cytotoxic chemotherapy in advanced disseminated breast carcinoma. *Journal of the Mount Sinai Hospital 33,* 1.

Greenspan, E. M. (1967). Combination anti-metabolite (methotrexate) and alkylating agent (thio-tepa) chemotherapy in advanced breast carcinoma. *Ob/Gyn Digest,* Nov. *51.*.

Greenwald, E. S. (1973). *Medical Outline Series, Cancer Chemotherapy,* 2nd edition, Medical Examination Publishing Co., Inc., New York.

*Hanham, I. W. F., Newton, K. A. and Westbury, G. (1971). Seventy-five cases of solid tumors treated by a modified quadruple chemotherapy regime. *British Journal of Cancer 25,* 462.

*Harvey, H. A., White, D. S. and Lipton, A. (1975). Five drug regimen plus asriamycin in metastatic breast cancer. *Proceedings of the American Society of Clinical Oncology 16,* 255.

Henderson, M. D., Buroker, T. R., Samson, M. K., Wood, D. W., Baker, L. H. and Vaitkevicius, V. K. (1975). Response of patients with carcinoma of the breast to hormonal therapy and combination chemotherapy. *Surgery, Gynecology, and Obstetrics 141,* 232.

Hoogstraten, B. and George, S. (1974). Adriamycin and combination chemotherapy in breast cancer: A Southwest Oncology Group Study. *Proceedings of the American Association for Cancer Research 15,* 70.

Jones, S. E., Durie, B. G. M. and Salmon, S. E. (1975). Combination chemotherapy with adriamycin and cyclophosphamide for advanced breast cancer. *Cancer 36,* 90.

Kaufman, S. and Goldstein, M. (1973). Combination chemotherapy in disseminated carcinoma of the breast. *Surgery, Gynecology, and Obstetrics 137,* 83.

Kiang, D. T. and Kennedy, B. J. (1975). The effect of short-term cyclophosphamide on estrogen therapy in breast cancer. *Proceedings of the American Association for Cancer Research 16,* 107.

Lefrak, E. A., Pitha, J., Rosenhelm, S., O'Bryan, R. M., Burgess, M. A. and Gottlieb, J. A. (1975). Adriamycin (NSC-123127) cardiomyopathy. *Cancer Chemotherapy Reports Part 3 6,* 203.

Leone, L. A. and Rege, V. (1973). Treatment of metastatic, recurrent, or inoperable carcinoma of breast with VCR/PRED/5-FU/MTX/CYCLO (Reg I) vs. VCR/PRED/5-FU (Reg II). *Proceedings of the American Association for Cancer Research 14,* 125.

Lokich, J. J. and Skarin, A. T. (1972). Five-drug combination chemotherapy for disseminated adenocarcinoma. *Cancer Chemotherapy Reports 56,* 761.

Nemoto, T. and Dao, T. L. (1971). 5-Fluorouracil and cyclophosphamide in disseminated breast cancer. *New York State Journal of Medicine 71,* 554.

Nemoto, T., Horton, J., Cunningham, T., Sponzo, R., Rosner, D., Diaz, R. and Dao, T. L. (1975). Update report: Comparison of combination chemotherapy (FCP) vs. adriamycin (ADM) vs. adrenalectomy (ADX) in breast cancer. *Proceedings of the American Association for Cancer Research 16,* 46.

Nowakowski, H., Rode, P. and Ruhstrat, K. (1971). Erfahryngen mit der Kombination von Äthinylöstradiol und Cyclophosphamid bei der Behandlung des progressiven metastasierenden Mammakarzinoms der Frau. *Deutsche Medizinische Wochenschrift 96,* 1855.

*Otis, P. T. and Armentrout, S. A. (1975). Combination chemotherapy in metastatic carcinoma of the breast: Results of a three-drug combination. *Cancer 36,* 311.

*Pouillart, P., Schwarzenberg, L. Amiel, J. L., Mathe, G., Huguenin, P., Morin, P., Baron, A., Laparre, C. and Parrot, R. (1975). Combinaisons chemotherapiques de drogues se potentialisant 1. Application au traitement des cancers du sein. *La Nouvelle Presse Medicale 4,* 713.

Presant, J. A. and Kolhouse, J. F. (1975). Adriamycin (A), BCNU(B), plus cyclophosphamide (C) in carcinoma of the breast and other malignancies. *Proceedings of the American Society of Clinical Oncology 16,* 232.

Ramirez, G., Strawitz, J. G., Wilson, W. L., Cornell, G. N., Madden, R. E. and the Central Oncology Group (1975); Multiple drug therapy in disseminated breast carcinoma—A randomized study. *Proceedings of The American Association for Cancer Research* [illegible], 33.

Rossi, A., Brambilla, C., Bonadonna, G. and Veronesi, U. (1975). Controlled study with L-PAM and 5-FU (IV or PO) plus or minus prednisone in advancing breast cancer. *Proceedings of the American Association for Cancer Research 16,* 189.

*Rosso, R., Brema, F. and Santi, L. (1973). Trattemento del carcinoma mammario avanzato con una associazione di vincristina, fluorouracile, methotrexate, ciclofosfamide e prednisone. *Tumori 59,* 163.

*Shingleton, W. W., Sedransk, N. and Johnson, R. O. (1971).

Systemic chemotherapy of mammary carcinoma. *Annals of Surgery 173,* 913.

Smalley, R. and Bornstein, R. (1975). C-A-F treatment for metastatic breast CA. *Proceedings of the American Society of Clinical Oncology 16,* 265.

Smalley, R. V., Murphy, S., Chan, Y-K. and Huguley, C. M. (1973). Comparison of two five-drug regimes vs. sequential chemotherapy in metastatic breast carcinoma. *Cancer Chemotherapy Reports 57,* 110.

*Spigel, S. C., Coltman, C. A. and Costanzi, J. J. (1973). Disseminated breast carcinoma: Treatment with combination chemotherapy *Archives of Internal Medicine 132,* 575.

Stott, P. B., Zelkowitz, L. and Tucker, W. G. (1973). Combination chemohormonal therapy for disseminated breast carcinoma. *Cancer Chemotherapy Reports 57,* 106.

*Stutz, F. H., Blom, J. and Tormey, D. C. (1974). Combination chemotherapy in disseminated carcinoma of the breast. *Oncology 29,* 139.

Talley, R. W., Vaitkevicius, V. K. and Leighton, G. A. (1965). Comparison of cyclophosphamide and 5-fluorouracil in the treatment of patients with metastatic breast cancer. *Clinical Pharmacology and Therapeutics 6,* 740.

Taylor, S. G., Canellos, G. P., Band, P. and Pocock, S. (1974). Combination chemotherapy for advanced breast cancer: Randomized comparison with single drug therapy. *Proceedings of the American Society of Clinical Oncology 15,* 175.

Taylor, S. G., Pocock, S. J., Shnider, B. I., Colsky, J. and Hall, T. C. (1975). Clinical studies of 5-fluorouracil + premarin in the treatment of breast cancer. *Medical and Pediatric Oncology 1,* 113.

Tormey, D. C. (1975). Adriamycin in breast cancer: An overview of studies. *Cancer Chemotherapy Reports (Part 3) 6,* 319.

Tormey, D., Falkson, G., Band, P., Blom, J. (1975a). Adriamycin and dibromodulcitol in metastatic breast cancer. *Proceedings of the American Association for Cancer Research 16,* 129.

Tormey, D. C., Waalkes, T. P., Ahmann, D., Gehrke, C. W., Zumwatt, R. W., Snyder, J. and Hansen, H. (1975b). Biological markers in breast carcinoma. I. Incidence of abnormalities of CEA, HCG, three polyamines, and three minor nucleosides. *Cancer 35,* 1095.

Tucker, W. G., Talley, R. W., Lane, M. and Bonnet, J. D. (1975). Treatment of adenocarcinoma with combinations of cyclophosphamide (NSC-26271), vincristine (NSC-67574), and 5-fluorouracil (NSC-19893). *Cancer Chemotherapy Reports 59,* 425.

*Van Dyk, J. J., Falkson, G. and Falkson, H. C. (1972). Bleomycin: A clinical evaluation of the agent on its own or in combination with mitomycin C. *South African Medical Journal 46,* 1921.

Wang, D. Y., Bulbrook, R. D., Hayward, J. L., Hendrick, J. C. and Franchimont, P. (1975). Relationship between plasma carcinoembryonic antigen and prognosis in women with breast cancer. *European Journal of Cancer 11,* 615.

Chapter

13

BASIL A. STOLL

Palliation by Castration or by Hormone Administration

The recent development of an assay for oestrogen receptor protein in human mammary cancer enables us to distinguish those women whose tumour has a very poor chance of response to a change in the existing endocrine balance. So far, however, we have no accurate guide as to the type of endocrine change most suitable for the circumstances existing in each individual patient. Any account of the practice of endocrine therapy in advanced breast cancer must therefore represent the personal experience of the clinician.

The policy of step-by-step endocrine therapy expressed in this section is based on the writer's personal experience and evaluation in the endocrine management of 1013 women with advanced mammary cancer. The details have been published previously (Stoll, 1969).

The endocrine management of women with disseminated mammary cancer will be considered under the following headings:

- Indications for endocrine therapy.
- Selecting the most suitable endocrine therapy.
- Endocrine therapy before the menopause.
- Endocrine therapy in perimenopausal women.
- Endocrine therapy in the older woman.
- Likely future developments.

INDICATIONS FOR ENDOCRINE THERAPY

Until recently it was generally accepted that an attempt at endocrine therapy was indicated when clinical evidence of widespread tumour dissemination appeared in the woman with mammary cancer. However, in the last few years, the markedly improved palliation rate which has been achieved from combination cytotoxic chemotherapy has led some to recommend that chemotherapy should be the primary method of choice (Ansfield et al., 1971; Greenspan, 1972; Sutton, 1973; Lee et al., 1974).

There is little need for confrontation on this issue. In most clinicians' experience the clinical circumstances will dictate the more suitable method, and cytotoxic and endocrine methods of palliation are

Table 1. The use of oestrogen receptor assay of the primary tumour or metastasis as a guide to the selection of patients for systemic therapy.

Oestrogen receptor assay *Primary*	*Metastasis*	*Systemic Treatment*
ER+	ER?	Endocrine therapy
ER?	ER+	Endocrine therapy
ER–	ER?	Immune/cytotoxic therapy
ER?	ER–	Immune/cytotoxic therapy

rarely competing treatments in the women with disseminated mammary cancer (Brunner et al., 1975). In addition, assay of oestrogen receptor protein in the tumour will permit selection of the woman unlikely to respond to endocrine therapy. The significance of oestrogen receptor assay of the primary growth or metastases is discussed in Chapter 8 and its application to the selection of patients for treatment is shown diagrammatically in Table 1.

Unfortunately there is no test with a similar ability to predict the likelihood of response to cytotoxic chemotherapy, but some writers have claimed that hormone insensitive tumours have an increased likelihood of response to cytotoxic agents. It is said that mammary cancers have an increased likelihood of responding to cytotoxic chemotherapy if they have failed to respond to oophorectomy (Talley et al., 1965; Samp and Ansfield, 1966) or to hypophysectomy (Edelstyn et al., 1968). Other authors on the other hand, deny that the nature of response to endocrine therapy bears any relationship to subsequent response to cytotoxic chemotherapy (Nemoto and Dao, 1971).

The extensive tumour burden present in advanced breast cancer is more unfavourable to cytotoxic chemotherapy than it is to endocrine therapy, and the reported response rate to combination chemotherapy seems to have plateaud at a level between 50% and 60% for a mean duration of 6 to 9 months. Some have expressed a hope of breaking through this barrier by combination with endocrine therapy (Brambilla et al., 1976), but there is so far, no convincing evidence that the response rate, either to endocrine ablation or to additive hormonal therapy, has been increased by the concomitant administration of presently available cytotoxic agents (see Chapter 12). If, as suggested above, the likelihood of response to cytotoxic and to endocrine modalities was indeed mutually exclusive, one would expect an unselected group with mammary cancer to show a higher rate of tumour regression from a combination of the two forms of therapy.

There is no evidence however, that oestrogen priming sensitizes breast cancer to cyclophosphamide administration (Meakin, 1970) and it has been reported that combining androgen with antimetabolite therapy may even diminish the response rate (Goldenberg et al., 1975). Whereas antimitotic agents act mainly in the proliferative phase, endocrine therapy may decrease the proportion of cells engaged in active mitosis. It has therefore been suggested that hormonal methods which *increase* the rate of proliferation of the tumour cells might be more useful in combination with cytotoxic therapy. This has obvious clinical dangers apart from the fact that it may encourage the development of clones which are resistant to cytotoxic agents (Boesen, 1974).

The well established practice of combining corticosteroid therapy with cytotoxic agents has, of course, a different rationale from that involving the use of sex steroids (see Chapter 8). An additive affect from a combination of corticosteroid and cytotoxic therapy was first reported in the case of lung metastases from mammary cancer (Stoll, 1960), and a combination of prednisolone with either fluorouracil or chlorambucil was later shown to double the regression rate expected from the latter alone (Freckman et al., 1964; Moore et al., 1967; Goldenberg et al., 1973). The addition of prednisolone to COMF cytotoxic therapy has in many series been claimed to lead to tumour regression in 60-90% of advanced breast cancers, in addition to providing subjective benefit.

Some cancer treatment centres have a tendency to "overkill" in the endocrine or cytotoxic management of women with advanced mammary cancer. There is no firm evidence that either endocrine manipulation or cytotoxic chemotherapy prolongs the life of the patient with advanced mammary cancer, except in the rare presence of a life-threatening complication such as hypercalcaemia. Therefore, our treatment must aim for the relief of the patient's symptoms and the cost in suffering must be commensurate with the possible benefits.

It is pointed out in Chapter 12 that combination cytotoxic therapy has doubled the response rate previously achieved with single agents, but that it also increases the potential for a wider spectrum of complications. "The mortality of combination regimes ranges from zero to ten per cent depending on the patient population, agents and dosages administered, and the experience of the oncologist." The conclusion is that in the pursuit of optimal palliation and maximal survival, a drug combination with a higher response rate for a short period does not, of necessity, provide a better treatment.

In selecting palliative treatment, whether endocrine or cytotoxic, the clinician must consider not only its response rate, but also the likely duration of survival in remission, its degree of completeness and the promptness with which it occurs. Against these four conjectural benefits of treatment must be set the likely morbidity and side effects of treatment, their effect on the patient's well-being and activity, and also their effect on her mood and outlook.

A decision based upon so many imponderables is easier to make when the patient has a severe symptom such as pain which requires urgent palliation. The decision is much more difficult however, if for example, the patient has small or non-symptomatic metastases in the skin, nodes, lungs or liver. Anticipatory treatment has a place under these conditions, but it must be based on informed experience and not given indiscriminately on a "prophylactic" basis, because breast cancer metastases often grow very slowly over a period of years.

Side effects and morbidity of treatment are usually unpleasant but the difficulty is often to compare the degree of unpleasantness to the individual patient. Does one offer the choice of loss of scalp hair as against the stimulation of facial hair growth? Or a choice of intermittent injections, nausea and malaise for months as against the short term morbidity of a major operation?

On the other hand, the side effects of some hormonal agents are sometimes beneficial and a positive advantage to the late cancer patient. Steroids such as corticosteroids (and often androgens and progestogens also) have an intrinsic ability to increase appetite and weight, and can lead to a subjective feeling of well being. These innate properties are not possessed by presently available cytotoxic agents.

SELECTING THE MOST SUITABLE ENDOCRINE THERAPY

As noted at the beginning of the chapter, an assay of the oestrogen receptor content of the tumour (see Chapter 8) will predict the likelihood of response to endocrine therapy. There are, however, also several clinical or biological indicators which may influence the choice of endocrine therapy for the individual patient.

Clinical Indicators

The age group of the patient is the most important of the factors deciding the choice of therapy. There is a fall in the incidence of breast cancer between the ages of 50 and 55 and it has been suggested that this may separate two distict biological types of mammary cancer with different morphological, immunological and endocrinological characteristics. The premenopausal type usually presents before the age of 50 and castration is the most effective method of endocrine treatment. After the age of 55, remission occurs most commonly from oestrogen or anti-oestrogen therapy, and these agents become increasingly more effective with advancing age. Patients whose disease shows progression during the 5 years following the menopause are the least responsive to present methods of endocrine therapy.

The next most important factor in deciding the choice of endocrine therapy is the duration of the recurrence-free interval between mastectomy and the first clinical evidence of recurrence or metastases. The longer the recurrence-free interval the more likely is the tumour to respond to castration, adrenalectomy, hypophysectomy or additive hormone therapy (Treves and Finkbeiner, 1958; Hellstrom and Franksson, 1958; Luft et al., 1958; Escher and Kaufman, 1963).

In terms of cell kinetics, a prolonged recurrence-free interval is thought to reflect a long doubling time and a low proportion of proliferating cells. This in turn may reflect two possibilities—either a genetically determined slowly dividing tumour, or a tumour which has been controlled by the immune or endocrine environment in the host. The latter may explain why almost the only patients who respond to endocrine therapy within five years after the menopause are those with a long recurrence-free interval. It is assumed that these are the patients in whom tumour growth has already been slowed up by the menopause; if bone metastases are present in such cases, they tend to show an osteosclerotic appearance (Stoll, 1969; Powles, 1977).

Doubling times are correlated with cytological and nuclear grading and well differentiated tumours are generally slowly growing. Adenocarcinoma of the breast however shows a very wide variation in growth fraction and the gross doubling times of breast cancers are usually not related to the histological type of the tumour. The tendency of a tumour to differentiate may depend (as does the rate of growth) both on genetically determined cell characteristics and on the effect of the immune or endocrine environment.

The third factor deciding the choice of endocrine therapy is the tissue which is predominantly affected by the metastases. In general, soft tissue metastases seem to offer the greatest likelihood of regression, response is less likely in the case of bone metastases and it is least likely for brain and liver metastases. But

in addition, each type of therapy is selective in its site response. Thus oestrogen, anti-oestrogen and progestogen therapy give their best results in the case of soft tissue metastases, androgen therapy and endocrine ablation in the case of bone metastases, and corticosteroids give the best palliation for visceral metastases.

Fourthly, the nature of response to previous endocrine therapy is important in deciding the choice of a second modality of treatment. One can predict that patients responding to castration will have a very high likelihood of responding later to adrenalectomy or hypophysectomy, provided that significant *objective* response was shown to castration. Relief of pain or lack of progression of a tumour following castration is not sufficient justification for a major operation such as adrenalectomy or hypophysectomy.

It should be noted that endocrine therapy and cytotoxic therapy are, *in some respects*, mutually exclusive with regard to factors influencing response. Women within 5 years after the menopause have a poor response rate to all forms of endocrine therapy, but the regression rate from cyclophosphamide and fluorouracil therapy is as high in this age group as in other age groups although this does not apparently apply to adriamycin therapy (see Chapter 12). Moreover, while a short recurrence-free period predicts a poor response to all forms of endocrine therapy, it has been shown in the case of cyclophosphamide and fluorouracil at least, that the regression rate from cytotoxic agents is twice as great when the period is less than 2 years than when it is more than 2 years (Ravdin and Eisman, 1967; Nemoto and Dao, 1971). Again, this does not appear to apply to adriamycin therapy.

The doubling rate of a tumour reflects the proportion of cells engaged in active growth and since most cytotoxic agents exert their major cancericidal effect during the proliferative cycle, one would expect the most susceptible tumours to be those with a rapid growth rate. A clinical manifestation of this contrast between cytotoxic and endocrine responsiveness is seen in the case of rapidly growing types of cutaneous infiltration such as "carcinoma en cuirasse" or "inflammatory" carcinoma of the breast. Whereas such tumours commonly regress on combination cytotoxic chemotherapy (Greenspan, 1972; Hanham et al., 1974), they rarely show response to endocrine therapy (Stoll, 1972).

Biological Indicators

The "discriminant function". It has been suggested that the proportion of androgenic to corticosteroid metabolites in the urine of the mammary cancer patient might be useful to predict the likelihood of a tumour responding to bilateral adrenalectomy or to hypophysectomy (Bulbrook et al., 1960). The predictive value of the findings was thought to be associated mainly with reduced androgen excretion (Miller and Durant, 1968), but the raised corticoid excretion also might play a part.

In the earlier reports, the discriminant was shown to distinguish patients with a 30% likelihood of response to major endocrine ablation from those with only a 13% chance of response (Atkins et al., 1968). The gap between the figures has narrowed in more recent surveys and the specificity of the test has also been questioned. Raised corticosteroid production in breast cancer patients has been shown to be associated with a poor outcome of the disease (Saez, 1974), while a reduced androgen excretion has been shown also in women with advanced non-mammary cancer, advanced hepatic disease or severe surgical stress (Durant and Miller, 1973). An unfavourable "discriminant" may therefore be an indicator of advanced disease.

In vitro assays. It has been suggested that response to hormonal manipulation can be predicted by observing the effect of hormones on the metabolism and morphology of breast cancer in tissue culture. The effect of the hormone on culture viability or on DNA synthesis can be shown in monolayer cultures (single cell aggregations), but to assess an effect on the function and morphology of the intact tissue, the integrity of the explant must be maintained in a short term organ culture.

It would seem unlikely that such *in vitro* response could predict the *in vivo* effect of hormonal administration. The proliferative kinetics both of tumour cell and stroma are different in the two instances. Moreover, the metabolic changes to which the hormone is subjected in the body and the homeostatic changes which it causes, cannot be reproduced under *in vitro* conditions.

Nevertheless, it has been reported by Burstein et al. (1971) that the effect of hormones on the uptake of tritiated thymidine in a monolayer suspension of breast cancer can be correlated with the clinical response of the tumour to endocrine therapy. In addition, the group led by Hobbs (1974) claims in a series of reports that testing of organ cultures for dependence on oestrogen, androgen or prolactin led to correct prediction of clinical response to endocrine therapy in 37 out of 40 patients.

Tumour sex chromatin. It was first suggested by Kimel (1957) that the proportion of breast cancer cells showing sex chromatin in the nucleus might

predict the likelihood of tumour response to oophorectomy or to androgen therapy. Sex chromatin is believed to represent the second X chromosome in the female somatic cell nucleus. Its presence in over 15% of tumour nuclei is regarded as normal for the female karyotype, while the presence of sex chromatin in less than 5% of tumour cell nuclei is termed a male karyotype.

Several reports since Bohle (1965) have confirmed his finding that tumours with a low sex chromatin content are less likely to respond to hypophysectomy, oophorectomy or androgen administration. A report by Perry (1972) compared the value of the sex chromatin count with that of the discriminant factor, and found the former more reliable in predicting response to hypophysectomy. The presence of the male karyotype is said to be associated with a poor prognosis, as well as with a low likelihood of response to endocrine manipulation (Kimel, 1957; Bohle, 1965). The explanation may be that sex chromatin is less easily recognised in anaplastic tumours. These would tend to be associated with a poor prognosis and possibly also with a lower likelihood of response to endocrine manipulation.

Hormonal Sensitivity and Clinical Response

Although a breast cancer shows biological evidence of hormonal sensitivity, it need not necessarily show clinical evidence of tumour regression after endocrine therapy; nor does the absence of regression signify lack of hormonal sensitivity. In most large series, a significant degree of tumour regression following endocrine manipulation is seen in about 25% of unselected patients and the following are the reasons that this represents only a small proportion of the tumours whose growth is actually affected by hormonal manipulation:

(1) Although a biological indicator or assay of oestrogen receptors may suggest sensitivity of the cancer to hormonal change, the response to endocrine therapy may be either inhibition or stimulation of growth. In fact, both effects could occur at the same time if more than one tumour clone is represented in the patient's tumour.

In the case of the postmenopausal patient given oestrogen or androgen therapy, there is often an increase in the size of soft tissue metastases, or an increase in the pain of bone metastases during the first three weeks of treatment. Yet, it is found in some of these cases, that if the patient persists in taking the hormone, it is followed by tumour regression later (Stoll, 1969). In the case of the premenopausal patient, oestrogen administration may stimulate the activity of breast cancer, but if the dose of diethyl stilboestrol is raised to 1 G daily, tumour regression may result (Kennedy, 1962).

The balance between inhibition and stimulation of tumour growth may be seen in the so-called "withdrawal response". Figure 1 graphically shows regression occurring three times over a period of five years as a result of intermittent oestrogen administration in an 81-year-old woman. After the third response, the oestrogen appeared to be stimulating the growth of the tumour and only when it was stopped did the tumour regress. Tumour stimulation can occur also following surgical endocrine ablation and has been reported both in a large adrenalectomy series (Wilson et al., 1958) and in a large oophorectomy series (Fracchia et al., 1969).

(2) As a result of specific site factors both inhibition and exacerbation of tumour growth may be seen in the patient at the same time. Figure 2 shows the response of a 62-year-old woman to oestrogen therapy. Her soft tissue metastases showed rapid regression but while they did so, new bone

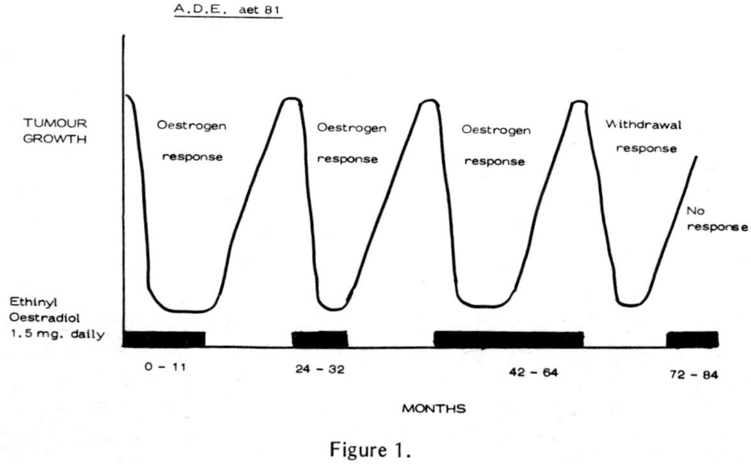

Figure 1.

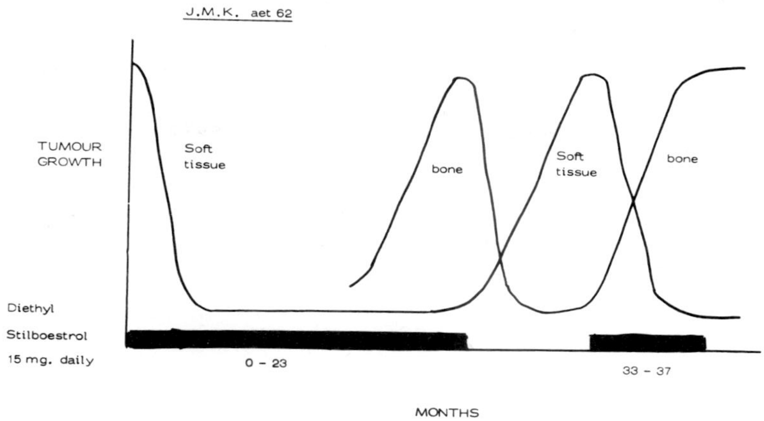

Figure 2.

metastases appeared and increased in size. When the oestrogen was stopped, the bone metastases regressed but the soft tissue tumour grew. The opposite occurred when the hormone was started again. Specific site factors are obviously involved, and the healing of bone metastases may involve an effect on local prostaglandin or calcitonin concentrations (Bennett et al., 1975; Powles, 1977).

(3) A third reason why the presence of hormone sensitivity may not predict clinical tumour regression following endocrine therapy, is that regression of a tumour requires that the rate of cell death shall exceed the rate of cell division. But the relationship between the two depends on a number of factors including the blood supply to the part (providing oxygen and nutrients), and the doubling time of the tumour cells. Even if cell division is considerably slowed by endocrine therapy, the death of adult cells may be so delayed that obvious reduction in tumour size does not occur.

This means that the degree and rate of regression can vary widely from tumour to tumour, even if the hormonal stimulus is similar. Yet, the widely accepted criteria of clinical regression require that the tumour measurements shall be reduced by at least one half. We find this degree of response in about 25% of cases, but there is another 20 to 30% of cases where the diameters of the tumour are reduced by something less than half. These tumours are showing evidence of biological sensitivity even if their degree of response is not acceptable to the clinician.

(4) The fourth reason why biological evidence of hormonal sensitivity does not always predict clinical regression is the variety in the methods of hormonal manipulation used and the differences between their mechanisms of action. This is discussed fully in Chapter 8.

ENDOCRINE THERAPY BEFORE THE MENOPAUSE

Until recently, castration either by surgery or by irradiation was practised in all premenopausal women presenting with recurrent or advanced mammary cancer. It is, however, better restricted to those women whose tumours possess a significant level of oestrogen receptor protein (ER+) if facilities for the assay are available. A similar selection of patients for castration is practised after hysterectomy or up to two years after the natural menopause, if serial assays of oestrogen excretion or of vaginal cytology suggest cyclical oestrogen secretion by the ovary.

Castration should be surgical if tumour growth appears to be rapid, or in the presence of urgent symptoms such as those associated with multiple bone metastases or visceral deposits. On the other hand, it is possible to use radiation castration if tumour growth is relatively indolent. The latter has been proved just as effective in ablating ovarian activity, but requires at least 3 months after irradiation before oestrogen excretion levels become minimal (Stoll, 1969). Although amenorrhoea may be delayed, tumour regression is sometimes seen earlier, suggesting that *complete* ablation of ovarian function is not necessary for the tumour to show response (see Chapter 8). On the other hand, tumour regression is sometimes delayed up to 5 or 6 months after radiation castration.

The regression rate reported from surgical castration in large series of mammary cancer patients is between 25 and 30% (Taylor, 1962; Hall et al., 1963; O'Bryan et al., 1974). There is no evidence that the results of castration are better in the case of histologically differentiated types of mammary cancer. Most reports agree that the results are worse

Table 2. Response to oophorectomy in advanced breast compared to that from "medical castration" by androgen therapy.

	Oophorectomy	Androgen
Regression rate (Pearson et al., 1965)	44%	13%
Mean duration regression (Hortling et al., 1962)	25 months	12 months

in women under the age of 35 than in those over the age of 35 (Taylor, 1962).

Androgen therapy will usually cause temporary amenorrhoea but "medical castration" using androgens is not advised as the primary method of endocrine therapy. Firstly, the dose required to cause amenorrhoea will almost inevitably lead to some symptoms of masculinisation. Secondly, in series where androgen therapy has been compared to surgical castration, it has yielded a much lower percentage and also a shorter duration of tumour regression (Table 2). There is also no advantage to be gained from combining androgen administration with castration as a routine, although in the case of women under the age of 35, I have found it to improve the usually poor response rate. The masculinising side effects may therefore be justified in such cases.

It is generally stated that response of mammary cancer to castration is more likely the longer the recurrence-free interval after primary treatment (Treves and Finkbeiner, 1958), but this is not confirmed in all series (Stoll, 1969; O'Bryan et al., 1974). The response rate to castration varies with the site of metastasis; bone metastases are the most likely to respond with sclerosis and relief of pain in over one third of cases, while soft tissue tumour in the breast, chest wall or nodes responds less often. Visceral metastases respond least frequently. While nodular metastases in the lung fields not uncommonly regress after castration, the lymphatic type of infiltration in the lung field rarely does.

In the very ill patient or in the presence of visceral or brain metastases, hypercalcaemia or leuco-erythroblastic anaemia, castration is best combined with corticosteroid therapy. High dosage of prednisone (at least 30 mg but up to 100 mg daily) is often required. However, the routine administration of corticosteroids at the time of castration, which has been suggested by some to simulate "adrenalectomy", is not recommended.

If oestrogen receptor assays are not available, response to castration is the best test we have of predicting later response to other forms of endocrine therapy especially adrenalectomy or hypophysectomy (see Chapter 14). There is a 3 to 4 fold greater likelihood of responding to major endocrine ablation in women who have responded to castration than in those who have failed to respond. As an alternative to adrenalectomy or hypophysectomy, tamoxifen (Nolvadex ®) or progestational agents such as norethisterone acetate (SH420®) or medroxyprogesterone acetate (Provera®) may be tried if soft tissue metastases predominate, while androgen may be tried if bone metastases predominate (see next section).

The Controversial Role of Androgen

Androgen therapy has been used widely as secondary hormonal therapy especially in the younger woman with advanced mammary cancer. Although regression of tumour is noted in only 20% of cases, the pain of bone metastases is relieved in over 80% of cases (Stoll, 1969). Moreover, a general sense of well being and increase in appetite and weight results in the majority of patients treated. Some clinicians however, oppose the use of androgen *under any circumstances* in mammary cancer, because of its tendency to cause masculinising symptoms. When challenged, it is nearly always found that their opinion is based on experience with older agents such as testosterone propionate or methyl testosterone.

It has been shown and confirmed (Stoll, 1958; Co-operative Breast Group, 1964) that the administration of fluoxymesterone (Halotestin®, Ultandren®) at a dosage of 20-30 mg daily by mouth will lead to similar regression rates to the older agents, and that when used for a trial period of 3 months, virilisation is almost never seen. If the agent leads to palliation, the patient can decide after 3 months whether the likely need for the use of a depilatory cream on the face is too high a price to pay for the relief which she has obtained. Several new androgenic agents have been introduced in recent years including 2α methyl dihydrotestosterone (Drolban® Masteril®) 7β17 dimethyltestosterone (Calusterone®, Methosarb®) and $\triangle$1 testololactone (Teslac®). In spite of early enthusiasm, none has proved both less virilising and more effective than fluoxymesterone in the palliation of mammary cancer (Gordan et al., 1972; Talley et al., 1973; Falkson et al., 1974).

After the menopause too, androgen is the most effective form of additive hormonal therapy for the treatment of bone metastases better even than anti-oestrogen therapy (Ward, 1976). Its stimulating effect on haemopoiesis is in contrast with the depressant

Table 3. Objective response rate to androgen therapy in 434 patients with advanced breast cancer, according to age group in relation to menopause and according to dominant site of metastases (Stoll, 1969).

		Total cases	*% showing regression*
Age group	Postmenopausal 0-5 years	212	10%
	Postmenopausal >5 years	222	24%
Site	Local soft tissue	149	16%
	Bonemetastases	204	19%
	Visceral metastases	81	11%
	Total	434	15%

effect of cytotoxic agents on an already damaged bone marrow. The effectiveness of androgen is relatively low in the immediate postmenopausal years (except in the treatment of osteosclerotic metastases) but it increases with age (Table 3). Particularly in the perimenopausal woman with widespread bone metastases, there is a danger of precipitating hypercalcaemia in the first few weeks of androgen therapy and it is important that regular serum calcium estimations should be carried out.

Because recalcification of bone metastases is not visible radiographically until after three months of therapy, a trial of androgen for at least three months has been found necessary in the past. However, recent reports suggest that measurement of biological tumour markers such as hydroxyproline/creatine (Roberts et al., 1975) or serial isotopic bone scans (Citrin et al., 1974) may in the future, be able to provide advance information on the likelihood of bone metastases healing under therapy.

ENDOCRINE THERAPY IN THE PERIMENOPAUSAL WOMAN

Several observers have shown prolongation of the recurrence-free interval after mastectomy in patients who are within 5 years after the menopause (Clemmesen, 1948; Smithers et al., 1952; AMA Committee, 1960). It has also been evident for many years that response to endocrine therapy of every type is least likely in this age group. The most likely explanation for these two observations is that human mammary cancer is composed of multiple clones, each with a different hormonal sensitivity; the growth of those cells which are sensitive to the endocrine homeostatic changes of the menopause will be inhibited in those women where the clinical development of the tumour spans the menopausal years. The cells which proliferate and gradually replace the tumour are therefore unlikely to respond to the types of hormonal manipulation at present in use.

In the case of cytotoxic therapy however, it is reported that the period within 5 years after the menopause yields a regression rate in mammary cancer as high as that in other age groups (Brunner, 1969) or even higher (Ravdin and Eisman, 1967; Nemoto and Dao, 1971). It is therefore obvious that to secure the highest possible regression rate in the first 5 years after the menopause, it is necessary to select therapy according to the characteristics of the patient and tumour.

There is no evidence that ER+ tumours in perimenopausal patients show a less than average response rate to endocrine therapy. A specimen of the tumour should therefore be examined for the presence of oestrogen receptor protein, and if ER+, an antioestrogen such as tamoxifen (Nolvadex®) is most likely to give a response (see p. 142). Alternatively, progestational agents such as norethisterone acetate (SH 420®) or medroxyprogesterone acetate (Provera®) may be used. Osteosclerotic bone metastases in this age group are usually hormone sensitive (see p. 135) and their pain will nearly always respond to androgen therapy. Hypophyseal ablation by the transnasal route can be considered later if there has been a temporary response to the additive hormone therapy.

If however, oestrogen receptor assay is not available, one has to be guided by clinical criteria. The perimenopausal patient with a short recurrence-free interval following mastectomy is unlikely to respond to any form of sex hormone therapy or to endocrine ablation, particularly if she has visceral metastases. Such cases are best treated by combination cytotoxic therapy (see Chapter 12) in conjunction with corticosteroid therapy.

The effect of corticosteroids in mammary carcinoma is quite unrelated to sex hormone sensitivity (Stoll, 1963), and their effect is to decrease oedema

Table 4. Objective response rate to oestrogen therapy in 407 patients with advanced breast cancer, according to age group in relation to menopause and according to dominant site of metastases (Stoll, 1969).

		Total cases	*% showing regression*
Age group	Postmenopausal 0-5 years	63	9%
	Postmenopausal >5 years	344	35%
Site	Local soft tissue	285	36%
	Bone metastases	62	7%
	Visceral metastases	60	28%
	Total	407	31%

around tumour deposits. They are, therefore, most valuable palliative agents for lung, brain or liver metastases, whatever the age of the patient. The ability of corticosteroid therapy to cause a subjective feeling of well-being and increase in appetite and weight is also most valuable, and its effect is often life-saving in the treatment of hypercalcaemia and leucoerythroblastic anaemia. However, remissions from corticosteroid therapy are usually short (between 6 and 9 months) and in this respect they resemble remissions from cytotoxic therapy.

ENDOCRINE THERAPY IN THE OLDER WOMAN

Treatment with oestrogen has long been advised as the primary step in the endocrine therapy of advanced mammary cancer in the older woman. In this age group, oestrogen therapy yields a higher rate of tumour regression than any other form of treatment, and more than 50% of women over the age of 70 will show response if they persist with oestrogen treatment. However, oestrogen therapy should not be instituted until after ovarian secretion has ceased, as reflected in serial oestrogen excretion estimations or vaginal smear assays. In practice, oestrogens may be prescribed safely if more than 5 years have elapsed since the menopause, or after hysterectomy if the patient is aged over 50.

The objective remission rate from oestrogen therapy was 31% overall in the writer's series of 407 cases (Stoll, 1969). As seen in Table 4, the remission rate increases markedly with increasing number of years after the menopause. Response is more likely also with a relatively longer recurrence-free interval. The average period before reactivation of the tumour is 16 months and survival is prolonged an average of 17 months in responding cases compared to non-responders. Since the responders include a higher proportion with a long recurrence-free period, it is possible that prolonged survival merely reflects a more slowly growing tumour.

Healing of even large ulcerated tumours, and regression of metastatic nodules and nodes is common in older women after oestrogen therapy. Regression of metastases in the lungs, pleura or peritoneum is often dramatic, but healing and sclerosis of bone metastases is much less common than it is from androgen therapy (see p. 139). Liver or brain metastases rarely respond to oestrogen therapy and are best treated by a combination of high dosage of corticosteroids associated with cytotoxic therapy.

The earliest sign of tumour regression usually appears within 4 to 6 weeks of initiating oestrogen therapy and a tumour cannot be regarded as unresponsive unless the drug trial is continued for at least 3 months. However, measurement of biological tumour markers may in the future, provide advance information on the likelihood of tumour regression (see Chapter 8). One of the remarkable features of oestrogen therapy is the so-called "withdrawal response". When tumour response to oestrogen administration is lost, it is found in 30% of cases that stopping the agent will lead to a second although shorter period of tumour regression. It is seen with other sex steroids also.

The synthetic oestrogen diethyl stilboestrol is usually given at a dose of 5 mg tds orally, although it has been shown in a randomized trial that 0.5 mg tds is just as efficacious (Stoll, 1969). Doses up to 1 G daily have been tested with no evidence of extra benefit, but markedly increased side effects. Ethinyl oestradiol is preferred by some and is usually given at a dose of 0.5 mg tds. In the presence of preliminary intolerance to either of these agents, Premarin®, a natural combination of conjugated oestrogens (mainly oestrone), is usually well tolerated at a dosage of 2.5 mg tds. When tolerance to oestrogen has been assured, treatment can be maintained by

intramuscular injection of oestradiol valerate 20 mg weekly.

Side effects from oestrogen administration are seen in 15 to 20% of women treated with oestrogen. Nausea and vomiting are the commonest symptoms and may be prevented either by giving the daily dose of oestrogen at night together with an antiemetic, or by building up the dose slowly to the required level. Fluid retention, swelling of the ankles and stress incontinence of micturition are not uncommon. Uterine bleeding is usually of the withdrawal type, but occasionally may be of a breakthrough character when it can be counteracted by *raising* the oestrogen dosage level.

In women whose tumours have responded to oestrogen therapy and then lost their response, secondary hormonal therapy is worth a trial. Progestational agents such as norethisterone acetate (SH 420®) or medroxyprogesterone acetate (Provera®) may be tried if soft tissue metastases predominate, or androgens if bone metastases predominate.

Anti-oestrogen Therapy

Oestrogen therapy has been used for 30 years with considerable success, in the treatment of the older patient with advanced mammary cancer. There is, however, every indication in the U.K. that anti-oestrogens such as tamoxifen (Nolvadex®) are going to replace it for this purpose. Anti-oestrogens are in general just as effective as oestrogens in this disease, but without the common disadvantages of gastro-intestinal intolerance and breakthrough or withdrawal bleeding. They have two additional advantages over oestrogen—they have not been shown to cause exacerbation of tumour growth and they may cause tumour regression even in the premenopausal patient.

Three anti-oestrogens have been reported in the clinical management of mammary cancer-clomiphene, nafoxidine and tamoxifen (Nolvadex®). The major case report on Clomiphene given at a dose of 100-250 mg orally daily, is by Brewin (1973). He noted regression in 42% of 110 cases and comments that the reponse was independent of the site of metastases, and better in the older age groups. The use of nafoxidine at a dose of 180-270 mg orally daily, has been reported by the EORTC Breast Group (1972), Bloom and Boesen (1974) and Heuson et al., (1975). The regression rates reported were 33% in 24 cases, 37% in 48 cases and 28% in 108 cases respectively, but a marked disadvantage is the frequent development of photosensitivity and ichthyosis of the skin.

The largest experience has been with tamoxifen (Nolvadex®) and the major reports emanate from the U.K. This agent is the *tran*-isomer of 1-(p-β-dimethyl-aminoethoxyphenyl) 1-2,diphenylbut-1-ene. It is a potent anti-oestrogen in several (but not all) mammalian species where it prevents replenishment of oestrogen receptors. While high dosage leads to a cornifying effect on the vaginal mucosa in some cases, the reason for this is not clear. The dose recommended for treatment of breast cancer is 20-40 mg orally daily in divided dosage (Cole et al., 1971; Ward et al., 1973, 1976; Band et al., 1976; Barrett, 1976).

All agree that side effects are very infrequent, and even then they are usually mild. Ward (1976) reports that only two out of 200 patients had to withdraw from drug trials and this compares with the 15% of patients who withdraw from oestrogen trials because of drug intolerance. Weight increase with some fluid retention, or hot flushes are reported in about 10% of cases but are mild and tend to subside with time. Nausea, headaches or vertigo are reported in about 5% of cases but can usually be controlled. A transient fall in the platelet count has been reported in a few patients (Ward et al., 1973; Band et al., 1976). Withdrawal or breakthrough uterine bleeding are normally not seen.

More than 50% decrease in tumour size has been reported in 22% of 46 cases (Cole et al., 1971), 32% of 187 cases (Ward, 1976), 44% of 41 cases (Band et al., 1976), and 60% of 59 cases (Barrett, 1976). The best responses are seen in soft tissue deposits but large liver and lung deposits often regress also. On the other hand, recalcification in bone metastases is only rarely reported, although stimulation of hyper-calcaemia has been reported (Patterson, 1976). The duration of response is usually about one year the mean being 11.4 months in the series of Barrett (1976). The response rate is rather less in patients within 5 years after the menopause than in older patients (Ward, 1976; Fiorentino, 1976), but response is recorded in three of 15 premenopausal patients mentioned in different series (Ward, 1976; Barrett, 1976; Willis, 1976).

Ward (1976) reports that a high proportion of patients failing to respond to tamoxifen, subsequently respond to oestrogen, androgen or progestogen (or *vice versa*) and the mechanism of response may be different. He also reports that patients who cease to respond to tamoxifen may achieve another response from the addition of agents such as levodopa or bromocriptine which lower serum prolactin levels.

The clinical response to anti-oestrogen resembles that due to oestrogen in that soft tissue and lung metastases are more likely to respond than are bone

metastases. The response may differ from that of oestrogen, in that it is not more likely in the presence of a long recurrence-free interval (Bloom and Boesen, 1973; Band et al., 1976).

LIKELY FUTURE DEVELOPMENTS

We have noted above that although only about one in four breast cancer patients shows clinical response to our present methods of endocrine manipulation, it is likely that the *majority* of breast cancers have some degree of hormonal sensitivity (see p. 137). A major improvement in the proportion of patients responding to endocrine therapy will come firstly, when we establish in each individual which of her endogenous hormones are stimulating mitotic activity in the tumour, and secondly, when we are able to inhibit or modify the effect of the hormones at the tumour level. Not only will the proportion of patients responding be increased but hopefully also the degree and duration of response; even possibly long enough for the patient to die of intercurrent disease. Hormonal control of disseminated breast cancer for five or more years is not uncommon even at present.

But to achieve these improvements, we will need a detailed knowledge both of the genetic characteristics of the tumour and also of the hormonal profile of the host, and treatment in each patient will need to be individualized. The homeostatic mechanisms which adjust to the administration of hormones or endocrine ablation are so complex in the human, that it is unlikely that any *one* hormonal manipulation will be able to cause inhibition of tumour growth in all patients.

For the immediate future, our possible advances can lie only in improving the selection of patients for treatment and in decreasing the morbidity of presently used methods. The approaches are as follows:

- Select the individuals with a high likelihood of responding to our available methods of hormonal manipulation.
- Plan monitored trials of hormonal therapy using biological tumour markers.
- Refine the present methods of hormonal manipulation.

With regard to the first method, we have been able to double the response rate to endocrine therapy by looking for evidence of oestrogen receptor protein in the tumour. Assay also of the other hormone receptors of the tumour cell will help to identify the genetic characteristics of each tumour, and thus select patients with a high likelihood of response to specific methods of endocrine manipulation (See Chapter 8).

The second method, involving the use of biological markers to monitor the course of a trial of therapy, will soon apply to all methods of treatment in breast cancer—surgical, radiation, endocrine, cytotoxic and immunological. Possible use in trials of adjuvant endocrine therapy is discussed in Chapter 8, but in advanced disease a change in the level of markers should provide early information as to the likelihood of tumour regression and will stop the clinician from persisting with useless treatment.

With regard to the third method of improving our approach to endocrine therapy, there have been considerable efforts made in recent years to develop selective pharmacological methods of hormonal ablation. To ablate *all* the trophic hormones of the pituitary and to burden the patient with cortisone/thyroid replacement for the rest of her life is obviously a crude approach. A "pharmacological hypophysectomy" could eliminate selected trophic hormones; but which hormones and how?

It has been made clear in a randomised controlled clinical trial (Table 5) that hypophysectomy is markedly superior to combined adrenalectomy and oophorectomy, both in the proportion of patients responding, the duration of remission and the duration of survival after treatment (Hayward et al., 1970). This suggests that there must be a pituitary trophic hormone other than gonadotrophin and ACTH which is important in controlling the growth of mammary cancer. It has been suspected for many years that prolactin plays this major role and that hormone sensitive mammary cancer is prolactin-dependent as well as being oestrogen-dependent.

This certainly applies in the case of the hormone sensitive DMBA-induced mammary cancer in rats, which resembles the human tumour closely in that it responds to oophorectomy, hypophysectomy, adrenalectomy, androgen and oestrogen administration. The rat tumour clearly shows inhibition of tumour growth after the administration of either levodopa or bromocriptine, both of which cause marked reduction in serum prolactin levels (Welsch

Table 5. Randomised prospective trial comparing objective remission from hypophysectomy to that of bilateral adrenalectomy in advanced breast cancer (Hayward et al., 1970).

	Bilateral adrenalectomy	*Hypophysectomy*
Total cases	77	70
Response rate	23%	36%
Mean remission	26.3 months	37.1 months
Mean survival of responders	31.6 months	40.8 months

and Meites, 1974). However, in the case of the human tumour, although both agents reduce the serum prolactin level, there is no clinical evidence of regression of mammary cancer after their administration (EORTC Breast Group, 1973; Stoll, 1973).

It is possible that in spite of similarities in their other responses, the prolactin/oestrogen ratio at the mammary cancer is more critical for response in the case of the human than it is in the rat. Alternatively, it may be the case in the human tumour that pituitary trophic hormones other than prolactin may be important. Human growth hormone may be involved, as tumours responding to prolactin in vitro are said to respond also to growth hormone (De Souza et al., 1975). Alternatively sebotrophic hormone may be involved (Goolamali and Shuster, 1975). This little known peptide may be allied to the melanocyte-stimulating hormone (MSH).

CONCLUSION

The ongoing search for new steroid derivatives, with both a greater effect on mammary cancer and lesser side effects on the host, has not been very successful. In spite of enthusiastic preliminary reports on androgens such as 2α methyl dehydrolestosterone, 7β17 dimethyltestosterone and Δ1 testololactone, it appears from current trials that none of these agents has both a better therapeutic effect and lesser side effects than the established androgen fluoxymesterone, introduced 20 years ago. However, the greatest advance in the field of additive hormone therapy is the recent introduction of the anti-oestrogen tamoxifen (Cole et al., 1971). This agent appears to yield the same regression rate as oestrogen but with almost negligible side effects, and apparently no danger of stimulating the growth of mammary cancer in the younger woman.

In the 25 years since the first hypophysectomy and adrenalectomy were carried out, there has been little improvement in the field except the introduction of the transethmoidal approach to the pituitary fossa (see Chapter 14). This provides the same degree of palliation as the more extensive operations with a much decreased morbidity.

The development of selective pharmacological hypophysectomy awaits more accurate knowledge of hypophyseal and hypothalamic control of mammary cancer in the human, and its application to the individual patient. When this is combined with assays of the various hormone receptors in the tumour cell, and assays of biological tumour markers in the body, we will be able to do more than palliate symptoms. We may be able to exert control over the spread of the disease and prolong life—a not inconsiderable aim for a disease which is believed to be widely disseminated in the majority of patients by the time it comes to primary treatment.

REFERENCES

AMA Committee on Research (1960). Androgens and estrogens in the treatment of disseminated mammary carcinoma. *J. Amer. Med. Assoc. 172,* 1271.

Ansfield, F. J., Ramiréz. G., Korbitz, G. C. and Davis, H. L. (1971). Five drug therapy for advanced breast cancer. Phase 1 Study. *Cancer Chemother. Rep. 55,* 183.

Atkins, H., Bulbrook, R. D., Falconer, M. A., Hayward, J. L., MacLean, K. C. and Schurr, P. H. (1968). Urinary steroids in the prediction of response to adrenalectomy or hypophysectomy. *Lancet 2,* 1261.

Band, P. R., Lerner, H., Israel, L. and Leung, B. (1976). In *Proceedings of Symposium on Hormonal Control of Breast Cancer.*

Barrett, A. (1976). In *Proceedings of Symposium on Hormonal Control of Breast Cancer.* Macclesfield.

Bennett, A., McDonald, A. M., Simpson, J. S. and Stamford, I. F. (1975). Breast cancer, prostaglandins and bone metastases. *Lancet 1,* 1218.

Bloom, H. J. G. and Boesen, E. (1974). Anti-oestrogens in treatment of breast cancer. Value of nafoxidine in 52 advanced cases. *Brit. Med. J. 2,* 7.

Boesen, E. (1974). Chemotherapy in breast cancer. *Proc. Roy. Soc. Med. 67,* 26.

Bohle, A. (1965). Significance of Barr bodies in mammary carcinoma. *Med. Welt. 23,* 1266, English abstract in *Cancer Chemother. Rep. 6,* 1345.

Brambilla, C., De Lena, M., Rossi, A., Valagussa, P. and Bonadonna, G. (1976). Response and survival in advanced breast cancer after two non-cross-resistant combinations. *Brit. Med. J. 1,* 801.

Brewin, T. B. (1973). Paper presented at 8th International Congress of Chemotherapy. Athens, September 1973.

Brunner, K. W. (1969). Combination chemotherapy of hormone resistant metastasising breast carcinoma. *Schweiz. Med. Wschr. 99,* 1298.

Brunner, K. W., Sonntag, R. W., Martz, G., Senn, H. J., Obrecht, P. and Alberto, P. (1975). A controlled study in the use of combined drug therapy for metastatic breast cancer. *Cancer 36,* 1208.

Bulbrook, R. D., Greenwood, F. C. and Hayward, J. L. (1960). Selection of breast cancer patients for adrenalectomy or hypophysectomy by determination of urinary 17 hydroxycorticosteroids and aetiocholanolone. *Lancet 1,* 1154.

Burstein, N. A., Kjellberg, R. N., Raker, J. W. and Shmidek, H. H. (1971). Human carcinoma of the breast in vitro, the effect of hormones. *Cancer 27,* 1112.

Citrin, D. L., Bessent, R. G., Tuohu, J. B., Greig, W. R. and

Blumgart, L. H. (1974). Quantitative bone scanning. A method of assessing response of bone metastases to treatment. *Lancet 2*, 1132.

Clemmesen, J. (1948). Carcinoma of breast. Results from statistical research. *Brit. J. Radiol. 21*, 583.

Cole, M. P., Jones, C.T.A. and Todd, I.D.H. (1971). A new anti-oestrogenic agent in late breast cancer. An early clinical appraisal of ICI 46474. *Brit. J. Cancer 25*, 270.

Co-operative Breast Cancer Group (1964). Testosterone propionate therapy in breast cancer. *J. Amer. Med. Assoc. 188*, 106.

De Souza, I., Morgan, L., Lewis, U. J., Raggatt, P. R., Salih, H. and Hobbs, J. R. (1974). Growth hormone dependency among human breast cancers. *Lancet 2*, 182.

Durant, J. A. and Miller, H. (1973). Non-specific factors that may influence significance of urinary excretion in breast cancer. *Brit. Med. J. 4*, 767.

Edelstyn, G., Gleadhill, C. and Lyons, A. (1968). Total hypophysectomy for advanced breast cancer. *Clin. Radiol. 19*, 426.

Escher, G. C. and Kaufman, R. J. (1963). Advanced breast carcinoma—factors influencing survival. *Acta Unio. Int. Contra. Canc. 19*, 1039.

E.O.R.T.C. Breast Cancer Group (1972). Clinical trial of nafoxidine and oestrogen antagonists in advanced breast cancer. *European J. Cancer 8*, 387.

E.O.R.T.C. Breast Cancer Group (1973). Clinical trial of Bromergocriptine in advanced breast cancer. *Europ. J. Cancer 9*, 657.

Falkson, G., van Dyk, J. J., van Eden, E. B., van der Merwe A. M. and Falkson, H. L. (1974). Calusterone, a poor substitute for fluoxymesterone in the treatment of advanced breast cancer. *Cancer Chemother. Rep. 58*, 939.

Fiorentino, M. (1976). In *Proceedings of Symposium on Hormonal Control of Breast Cancer.* Macclesfield.

Fracchia, A. A., Farrow, J. H., de Palo, A. J. et al. (1969). Castration for primary inoperable and recurrent breast cancer. *Surg. Gynec. Obst. 128*, 1226.

Freckman, H. A., Fry, H. L., Mendez, F. L. and Maurer, E. R. (1964). Chlorambucil/prednisone therapy for disseminated breast cancer. *J. Amer. Med. Assoc. 189*, 23.

Goldenberg, I. S., McMahan, C. A., Escher, G. C., Volk, H., Ansfield, F. J. and Olson, K. B. (1973). Secondary chemotherapy of advanced breast cancer. *Cancer 31*, 660.

Goldenberg, I. S., Sedransk, N., Volk, H., Segaloff, A., Kelley, R. M. and Haines, C. R. (1975). Combined androgen and antimetabolite therapy of advanced female breast cancer. *Cancer 36*, 308.

Goolamali, S. K. and Shuster, S. (1975). A sebotrophic stimulus in benign and malignant breast disease. *Lancet 1*, 428.

Gordan, G. S., Wessler, S. and Avioli, L. V. (1972). Calusterone therapy for advanced breast cancer. *J. Amer. Med. Assoc. 219*, 483.

Greenspan, E. M. (1966). Combination cytotoxic chemotherapy in advanced disseminated breast carcinoma. *J. Mt. Sinai Hosp. N.Y. 33*, 1.

Greenspan, E. M. (1972). Combination chemotherapy for advanced mammary carcinoma; a twelve year experience. *J. Mt. Sinai Hosp. N.Y. 39*, 435.

Hall, T. C., Dederick, M. M., Nevinny, H. B. and Muench, H. (1963). Prognostic value of response of patients with breast cancer to therapeutic castration. *Cancer Chemother. Rep. 31*, 47.

Hanham, I. W. F., Newton, K. A. and Westbury, G. (1971). Seventy five cases of solid tumour treated by a modified quadruple chemotherapy regime. *Brit. J. Cancer 25*, 462.

Hayward, J. L., Atkins, H. J. B., Falconer, M. A., MacLean, K. S., Salmon, L. F. W., Schurr, P. H. and Shaheen, C. H. (1970). Clinical trials comparing transfrontal hypophysectomy with adrenalectomy and with transethmoidal hypophysectomy. In *Second Tenovus Workshop on Breast Cancer.* Ed. C. A. F. Joslin and E. N. Gleave, Cardiff.

Hellstrom, J. and Franksson, C. (1958). Adrenalectomy in cancer of the breast. In *Endocrine Aspects of Breast Cancer,* p. 5. (Ed. A. R. Currie and C. F. W. Illingsworth). Edinburgh: Livingstone.

Henderson, M. D., Buroker, T. R., Samson, M. K. et al. (1975). Response of patients with carcinoma of the breast to hormonal therapy and combination chemotherapy. *Surg. Gynec. Obst. 141*, 232.

Heuson, J. C., Engelsmann, E., Blonk-Van der Wijst, J. et al. (1975). Comparative trial of nafoxidine and ethinyloestradiol in advanced breast cancer. *Brit. Med. J. 2*, 711.

Hobbs, J. R., de Souza, I., Salih, H. and Raggatt, P. (1974). Selection of hormone dependent breast cancers. *Brit. J. Surg. 61*, 785.

Kennedy, B. J. (1962). Massive estrogen administration in premenopausal women with metastatic breast cancer. *Cancer 15*, 641.

Kimel, V. M. (1957). Clinical cytological correlations of mammary carcinoma based upon sex chromatin counts. *Cancer 10*, 922.

Lee, J. M., Abeloff, M. D., Lenhard, R. E. and Baker, E. R. (1974). An evaluation of five-drug combination chemotherapy in the management of recurrent carcinoma of the breast. *Surg. Gynec. Obst. 138*, 77.

Luft, R., Olivecrona, H., Ikkos, D., Nilsson, L. B. and Mossberg, H. (1958). Hypophysectomy in the management of metastatic carcinoma of the breast. In *Endocrine Aspects of Breast Cancer,* p. 27 (Eds A. R. Currie and C. F. W. Illingworth). Edinburgh: E. & S. Livingstone.

Meakin, J. W. (1970). Effect of chemotherapeutic agents on hormone dependent neoplasms and tissues. *Ann. Rep. Ontario Cancer Res. Found.* p. 151.

Miller, H. and Durant, J. A. (1968). The value of urine steroid hormone assays in breast cancer. *Clinical Biochemistry 1*, 286.

Moore, F. D., Woodrow, S. I., Aliopoulios, M. A. and Wilson, R. E. (1967). Carcinoma of the breast. A decade of new results with old concepts. *New Engl. J. Med. 227*, 411 and 460.

Nemoto, T. and Dao, T. L. (1971). 5-Fluorouracil and cyclophosphamide in disseminated breast cancer. Relationship between chemotherapy and hormonal therapy. New York. *J. Med. 71*, 554.

O'Bryan, R. M., Gordan, G. S., Kelley, R. M., Ravdin, R. G., Segaloff, A. and Taylor, S. G. (1974). Does thyroid substance improve response of breast cancer to surgical castration? *Cancer 33*, 1082.

Patterson, J. S. (1976). In *Proceedings of Symposium on Hormonal Control of Breast Cancer.* Macclesfield.

Perry, M. (1972). Evaluation of breast tumour sex chromatin (Barr body) as an index of survival and response to pituitary ablation. *Brit. J. Surg. 59*, 731.

Powles, T. J. (1977). Factors influencing metastasis in bone. In *Secondary Spread in Breast Cancer,* (Ed. B. A. Stoll) London and Chicago: Heinemann Medical, and Year Book Medical.

Ravdin, R. G. and Eisman, S. H. (1967). Disseminated breast cancer; relationship of response to endocrine manipula-

tion, Cytoxan and Fluorouracil. In *Current Concepts of Breast Cancer,* p. 200 (Eds A. Segaloff, K. K. Meyer and S. Debakey). Baltimore: Williams and Wilkins.

Roberts, J. G., William, M., Henk, J. M., Bligh, A. S. and Baum, M. (1975). The hypronosticon test in breast cancer. *Clin. Oncol. 1,* 33.

Saez, S. (1974). Corticotrophin secretion in relation to breast cancer. In *Mammary Cancer and Neuroendocrine Therapy,* p. 101 (Ed. B. A. Stoll). London: Butterworth.

Samp, R. J. and Ansfield, F. J. (1966). Breast cancer treated with fluorouracil. Survival studies in advanced stage. *J. Amer. Med. Assoc. 198,* 724.

Smithers, D. W., Rigby-Jones, P., Galton, D. A. G. and Payne, P. N. (1952). Cancer of the breast—a review. *Brit. J. Radiol. Suppl. 4,* 1.

Stoll, B. A. (1958). Fluoxymesterone (Halotestin) in advanced breast carcinoma. *Med. J. Aust. 1,* 70.

Stoll, B. A. (1960). Nitromin and corticosteroids in the treatment of advanced cancer. *Acta Unio Int. Contra Canc. 16,* 919.

Stoll, B. A. (1963). Corticosteroids in the therapy of advanced mammary cancer. *Brit. Med. J. 2,* 210.

Stoll, B. A. (1969). *Hormonal Management in Breast cancer.* Pitman Medical and Lippincott, London and Philadelphia.

Stoll, B. A. (1972). *Endocrine Therapy in Malignant Disease,* (Ed. B. A. Stoll). London: W. B. Saunders.

Stoll, B. A. (1972). Breast cancer and catecholamines—a hypothesis. *Lancet 1,* 431.

Sutton, M. L. (1973). Evolution of a practical policy for chemotherapy of carcinoma of the breast. *Proc. Roy. Soc. Med. 66,* 26.

Talley, R. W., Vaitkevicius, V. K. and Leighton, G. A. (1965). Comparison of cyclophosphamide and 5-fluorouracil in the treatment of patients with metastatic breast cancer. *Clin. Pharmacol. Ther. 6,* 740.

Talley, R. W., Haines, C. R., Waters, M. N., Goldenberg, I. S., Olson, K. B. and Bisel, H. F. (1973). A dose response evaluation of androgens in the treatment of metastatic breast cancer. *Cancer 32,* 315.

Taylor, S. G. (1962). Endocrine ablation in disseminated mammary carcinoma. *Surg. Gynec. Obstet. 68,* 452.

Treves, N. and Finkbeiner, J. A. (1958). An evaluation of therapeutic surgical castration in the treatment of metastatic, recurrent and primary inoperable mammary carcinoma in women. *Cancer 11,* 421.

Ward, H. W. C. (1973). Anti-oestrogen therapy for breast cancer; A trial of tamoxifen at two dose levels. *Brit. Med. J. 1,* 13.

Ward, H. (1976). In *Proceedings of Symposium on Hormonal Control of Breast Cancer.* Macclesfield.

Willis, K., London, D. R. and Butt, W. R. (1976). In *Proceedings of Symposium on Hormonal Control of Breast Cancer.* Macclesfield.

Wilson, R. E., Jessiman, A. G. and Moore, F. D. (1958). Severe exacerbation of cancer of the breast after oophorectomy and adrenalectomy. *New Engl. J. Med. 258,* 312.

Welsch, C. W. and Meites, J. (1974). Neuroendocrine control of murine mammary carcinoma. In *Mammary Cancer and Neuroendocrine Therapy,* p. 25 (Ed. B. A. Stoll). London: Butterworth.

Chapter

14

P. E. ROBIN AND G. A. DALTON

The Role of Major Endocrine Ablation

Though as early as 1896 Beatson described oophorectomy as a form of endocrine ablation for carcinoma of the breast, major endocrine ablation (MEA) had to await the availability of cortisone for hormone replacement. In 1952, Huggins and Bergenstal reported the results of total adrenalectomy with cortisone substitution in the treatment of advanced breast carcinoma, and Perrault et al. (1952), Hirsch (1952) and Luft et al. (1952, 1953) were almost simultaneous in reporting the effect of transcranial hypophysectomy for the same disease.

The purpose of MEA is expressed simplistically by suggesting that procedures which deprive the patient of hormones upon which her breast carcinoma may be dependent, can result in the arrest or regression of that tumour. Because of the observed tumour response to oophorectomy and because oophorectomy is known to reduce the serum levels and excretion of oestrogen, it had been assumed that removal of the main extra-ovarian source of oestrogens would have a complementary effect. Adrenalectomy directly, and pituitary destruction indirectly, reduce or even abolish the extra-ovarian oestrogen production. In the case of pituitary ablation, residual oestrogen secretion by the ovaries is also abolished.

The complexity of MEA arises mainly in regard to its effect on the pituitary and the hormones related to it. Experimental work in the field of the pituitary gland is fraught with considerable problems involving interspecies differences in both function and anatomy. Attempts to assess the mechanism of pituitary destruction in causing regression of mammary cancer must therefore rely heavily on clinical findings. Because of the considerable variation in patient selection methods, timing of operation, extent of disease and assessment of results, the role of MEA is still subject to controversy. The variety of available methods makes the choice even more confusing for the clinician.

BILATERAL TOTAL ADRENALECTOMY

This operation may be performed either from a posterior approach (in effect two operations, usually

Table 1. Mortality of Adrenalectomy.

Reference	*Number*	*%*
Atkins et al. (1960)	79	8.9%
Byron (1967)	339	4.0%
Westbury (1967)	437	4.8%
Dargent (1970)	–	10.0%
Calderola et al. (1971)	118	1.7%
Fracchia et al. (1971)	500	4.0%
Horsley et al. (1971)	113	0.8%
Nash and Robbins (1973)	241	1.2%
Ratzkowski et al. (1973)	173	25.0%

Table 2. Results of Bilateral Adrenalectomy.

Reference	*Number*	*Response Rate*
Pearson and Ray (1959)	86	54.0%
Dao et al. (1961)	19	44.0%
McDonald (1962)	690	28.4%
Notter and Melander (1967)	901	28.4%
Westbury (1967)	437	49.0%
Prohaska (1967)	556	49.0%
Dao (1967)	405	40.0%
Fracchia et al. (1967)	500	36.0%
Byron (1967)	339	35.0%
Wilson et al. (1969)	164	58.0%
Harris et al. (1969)	64	33.0%
Hayward (1970a)	77	23.0%
Schmidt et al. (1971)	573	30.0%
Ratzkowski et al. (1973)	114	32.0%

staged) or transabdominal (with or without oophorectomy). The posterior approach is in some ways safer but more laborious (Wilson et al., 1969) but some (Fracchia et al., 1967; Harris and Spratt, 1969) prefer the abdominal approach. Nash and Robbins (1973) compared both methods, showing that while there is little difference in mortality in their hands, the posterior approach takes longer with greater blood loss and a markedly higher pulmonary complication rate.

The reported mortality rate in different series varies widely from 1.2% to 25% (see Table 1), and is influenced greatly by the general condition of the patient when accepted for surgery. Mortality related directly to the operation is now between 1% and 4% (Fracchia et al., 1967, 1971) but rates differ depending on whether it is taken to include only deaths strictly related to surgery, or deaths in hospital or deaths within a defined period. Abdominal adrenalectomy may be contraindicated in the presence of abdominal metastases, and also in the presence of extensive pulmonary and pleural involvement. The latter carries the highest mortality (Westbury, 1967).

A variation of importance in bilateral adrenalectomy is the implantation of one adrenal into the spleen (Dargent et al., 1967). The purpose was to reduce the problems of steroid replacement while at the same time destroying adrenal oestrogens in the liver. Its success was limited in that many of those who initially did not require cortisone replacement came to need it later. In addition, the need for splenectomy in 20% of adrenalectomies (Nash and Robbins, 1973) makes implantation into the spleen impossible in a number of cases.

Other methods (Zimmermann et al., 1972) have not progressed beyond experiment. "Medical adrenalectomy" by corticosteroid administration does not compare at all favourably (Dao et al., 1961), though Lipton and Santen (1974) claim improvement from its combination with aminoglutethimide. Adrenalectomy can be combined with 5-fluorouracil therapy (Hall and Wilson, 1966) but the advantage is unclear. Accessory adrenal tissue has been postulated as a source of persistent oestrogen excretion after adrenalectomy (Juret, 1966a) though Symington et al. (1958) could find no such tissue.

Immediate complications of the operation are relatively frequent; Fracchia et al. (1967) reported an incidence of 40% among 500 patients while Nash and Robbins (1973) reported 18% among 241 patients. The only persistent problem is wound herniation, and prolonged morbidity among those who survive adrenalectomy is not high. Cortisone acetate is required but rarely fluorocortisone. However, such patients are relatively "brittle", in that illness and other disturbance may upset the steroid maintenance balance (Roberts, 1970).

Tumour response rates which have been reported vary between 23% and 58% (Table 2) depending on the physical condition and age of the patients selected, the extent of the disease and the post-operative mortality. The response rate depends also on the criteria of response utilised, including whether subjective or objective response is demanded; generally the subjective response rate is higher than the objective rate.

That good palliation results in some patients is certain, and that some subjective relief occurs in some cases where objective remission is absent is likewise accepted. However, while most earlier series tended to suggest objective remission in about half the cases, more stringent evaluation has reduced this figure to around 30% (McDonald, 1962; Hayward, 1970a). Adrenalectomy leads to an increase in life expectancy in those cases where palliation occurs (Dao, 1967; Schmidt et al., 1971).

Table 3. Mortality of Transfrontal Hypophysectomy.

Reference	*Number*	*%*
Pearson and Ray (1959)	88	4.6%
Dunbar (1967)	343	1.2%
Boesen and Smith (1967)	45	11.0%
Edelstyn et al. (1968)	70	17.0%
Kennedy and French (1965)	71	5.6%

TRANSFRONTAL HYPOPHYSECTOMY

The neurosurgical approach to the pituitary has been used since the beginning of the century in the management of pituitary tumours. Following a head shave, a frontal bone flap is elevated and retraction of the cortex permits an approach to the pituitary, close to the optic nerves and chiasma and the arteries of the circle of Willis. The pituitary stalk can be sectioned and the pituitary removed by suction or curettage.

Mortality rate of the operation varies with different series, between 17% and 1.2% (Table 3) in a number of published series. Juret (1966b) regards the true operative mortality as 4% and this corresponds with most series, if the later deaths not related to surgery (i.e. due to cancer) are excluded.

The list of complications of transfrontal hypophysectomy was originally quite daunting. While diabetes insipidus is common, it is usually transitory and mild. Anosmia is not uncommon, its frequency being variously described as 11% (Fracchia, 1971) and 50% (Juret, 1966b). On the other hand, serious problems such as visual loss or field deficit occur in only a small proportion of cases, variously reported as 9% (Fracchia et al., 1971), 3% (Edelstyn et al., 1968) and 0.6% (Dunbar, 1967).

The reported tumour response rate varies in the same way as that of adrenalectomy, from 24%-41% (Table 4). The Joint Committee (1961) and McDonald (1962) suggested guidelines and assessed a collected series of hypophysectomies, giving 32.6% as the average response rate. Survival time has been shown to be increased in responding cases (Juret, 1966b; Boesen and Smith, 1967; Atkins, 1974).

Edelstyn et al. (1968) reported surgical transfrontal hypophysectomy with ^{90}Y wax packed into the fossa in 102 cases. The results of this were conderably better than in 70 cases of surgical excision alone, but at the cost of increased morbidity. In the cases where ^{90}Y wax was used, serious ocular problems were nearly three times as common as when hypophysectomy alone was performed.

Table 4. Results of Transfrontal Hypophysectomy.

Reference	*Number*	*Response Rate*
Pearson and Ray (1959)	109	35.0%
McDonald (1962)	340	33.0%
Dunbar (1967)	343	41.0%
Edelstyn et al. (1968)	70	24.0%
Wilson et al. (1969)	164	40.0%
Hayward (1970a)	70	36.0%
Fracchia et al. (1971)	103	35.0%

TRANSSPHENOIDAL (SURGICAL) HYPOPHYSECTOMY

The rhinological approach to the pituitary dates initially from the beginning of the century but was not widely accepted for excision of the normal pituitary until reported by Hamberger et al. (1961), Riskaer et al. (1961) and Bateman (1962). The procedure differs marginally in the hands of different surgeons—Bateman (1962) used the mid-line septal approach, Hamberger et al. (1961) preferred the transantral route, while the method commonly adopted is a transethmoidal exposure, but using the nose for instrumentation (Riskaer et al., 1961; James, 1964; Kapur and Dalton, 1969). The precise method is important only to the extent that it allows total excision.

It differs from the neurosurgical procedure in that no craniotomy is performed and thus it does not need any particularly sophisticated facilities other than an operating microscope. Inherent in the procedure is the fact that the level at which the pituitary stalk is avulsed is usually lower than in the transcranial approach; on the other hand the pituitary fossa can be visualised more or less completely. The only contraindications are overt nasal sepsis, a sphenoid obliterated by secondary tumour (Robin et al., 1975) and intercavernous sinuses so extensive as to mask the fossa (an extremely rare occurrence).

The mortality of the procedure varies from 1.2% to 7.1% in published series (Table 5). In 158 operations performed for breast cancer which were reviewed in 1972 (of which 108 were reported by Robin et al. 1975), only two died as a result of surgery. Of operations for pituitary tumours (Williams, 1974; Dalton, 1974; Richards et al., 1974) only two of 136 died. The operation carries an intrinsic mortality probably lower than that of other forms of surgical hypophysectomy.

Morbidity can be compared to that of transfrontal surgery. While the incidence of diabetes insipidus is

similar and is as transient, anosmia is rare (Harrold et al., 1968; Fracchia, 1971). The incidence of ocular complications is lower in the transsphenoidal procedure—0.04% according to Harrold et al. (1968). On the other hand, meningitis seems slightly more frequent, being reported in 5% (Harrold et al., 1968) and 3% (Fracchia et al., 1971). Cerebrospinal fluid rhinorrhoea also is more common in transsphenoidal hypophysectomy than by the transcranial route (Fracchia et al., 1971), but rarely is it of serious significance (Kapur and Dalton, 1969).

The available results from transsphenoidal hypophysectomy are limited but response rates in breast cancer range from 24% to 47% (Table 6). There is evidence that transsphenoidal hypophysectomy prolongs life in responding cases (Harrold et al., 1968; Robin et al., 1975). Response rates are claimed by some to reflect completeness of surgery, and there is a broad correlation with the degree of diabetes insipidus (Bateman, 1962; Reed and Pizey, 1967; Kapur and Dalton, 1969).

Transsphenoidal hypophysectomy is a procedure with few contra-indications and although there is a long list of possible complications in the post-operative period (as there are for the transfrontal procedure), each is individually uncommon and rarely of serious significance.

Table 5. Mortality of Transsphenoidal Hypophysectomy.

Reference	*Number*	*%*
Escher (1967)	85	7.1%
Harrold et al. (1968)	258	5.8%
Fracchia et al. (1971)	100	2.0%
Williams (1974)	56	1.8%
Dalton (1974)	40	0.0%
Richards et al. (1974)	86	1.2%

Table 6. Results of Transsphenoidal Hypophysectomy.

Reference	*Number*	*Response Rate*
Bateman (1962)	35	33.0%
Escher (1967)	35	37.0%
Reed and Pizey (1967)	92	47.0%*
Harrold et al. (1968)	258	
Kapur and Dalton (1969)	63	32.0%
Fracchia et al. (1971)	100	33.0%
Robin et al. (1975)	108	24.0%

* subjective and objective.

HYPOPHYSEAL DESTRUCTION BY IMPLANTATION OF RADIOACTIVE ISOTOPES

The greatest challenge to hypophysectomy has come from implantation of radioactive isotopes. This procedure generally uses the transnasal transsphenoidal route, although Edelstyn et al. (1968) used ^{90}Y wax in combination with excision via the transfrontal route. Transnasal implant is a method applicable in poor risk patients (Juret, 1966b).

Initially, Radon or ^{198}Au (a gamma emitter) was used with moderate success, but among 45 cases 18% had severe visual loss and 4.5% had late CSF rhinorrhoea. This risk of visual loss was unacceptable and subsequently, insertion of ^{90}Y under full radiological control with stereotaxis, and using a screw to seal the pituitary fossa improved the method (Forrest et al., 1959). The mortality was 6.5%, incidence of visual loss 4% and CSF rhinorrhoea 7%.

Complications, initially very high (Forrest et al., 1959), are now said to be reduced, yet Notter and Melander (1967) had CSF rhinorrhoea in 30%, meningitis in 14%, and deaths from this cause alone in 4%. The mortality from implantation of ^{90}Y seems to be low, varying from 0.2% to 5% in reports (Table 7), and is probably no greater than that of transsphenoidal hypophysectomy. The complications are generally ocular and CSF rhinorrhoea, and in the latter, meningitis is a very significant risk.

The response rates to implantation with radioactive isotopes vary between 19% and 38%, similar to other methods of MEA (Table 8.). Generally the

Table 7. Mortality of ^{90}Y Implantation.

Reference	*Number*	*%*
Forrest et al. (1959)	95	5.0%
Notter and Melander (1967)	100	4.0%
Scheer (1967)	457	0.2%

Table 8. Results of Implantation.

Reference	*Number*	*Response Rate*
Notter (1959)	48	33.0%
Juret (1961, 1966b)	75	38.0%
Scheer (1967)	467	19.0%
Notter and Melander (1967)	100	32.0%
Edelstyn et al. (1967) (surgery plus ^{90}Y)	102	57.0%

results appear to be similar though perhaps slightly inferior to surgical excision, though in the opinion of Roberts (1970) implantation is superior.

Other Methods of Pituitary Destruction

Cryohypophysectomy This not very widely used method described by Conway and Collins (1969) and Norrell et al. (1970) seems, on the little evidence available, to be comparable in its problems and effects with other methods. Ocular complications are generally transient, and can be monitored during the procedure under local anaesthetic (Norrell et al., 1970). Other complications are similar to those following surgery and results may be comparable (Conway and Collins, 1969), though the degree of ablation of pituitary is possibly less. Postoperative mortality may also be less.

Pituitary stalk section (Ehni and Eckles, 1959) is perhaps slightly simpler than transfrontal hypophysectomy. It may carry similar complications with a lower remission rate.

Ultrasonic destruction (Arslan, 1968) is said by the author to have excellent results with negligible risk of complications, but has never been accepted elsewhere with any enthusiasm.

Radiofrequency (heat destruction) has also been described (Zervas, 1965) but never adopted by others.

External irradiation has been proposed by Lawrence (1967) and Backlund et al. (1972), but though results similar to other methods have been claimed, special (and costly) apparatus is required. There is not yet sufficient information to assess the value of this technique.

DEGREE OF PITUITARY ABLATION

Discussion of the relative values of hypophyseal ablation techniques has revolved mainly around the mortality, the morbidity, and the remission rates. That the tumour remission rate is related to the degree of pituitary destruction is a logical assumption but the evidence is conflicting. Though it has been indicated by some (Pearson and Ray, 1959; Hayward, 1970b; Theoglides et al., 1974) that total destruction of the gland is not necessary for tumour response to take place, others suggest a correlation between increased destruction and a greater likelihood of response (Notter, 1959; Notter and Melander, 1967; Juret and Hayem, 1960). Studies of the sella after death have been undertaken after implantation in a few cases (Forrest et al., 1959) and have demonstrated varying degrees of destruction. Of the implantation methods, ^{90}Y with stereotaxis and screw seal was found the most effective. Norrell et al. (1970) demonstrated the varying degrees of destruction achieved in cryohypophysectomy.

However, the more usual assessments have been by hormone studies, initially by assessing iodine uptake (Juret, 1966b), but later the levels of pituitary hormones. Hayward (1970b) indicated that most ablative procedures will reduce hormones to a low level but significant residual levels can remain. According to Theoglides et al. (1974) growth hormone levels are the best index of pituitary ablation and of 14 cases studied all had suppression of growth hormone (in response to arginine infusion) after transfrontal hypophysectomy. Roberts (1970) reports the degree of ablation to be similar in ^{90}Y and transsphenoidal hypophysectomy. Our own studies demonstrate uniform hormonal ablation after transsphenoidal hypophysectomy in 11 patients. The completeness of excision may be loosely reflected in the degree of diabetes insipidus. This has been confirmed by many (Bateman, 1962; Reed and Pizey, 1967; Harrold et al., 1968; Kapur and Dalton, 1969; Robin et al., 1975).

Incomplete removal of the pituitary is a deficiency apparently inherent in all methods. Transfrontal procedures may not allow complete inspection of the pituitary fossa, but permit section of the stalk at any level. Simple stalk section does not attempt to remove pituitary tissue but interrupts the portal system carrying releasing hormones from the hypothalamus to the adenohypophysis. Radioactive isotopes are implanted without precise knowledge of the exact shape of the pituitary, and an irregular shape makes it difficult to achieve a uniform dose for destruction without complications.

Implantation of ^{90}Y wax in the fossa after excision (Edelstyn et al., 1968) was intended to destroy residual gland tissue, but a higher tumour response rate was obtained at a cost of serious complications. Transsphenoidal hypophysectomy generally allows the most complete visualisation of the fossa, though there are sometimes difficulties. The persistence of functioning tissue can perhaps be explained by the pharyngeal hypophysis and this can possibly be removed in addition (Richards and Evans, 1974).

RELATIVE VALUES OF MEA TECHNIQUES

Because of the failure to correlate hormonal assays with response to endocrine ablation, we inevitably

Table 9. Relative Values of Major Endocrine Ablation.

Reference	Response		Remission time	
	Hypophysectomy	Adrenalectomy	Hypophysectomy	Adrenalectomy
Pearson and Ray (1959)	56.0%	53.8%	greater	less
Atkins et al (1960)	no sig. diff.	no sig. diff.		
Joint Committee (1961)	no sig. diff.	no sig. diff.		
McDonald (1962)	32.6%	23.4%		
Notter and Melander (1967)	22.7%	24.2%		
Wilson et al (1969)	40.0%	58.0%		
*Hayward (1970a)	36.0%	23.0%	41 months	32 months
Roberts (1970) (^{90}Y)		greater (trend)		

* controlled trials.

return to the comparison of clinical material in an attempt to decide which is the most useful method (Table 9).

Many observations have been made concerning the superiority or otherwise of hypophysectomy over adrenalectomy. In spite of lack of randomisation, there is a definite trend in favour of hypophysectomy, though with exceptions (Wilson et al., 1969). Moreover, the randomised controlled studies of Hayward (1970a) and Atkins (1974) are unequivocal in showing that transfrontal hypophysectomy is significantly superior to adrenalectomy in response rate and extension of life. An early controlled trial on the relationship of transsphenoidal to transfrontal hypophysectomy (Hayward 1970a) had to be interrupted because of the high morbidity rate experienced by the first few cases submitted to the transsphenoidal approach. However, more recent reports by the same group suggest that the palliative results are very similar.

As with most operations, morbidity is reduced with experience whichever procedure is adopted (Pearson and Ray, 1959; Harrold et al., 1968), and transsphenoidal hypophysectomy is undoubtedly more acceptable and "less of an ordeal" to the patient (Hayward, 1970a). The results of ^{90}Y and transsphenoidal hypophysectomy do not differ significantly (Roberts, 1970). It is likely that the results of all forms of hypophysectomy are difficult to distinguish, but there is a theoretical advantage to the transsphenoidal route in that tissue ablation is thorough, and visualisation of the fossa is greatest.

Though hypophysectomy and adrenalectomy are usually compared by their objective regression rates, the operations are performed in many cases in the hope of relieving pain, especially that of bone metastases. The relief of pain following hypophysectomy may be almost instantaneous, and may be related to the section of the pituitary stalk (Juret et al., 1966b) because it has been described even in cancers not otherwise regarded as hormone dependent. This rapid relief of pain is found less frequently with adrenalectomy (Juret, 1966a).

SELECTION AND PREDICTION

The multiplicity of predictive tests in the past was testimony to their inadequacy. Generally their use will indicate the group in which a higher or lower rate of response by the tumour can be expected, yet it is not of absolute value in any individual. Bulbrook et al. (1960) by their "discriminant" indicated the possibility that the hormonal environment of the host might indicate hormone dependent tumours. More recently however, many groups of observers including Leung et al. (1974) relate tumour response to the presence of oestrogen receptors in the tumour (see Chapter 13). In vitro tests of the tumour sensitivity to hormones may be promising if the work of Hobbs et al. (1973) is substantiated.

Because of these difficulties, clinical factors are of importance. Robin et al. (1975) found the relationship of response to the menopause a complicated one, but Harrold et al. (1968) found the age group shortly preceding the menopause unrewarding. The general concensus would be represented by Juret (1966b) who suggested that premenopausal women and those some length of time post-menopausal were more likely to respond, while perimenopausal patients did not respond frequently.

The importance of the site of disease has been another subject of dispute. There is general agreement that bone deposits respond well (Juret 1966a,,b; Pearson and Ray, 1959; Prohaska, 1967; Fracchia et al., 1967; Harrold et al., 1968). Pleuropulmonary and cutaneous deposits are also regarded as favourable sites (Juret 1966a, b; Prohaska, 1967; Harrold et al.

1968), while central nervous system, hepatic, visceral and marrow deposits respond poorly (Fracchia et al., 1967; Juret, 1966a, b; Westbury, 1967). Many do not regard the site of metastasis as particularly important (Westbury, 1967; Wilson et al., 1969; Robin et al. 1975), but regard the degree of dissemination as more relevant than the individual site. There does indeed appear to be a stage or degree of dissemination beyond which little or nothing will have a favourable effect.

Response to oophorectomy is usually regarded as a good predictive guide (Schmidt et al., 1971; Juret, 1966a, b) but this guide is not often available. The timing of MEA has been the subject of several studies. Neither adrenalectomy (Dao et al., 1968; Hayward, 1970a), nor ^{90}Y implantation (Forrest et al., 1968), nor hypophysectomy (Atkins et al., 1966) have shown any significant advantage if performed "prophylactically" early in the course of the disease.

There is general agreement that those patients with a long recurrence-free interval have a longer tumour remission. Such patients would therefore show a higher response rate if remission for a definite time period (e.g. 3 or 6 months) was insisted on (Pearson and Ray, 1959; Byron, 1967; Conway and Collins, 1969; Horsley et al., 1971; Juret, 1966a, b). It may be more reasonable therefore, to consider the length of response in relation to the rate of growth of the underlying disease process (Robin et al., 1975).

There is no general agreement as to the significance to be attached to previous response to hormone therapy. It is suggested (Juret, 1966a; Harrold et al., 1968; Westbury, 1967) that where there has been a response, MEA will be more likely to give a further response. However, rejection of those patients without previous response to hormones may exclude a significant number of potential responders (Byron, 1967). Age in relation to the menopause, discriminant function, site of disease, physical condition, may all influence the consideration of MEA, but even the most unlikely responder can hardly be refused if severe generalised pain is the main indication for MEA (Wilson et al., 1969).

CONCLUSION

It is evident from the foregoing description and development of MEA that these procedures have a part to play in the management of advanced breast cancer. Each procedure is palliative and the aim must be a reduction of symptoms (with in some cases increased life expectancy), while incurring the minimum of suffering from the procedure itself.

The choice of method often depends on availability. Most hospital centres have capable general surgeons who are prepared to perform adrenalectomy. Many hospital centres have access to rhinological services, but there is no doubt that a degree of familiarity with the operation is desirable in the surgeon carrying out transsphenoidal hypophysectomy. Neurosurgical facilities are often less accessible and the operation is, relatively, somewhat of an ordeal. Radiotherapeutic services for implantation techniques are limited and in addition, ^{90}Y implantation needs the support of rhinological surgery.

The applicability of each method is limited by the general condition and occasionally by the anatomy of the patient. Many patients are very ill, and not infrequently unsatisfactory for adrenalectomy. Whereas transfrontal procedures also require a moderately fit subject, transsphenoidal hypophysectomy can be used in those severely ill, while ^{90}Y implantation can be carried out in almost any circumstances.

There is firm evidence that hypophysectomy is more effective than adrenalectomy and a probability that radioactive implant is slightly less efficacious than excision. Of pituitary operations, transsphenoidal manoeuvres are the most acceptable to the patients. The combination of all these factors, availability, applicability, efficacy and acceptability, suggests that transsphenoidal hypophysectomy in a reasonably experienced unit is the method of choice, but this does not imply that other methods may not have definite advantages in some circumstances.

Selection of cases is possibly the most difficult problem. Some factors attract no dispute. A favourable response to previous oophorectomy, a long recurrence-free interval, and a positive oestrogen receptor assay in the tumour, all indicate a high likelihood of tumour regression. Conversely, severely ill cases with rapidly progressive disease, unfavourably sited metastases, and unfavourable results to predictive tests may yield poor results. The situation in the majority of cases is not so clearly definable because of conflicting evidence concerning the influence of factors such as age in relation to the menopause, site of metastases, and previous response to hormonal treatment.

Some patients are in such desperate straits with pain or other symptoms that any attempt at palliation would be justifiable, however slim the chance of response. On the other hand some with favourable indicators could be so disabled that prolongation of life would be unkind. The final decision, though aided by measurable parameters, will depend on the

philosophy of the surgeon or therapist, or even more important that of the patient. Scientific knowledge must not deter us from the fact that palliation is related primarily to the sufferer.

REFERENCES

Arslan, M. A. (1968). Ultrasonic selective hypophysectomy. Proceedings of the Royal Society of Medicine. *61,* 7.

Atkins, H. (1974). The treatment of breast cancer. Proceedings of the Royal Society of Medicine. *67,* 277.

Atkins, H., Falconer, M. A., Hayward, J. L., McLean, K. S. and Schurr, P. H. (1966). The timing of adrenalectomy and of hypophysectomy in the treatment of breast cancer. *Lancet 1,* 827.

Atkins, H. J. B., Falconer, M. A., Hayward, J. L., McLean, K. S., Schurr, P. H. and Armitage, P. (1960). Adrenalectomy and hypophysectomy for advanced cancer of the breast. *Lancet 1,* 1148.

Backund, E. O., Rahn, T., Sarby, B., De Schryver, A. and Wennerstrand, J. (1972). Closed stereotaxic hypophysectomy by means of ^{60}Co gamma radiation. *Acta Radiologica (Ther) 11,* 545.

Bateman, G. H. (1962). Transsphenoidal hypophysectomy. *Journal of Laryngology and Otolaryngology 76,* 442.

Beatson, G. T. (1896). On the treatment of inoperable cases of carcinoma of the mamma: suggestions for a new method of treatment, with illustrative cases. *Lancet 2,* 104 and 162.

Boesen, E. and Radley Smith, E. J. (1967). Pituitary ablation for patients with disseminated breast cancer. In *Major Endocrine Surgery in the Treatment of Carcinoma of the Breast in Advanced Stages,* p. 85 (Ed. M. Dargent and C. Romieu). Lyon: Simep Editions.

Bulbrook, R. D., Greenwood, F. C. and Hayward, J. L. (1960) Selection of breast cancer patients for adrenalectomy or hypophysectomy by determination of urinary 17-hydroxycorticosteroids and aetiocholanolone. *Lancet 1,* 1154.

Byron, R. L. (1967). Bilateral adrenalectomy in advanced breast cancer. In *Major Endocrine Surgery for the Treatment of Carcinoma of the Breast in Advanced Stages,* p. 33 (Ed. M. Dargent and C. Romieu). Lyon: Simep Editions.

Calderola, L., Badellino, F. and Molinatti, A. M. (1971). Ovariectomie avec surrenalectomie bilaterale pour cancer du sein au stade advance. *La Presse Medicale 2,* 1743.

Conway, L. W. and Collins, W. F. (1969). Results in transsphenoidal cryohypophysectomy for carcinoma of the breast. *New England Journal of Medicine 281,* 1.

Dalton, G. A. D. (1974). Transsphenoidal hypophysectomy for pituitary tumours. Proceedings of the Royal Society of Medicine *67,* 885.

Dao, T. (1967). Survival experience following adrenalectomy and hormone therapy in advanced mammary cancer. In *Major Endocrine Surgery for the Treatment of Carcinoma of the Breast in Advanced Stages,* p. 9 (Ed. M. Dargent and C. Romieu). Lyon: Simep Editions.

Dao, T. L., Nemoto, T. and Bross, I. (1968). A controlled randomised comparative study of early and late adrenalectomy in women with advanced breast cancer. In *Prognostic Factors in Breast Cancer,* p. 177 (Ed. A. P. M. Forrest and P. B. Kunkler). Edinburgh: Livingstone.

Dao, T. L., Tan, E. and Brooks, V. (1961). A comparative evaluation of adrenalectomy and cortisone in the treatment of advanced mammary carcinoma. *Cancer 14,* 1259.

Dargent, M. (1970). Carcinoma of the breast. *Aktuelle Probleme in der Chirurgie 14,* 731.

Dargent, M., Mayer, M. and Lombard R. (1967). Modalites techniques de la chirurgie surrenalienne: surrenalectomie bilaterale d'emblee ou en deux temps. Transplantation surreno-splenique. In *Major Endocrine Surgery for the Treatment of Carcinoma of the Breast in Advanced Stages,* p. 61 (Ed. M. Dargent and C. Romieu). Lyon: Simep Editions.

Dunbar, H. S. (1967). Hypophysectomy for advanced breast cancer. In *Major Endocrine Surgery for the Treatment of Carcinoma of the Breast in Advanced Stages,* p. 33 (Ed. M. Dargent and C. Romieu). Lyon: Simep Editions.

Edelstyn, G., Gleadhill, C. and Lyons, A. (1968). Total hypophysectomy for advanced breast cancer. *Clinical Radiology 19,* 426.

Ehni, G. and Eckles, N. E. (1959). Interruption of the pituitary stalk in patients with mammary carcinoma. *Journal of Neurosurgery 16,* 628.

Escher, F. (1967). Technique et resultats de l'hypophysectomie transethmoidosphenoidale pour cancer du sein advance. In *Major Endocrine Surgery in the Treatment of Carcinoma of the Breast in Advanced Stages,* p. 109 (Ed. M. Dargent and C. Romieu). Lyon: Simep Editions.

Forrest, A. P. M., Blair, D. W., Peebles-Brown, D. A., Stewart, H. J., Sandison, A. T., Harrington, R. W., Valentine, J. H. and Carter, P. T. (1959). Radio-active implantation of the pituitary. *British Journal of Surgery 47,* 61.

Forrest, A. P. M., Stewart, H. J., Benson, A., Kerr, H., Jones, V., Kunkler, P. B. and Campbell, H. (1968). Controlled studies in advanced breast cancer. In *Prognostic Factors in Breast Cancer,* p. 186 (Ed. A. P. M. Forrest and P. B. Kunkler). Edinburgh: Livingstone.

Fracchia, A. A., Farrow, J. H., Miller, T. R., Tollefsen, R. H., Greenburg, E. J. and Knapper, W. H. (1971). Hypophysectomy as compared to adrenalectomy for advanced breast cancer. *Surgery, Gynecology and Obstetrics 133,* 241.

Fracchia, A. A., Randall, H. T. and Farrow, J. H. (1967). The results of adrenalectomy in advanced breast cancer in 500 consecutive patients. *Surgery, Gynecology and Obstetrics 125,* 747.

Hall, T. C. and Wilson, R. E. (1966). Safe and effective method of administering 5FU to adrenalectomised patients. *Surgery, Gynecology and Obstetrics 123,* 978.

Hamberger, C. A., Hammer, G., Norlen, G. and Sjogren, B. (1961). Transsphenoidal hypophysectomy. *Archives of Otolaryngology 74.* 2.

Harris, H. S., Jr. and Spratt, J. S. (1969). Bilateral adrenalectomy in metastatic mammary carcinoma—an analysis of 64 cases. *Cancer 23,* 145.

Harrold, B. P., Cates, J. E. and James, J. A. (1968). Treatment of advanced breast cancer by transsphenoidal hypophysectomy. *British Journal of Cancer 22,* 19.

Hayward, J. L. (1970a). Clinical trials comparing transfrontal hypophysectomy with adrenalectomy and with transethmoidal hypophysectomy. In *Clinical Management of Advanced Breast Cancer,* p. 50 (Ed. C. A. F. Joslin and E. N. Gleave). Cardiff: Second Tenovus Workshop.

Hayward, P. (1970b). The adrenals and the pituitary. In *Recent Results in Cancer Research,* p. 33. London: Heinemann.

Hirsch, O. (1952). Symptoms and treatment of pituitary tumours. *Archives of Otolaryngology 55,* 268.

Hobbs, J. R., Salim, H., Flax, H. and Brander, W. (1973). Prolactin dependence in human breast cancer. *Proceedings of the Royal Society of Medicine 66,* 866.

Horsley, J. S., Alrich, E. M., Sears, H. F. and Wright, C. B. (1971). Adrenalectomy for metastatic mammary cancer. *Annals of Surgery 173,* 906.

Huggins, C. and Bergenstal, D. M. (1952). Inhibition of human mammary and prostatic cancer by adrenalectomy. *Cancer Research 12,* 134.

James, J. A. (1964). Hypophysectomy in general medicine and surgery. *Journal of the Royal College of Surgeons in Ireland 1,* (2). 83.

Joint Committee on Endocrine Ablative Procedures in Disseminated Mammary Carcinoma (1961). *Journal of the American Medical Association 175,* 787.

Juret, P. (1966a). Bilateral adrenalectomy. In *Endocrine Surgery in Human Cancers,* p. 58. Thomas, Springfield.

Juret, P. (1966b). Hypophysectomy. In *Endocrine Surgery in Human Cancers,* p. 142. Thomas, Springfield.

Juret, P. and Hayem, M. (1961). Implantation de material radioactif intrahypophysaire (^{198}Au et ^{90}Y) dans les cancers du sein metastatiques. *Revue Francaise d'Etudes Cliniques et Biologiques 6,* 19.

Kapur, T. and Dalton, G. A. D. (1969). Transsphenoidal hypophysectomy for metastatic carcinoma of the breast. *British Journal of Surgery 56,* 332.

Kennedy, B. J. and French, L. (1965). Hypophysectomy in advanced breast cancer. *American Journal of Surgery 110,* 411.

Lawrence, J. H. (1967). Heavy particle irradiation to the pituitary in metastatic breast cancer. In *Major Endocrine Surgery in the Treatment of Cancer of the Breast in Advanced Stages,* p. 89 (Ed. M. Dargent and C. Romieu). Lyon: Simep Editions.

Leung, B. S., Krippaehne, W. W. and Fletcher, W. S. (1974). Prognostic value of oestrogen receptors to endocrine ablation in cancer of the breast. *Surgery Gynecology and Obstetrics 139,* 525.

Lipton, A. and Santen, R. J. (1974). Medical adrenalectomy using aminoglutethamide and dexamethasone in advanced breast cancer. *Cancer 33,* 503.

Luft, R. and Olivecrona, H. (1953). Experiences with hypophysectomy in man. *Journal of Neurosurgery 10,* 301.

Luft, R., Olivecrona, H. and Sjogren, B. (1952). Hypotysectomi pa narriska. Quoted in Luft, R. and Olivecrona, H. (1953).

McDonald, I. (1962). Endocrine ablation in disseminated mammary carcinoma. *Surgery, Gynecology and Obstetrics 115,* 215.

Nash, A. C. and Robbins, G. F. (1973). The operative approach to the left adrenal gland. *Surgery, Gynecology and Obstetrics 137,* 670.

Norrell, H., Alves, A. M., Winternitz, W. W. and Maddy, J. (1970). A clinicopathologic analysis of cryohyphysectomy in patients with advanced cancer. *Cancer 25,* 1050.

Notter, G. (1959). A technique for destruction of the hypophysis using ^{90}Y spheres. *Acta Radiologica Supplement 184,* 1.

Notter, G. and Melander, O. (1967). Pituitary implantation with ^{90}Y in the treatment of advanced breast cancer. In *Major Endocrine Surgery in the Treatment of Carcinoma of the Breast in Advanced Stages,* p. 113 (Ed. M. Dargent and C. Romieu). Lyon: Simep Editions.

Pearson, O. H. and Ray, B. S. (1959). The results of hypophysectomy in the treatment of metastatic mammary cancer. *Cancer 12,* 85.

Perrault, M., LeBeau, J., Klotz, B., Sicard, J. and Clavel, B. (1952). L'hypophysectomie totale dans le traitment de cancer du sein. Premier cas francais, avenir de la methode. *Therapie 7,* 290.

Prohaska, J. (1967). Mammary carcinoma metastases—response to endocrine ablative surgery. In *Major Endocrine Surgery in the Treatment of Cancer of the Breast in Advanced Stages,* p. 37 (Ed. M. Dargent and C. Romieu). Lyon: Simep Editions.

Ratzkowski, E., Adler, B. and Hochman, A. (1973). Survival time and treatment results of patients with disseminated breast cancer especially after adrenalectomy and hypophysectomy. *Oncology 28,* 385.

Reed, P. I. and Pizey. N. C. D. (1967). Transsphenoidal hypophysectomy in the treatment of advanced breast cancer. *British Journal of Surgery 54,* 369.

Richards, S. H. and Evans, I. T. G. (1974). The pharyngeal hypophysis and its surgical significance. *Journal of Laryngology and Otology 88,* 937.

Richards, S. H., Thomas, J. P. and Kilby, D. (1974). Transethmoidal hypophysectomy for pituitary tumours, *Proceedings of the Royal Society of Medicine 67,* 889.

Riskaer, N., Fog, C. U. M. and Hommelgaard, T. (1961). Transsphenoidal hypophysectomy in metastatic cancer of the breast. *Archives of Otolaryngology 74,* 483.

Roberts, M. M. (1970). A comparison of transethmoidal hypophysectomy and ^{90}Y implant and adrenalectomy. In *Clinical Management of Advanced Breast Cancer,* p. 54 (Ed. C. A. F. Joslin and E. N. Gleave). Cardiff: Second Tenovus Workshop.

Robin, P. E., Powell, D. J., Waterhouse, J. A. H. and Dalton, G. A. (1975). Transsphenoidal hypophysectomy in disseminated carcinoma of the breast. *British Journal of Surgery 62,* 85.

Scheer, K. (1967). Technique and results of radioactive pituitary implants in cases of advanced breast carcinoma. In *Major Endocrine Surgery in the Treatment of Carcinoma of the Breast in Advanced Stages,* p. 94 (Ed. M. Dargent and C. Romieu). Lyon: Simep Editions.

Schmidt, M., Nemoto, T., Dao, T. and Bross, I. D. J. (1971). Prognostic factors affecting adrenalectomy in patients with metastatic cancer of the breast. *Cancer 27,* 1106.

Symington, T. L., Grant, J., O'Donnel, U. J., Carr, I. A. and Forrest, A. P. M. (1958). Post mortem studies on the adrenals. In *Endocrine Aspects of Breast Cancer,* p. 115 (Ed. A. R. Currie). Edinburgh: Livingstone.

Theoglides, A., Lindall, A. W. and Norelli, E. (1974). Growth hormone after transsphenoidal hypophysectomy. *Journal of the American Medical Association 227,* 1258.

Westbury, G. (1967). Adrenalectomy for breast cancer. In *Major Endocrine Surgery in the Treatment of Cancer of the Breast in Advanced Stages,* p. 31 (Ed. M. Dargent and C. Romieu). Lyon: Simep Editions.

Williams, R. A. (1974). Transsphenoidal hypophysectomy for acromegaly. *Proceedings of the Royal Society of Medicine 67,* 881.

Wilson, R. E., Piro, A. J., Aliapoulios, M. A. and Moore, F. D. (1969). Evaluation of adrenalectomy and hypophysectomy in the treatment of metastatic cancer of the breast. *Cancer 24,* 1322.

Zervas, N. T. (1965). Technique of radiofrequency hypophysectomy. *Confinica Neurologica 26*, 157.

Zimmermann, C. E., Kettyle, W. M., Eisenberg, H. R., Spark, R., Rosoff C. B. and Cohen, R. B. (1972). Transvenous adrenalectomy. *Journal of Surgical Research 12*, 124.

Chapter

15 ROBERT G. TWYCROSS

Care of the Terminal Patient

"It was like a miracle to me, the relief I felt; free from pain the first week and the gradual cure of the sickness, and at last eating the first time for weeks. Now I go home walking again. Indeed, I am truly thankful".

(Extract from letter by Mrs. V. N.).

The following discussion is based on the management of breast cancer in a hospital devoted to terminal care—St. Christopher's Hospice, London. Nevertheless, it is applicable to the management of the terminal cancer patient in other circumstances—whether at home or in a general hospital.

It is notoriously difficult to estimate the prognosis in the patient with advanced breast cancer. We firmly believe that unrelieved pain in the late cancer patient will cause a worsening of the condition and lead to an earlier death. If however, pain is relieved the patient may improve considerably and live for months or even years. This means that severity of pain, rather than short expectation of life, should be the criterion for the prescription of a narcotic analgesic.

CONTROL OF PAIN

The main reason for poor pain control is probably a failure by the doctor to understand the nature of pain. The perception of the physical sensation is always modified by the patient's emotional reaction to it. In other words, pain is not simply a sensation; it is a psychosomatic experience. This means that attention must be paid to non-pharmacological factors that affect pain threshold as well as to the correct use of analgesic and other drugs (Table 1).

Pain associated with advanced cancer is usually persistent, even if variable in intensity and, unlike acute pain, is a situation rather than an event. It is impossible to predict when it will end; usually it gets worse rather than better; appears meaningless; and frequently expands to occupy the patient's whole attention, isolating her from the world around. When that happens, life is no longer worth living.

Undoubtedly much suffering is caused by "depersonalization". Although it is her illness, the patient is not consulted about anything; her cooperation is not sought. Resentment at everything and with everyone begins to build up, symptoms tend to multiply and worsen—all because the patient is not treated as a person.

This point was illustrated in the case of a patient

Table 1. Factors that modify pain threshold.

Threshold lowered (↓)		Threshold raised (↑)
Discomfort		Relief of symptoms
Insomnia		Sleep
Fatigue		Rest
Anxiety		Sympathy
Fear	Threshold	Understanding
Anger	lowered	Diversion	Threshold raised
Sadness		
Depression		
Mental isolation		
Introversion		Analgesics
		Anxiolytics
(Past experience)		Antidepressives

with skeletal metastases from disseminated breast cancer whose pain remained unrelieved despite the use of narcotic analgesics (Special Correspondence, 1971). A suggestion was made that the pain was intractable as the woman was angry with her doctors and relatives because they would neither admit that she was dying nor discuss the problems this created. This proved to be the right explanation; a full and frank discussion resulted in a dramatic improvement in her mental state and she no longer complained of pain.

A diagnosis of cancer does not necessarily mean that the malignant process is responsible for the patient's pain and as always, diagnosis must precede treatment. Constipation, peptic ulcer, bedsores, cystitis or musculoskeletal pain may prove to be the cause of pain and demand specific treatment.

Bone Pain

Skeletal metastases are the main or only cause of pain in about two-thirds of those with this symptom, a feature which distinguishes advanced breast cancer from most other forms of terminal malignancy. As bone pain is not always relieved by analgesics alone, it may be necessary to use several measures simultaneously to obtain relief. These may either be measures that modify tumour growth (hormone therapy, oophorectomy, adrenalectomy, pituitary ablation, chemotherapy, radiation) or anti-inflammatory agents (indomethacin, ibuprofen, prednisolone). However, as the cancer progresses and attempts to palliate the disease become less effective, the use of analgesics and other measures to elevate the pain threshold become more important.

Internal fixation or the insertion of a prosthesis should always be considered if a pathological fracture occurs. Such measures obviate the need for prolonged bedrest and pain is usually relieved. In the writer's series, median survival after the first or only fracture was five months, ranging from two months to four years; a similar figure has been reported by both Marcove and Yang (1957) and Galasko (1972). The decision whether or not to treat surgically depends on the patient's general condition; unlike the case of bronchial carcinoma, pathological fracture in breast cancer is not generally a terminal event.

Recently, it has been suggested that when pathological fracture is likely, long bones should be nailed prophylactically, as this is simpler than the internal fixation of an established displaced fracture, and less disturbing for the patient. Prophylactic nailing facilitates nursing and usually results in considerable reduction of pain. Moreover, even if a fracture occurs after the nailing it can be virtually symptomless. Parrish and Murray (1970) described the indication for prophylactic internal fixation as increasing pain combined with destruction of more than 50% of the cortex. When more than half the cortex has been destroyed, deformity takes place on weight-bearing and causes pain in a similar manner to a stress fracture; this is prevented by internal fixation.

Fidler (1973) reviewed 19 fractures through metastases, 18 of them in the femur. He confirmed that fracture was unlikely when less than 25% of the cortex had been eroded, but that with over 75% involvement the bone was so weak as often to fracture spontaneously. Further, he emphasized that, although pain may draw attention to a metastasis, it was not helpful in deciding whether a fracture was likely. In fact only half his patients had pain before the fracture. He concluded that destruction of 50% of the cortex was an indication for prophylactic internal fixation and cited nine such operations. In one, the femur fractured during surgery, but in none did a pathological fracture follow the operation.

A more elaborate technique has been described for use when bone destruction is widespread or when the fracture is close to the end of the bone and adequate fixation by nail is not possible (Harrington et al., 1972); lesions are first treated by excision and curettage, and then by appropriate internal fixation and the simultaneous insertion of an acrylic cement into the bone-defect. However, because of the possibility of tumour dissemination, curettage is probably not advisable in the majority of cases. The selective use of acrylic cement without curettage will still allow the fixation of fractures that would otherwise not be manageable (Editorial, 1973).

ANALGESICS

Patients should not constantly be taking tablets or receiving injections and a four-hour interval between

doses should be regarded as the norm though occasionally a shorter period may be necessary. Pain is a potent "antanalgesic" and to allow the pain to re-emerge before administering the next dose not only causes unnecessary suffering but encourages tolerance. Accordingly, "four-hourly as required" has no place in the treatment of persistent pain.

Whatever its aetiology, chronic pain requires regular preventive therapy. The aim is to titrate the level of analgesia against the patient's pain, gradually increasing the dose until the patient is pain-free. The next dose is given before the effect of the previous one has worn off and, therefore, before the patient may think it necessary. It is thus possible to erase the memory and fear of pain. Many patients do not require a dose at 2 a.m. though, if necessary, a patient is wakened to take it rather than let her wake later complaining of pain.

If an analgesic ceases to be effective the patient should be transferred to a stronger alternative. In many cases this will be a narcotic analgesic. "Maximum" or "recommended" doses, derived mainly from postoperative parenteral single-dose studies, are not generally applicable to the treatment of chronic pain. Patients prescribed a narcotic analgesic should be questioned about nausea and vomiting and either have an antiemetic prescribed simultaneously, or the need for such an agent reviewed two or three days later. A patient will not continue to take an analgesic if it results in nausea or vomiting.

Choice of analgesic

Unless the pain is severe, non-narcotic analgesics should be tried initially. Many patients can tolerate up to 1200 mg of aspirin four-hourly, obtaining relief denied to them at the more conventional 600 mg dose. For those unable to tolerate aspirin, paracetamol may be used. If these are not effective the weak narcotic analgesics, codeine and propoxyphene (Doloxene® Darvon®) are prescribed, usually in combination with aspirin or paracetamol.

Pentazocine (Fortral®, Talwin®) and pethidine (Demerol®) have little place in treatment of chronic pain. By mouth, 50 mg of pentazocine is less potent than two tablets of the weaker narcotic analgesics (Robbie and Samarasinghe, 1973). Furthermore, the proportion of patients experiencing psychotomimetic side-effects is unacceptably high when there are safer alternatives (Wood et al., 1974). Although such side-effects tend to be dose-related, they have been observed after even small doses by mouth. Similarly, orally administered pethidine should not be regarded as a potent analgesic and, by injection, acts only for some two to three hours.

Table 2. Analgesic ladder

Pain	*Analgesics*	
Mild	Aspirin, paracetamol	increasing potency ↓
Moderate	Codeine, propoxyphene, dipipanone, papaveretum	
Severe	Diamorphine, morphine, levorphanol, phenazocine	

Papaveretum (Omnopon®, Pantopon®) and dipipanone are useful intermediates between codeine- and propoxyphene-containing preparations and morphine (Table 2). Dipipanone is available in the U.K. only in combination with cyclizine (Diconal®), but there is no evidence that it causes more nausea than other narcotics. Levorphanol (Dromoran®) and phenazocine (Narphen®) should be regarded as alternatives to morphine and diamorphine. By mouth, on a weight for weight basis, both are approximately three times more potent than diamorphine. Because of its longer duration of action, phenazocine may be given six or eight-hourly. This makes it a useful preparation if a four-hourly regimen is impractical or inconvenient.

Methadone (Physeptone®) which has a plasma half-time of more than 50 hours (Verebely et al., 1975), is also useful in such circumstances. Diamorphine and morphine, with a plasma half-time of about 2.5 hours (Brunk and Delle, 1974), are, however, better for very ill patients; when a constant dose is given they do not accumulate in the body to the same extent as methadone and the risk attached to their use is correspondingly less.

The top of the analgesic ladder has not been reached simply by prescribing diamorphine or morphine. Both may be given in a wide range of oral doses, from 5 to 100 mg every four hours, after which injections can be used. In Britain diamorphine and morphine are usually administered in an elixir with cocaine, and it should be remembered that because of their limited shelf life, unused solutions containing diamorphine should be discarded after four weeks. Alternatively, aspirin and opium (Nepenthe) may be used; each 1 ml of undiluted Nepenthe contains about 10 mg of morphine.

By mouth, diamorphine is about one and a half times more potent than morphine; it is rapidly metabolised *in vivo*, firstly to monoacetylmorphine and then to morphine (Way et al., 1965). Thus diamorphine and morphine have similar actions and unwanted effects. Nevertheless, as diamorphine is considerably more soluble than morphine—100 mg

Table 3. Common symptoms in 126 patients admitted consecutively with advanced breast cancer.

Symptom	*%*
Pain	66
Anorexia	55
Weight loss	50
Dyspnoea	49
Weakness	44
Nausea and Vomiting	40
Constipation	37
Lymphoedema of arm	26
Ulceration	17

will dissolve in 0.2 ml—freeze-dried ampoules of diamorphine hydrochloride are recommended when regular injections are required.

It should be emphasized that most patients can be maintained on oral medication. The main indication for parenteral administration, apart from the last few hours of life, is intractable nausea and vomiting despite the prescription of antiemetic. The need for injections may sometimes be avoided by using analgesic suppositories, such as oxycodone pectinate 30 mg (Proladone®), one or two every six to eight hours, or by giving phenazocine tablets sublingually (Brown, 1966). Alternatively, round-the-clock relief may be maintained by using a microcrystalline suspension of morphine, two or three times a day.

Adjuvant Treatment

Although pain is the commonest symptom requiring treatment in the terminal patient, other symptoms also may require considerable attention (Table 3). Nausea and vomiting are common in advanced breast cancer and the use of a narcotic analgesic may precipitate or exacerbate these symptoms, particularly if the patient is ambulant (Comroe and Dripps, 1948). A phenothiazine (generally prochlorperazine-Stemetil®, Compazine®) is generally prescribed routinely with diamorphine. It acts not only as an antiemetic but also supplements the sedative effect of the narcotic analgesic. This is replaced by chlorpromazine or, occasionally, methotrimeprazine in patients with an appreciable psychological component to their pain—for example, the woman who feels that her fungating breast cancer is jeopardizing her relationship with her husband, or the patient experiencing both pain and dyspnoea who fears death by suffocation. Chlorpromazine or promazine are also used to control confusion, delirium, or psychotic manifestations. With patients who are both elderly and debilitated it is wise to prescribe not more than 12.5 mg of chlorpromazine initially, to be administered every four hours with the narcotic analgesic.

A quarter of the patients are also prescribed either a tricyclic antidepressant or a benzodiazepine tranquillizer. Generally speaking, the latter are used for short periods to help patients at times of severe anxiety, while the former are used for longer periods if the patient becomes depressed. This occurs more frequently in patients who have a prolonged terminal phase. Other measures that may be effective in special circumstances are listed in Table 4.

The value of diversional activity should not be forgotten. It ranges from backrubs to occupational therapy, talking books, access to radio and television and someone to talk to. Pain feels worse when it occupies the patient's whole attention. Diversional activity does much more than just "pass the time": it also diminishes the pain.

Unwanted effects of treatment

When a narcotic-phenothiazine combination is prescribed, the patient may feel sleepy initially but this

Table 4. Additional analgesic measures.

Site of pain	*Mechanism*	*Consider*
Breast	Ulceration of primary or cutaneous recurrence → secondary infection	Antibiotic
Arm	Gross lymphoedema	Diuretic or compression machine
Liver	Gross enlargement due to metastases	Glucocorticosteroid
Head	Brain metastasis → raised intra-cranial pressure	Glucocorticosteroid
Arm Trunk Leg	Nerve involvement	Intrathecal nerve-block

usually diminishes after two or three days. Persistent drowsiness is unusual and appears to be related more to a state of advanced debility than to the use of narcotic analgesics. The writer has found no significant correlation between the dose administered and mobility of the patient.

Respiratory depression is rarely seen in association with oral medication, especially when the dose in individually determined. Even so, many doctors are reluctant to use narcotic analgesics, particularly diamorphine or morphine, because they fear that the patient will become addicted. But, psychological addiction—a compulsion or overpowering drive to take a drug to experience its psychological effects—does not occur when pain control is part of a pattern of total care.

Occasionally a newly arrived patient appears to be addicted, demanding "an injection" every two or three hours. Typically such a patient has a long history of poor pain control and will for several weeks have been receiving fairly regular (four-hourly as required), but inadequate, injections of one or more narcotic analgesics. Given time, it is usually possible to control the pain adequately, prevent clock-watching and demanding behaviour, and, sometimes, transfer the patient to an oral preparation. But even in such a case it cannot be said that the patient is addicted; she is not demanding the narcotic in order to experience its psychological effect but to be relieved from pain for at least an hour or two.

Physical dependence probably develops in most patients treated for more than two or three weeks with a narcotic analgesic, but it does not prevent the gradual downward adjustment of dose nor the complete curtailment of treatment should either become clinically feasible (Twycross, 1974). Apart from dextromoramide (Palfium®) tolerance is not a problem when potent analgesics are used in the way described.

ALIMENTARY SYMPTOMS

Dry Mouth

Many patients, if asked, complain of a dry mouth. While it may be an indication of hypercalcaemia, it is more usually multifactorial in aetiology (Table 5). Control of nausea and vomiting, encouraging the patient to drink more (what is her favourite beverage?), and treating moniliasis if present, will go a long way to easing the discomfort. In some patients who are sensitive to the anticholinergic effects of psychotropic and other drugs, it may be possible to modify their medication.

When modification is either not possible or fails to relieve, measures to stimulate the flow of saliva and/or to lubricate the mouth should be considered, including smoking, chewing gum, sucking acid (lemon) drops or ice chips, sucking glycerine and blackcurrent lozenges, avoidance of dry food.

Other treatments include the use of vitamin C effervescent tablets in a glass of water with meals, and also a mixture of one part simple syrup with four parts olive oil and a few drops of lemon essence, to use as a lubricant for the mouth two or three times daily (Anonymous, 1971). Regular oral toilet is especially necessary in the very ill.

Nausea and Vomiting

Half the patients reviewed complained of nausea and/or vomiting (Table 3). Anxiety and unrelieved pain increase the likelihood of these symptoms occurring. The underlying cause in breast cancer is, however, almost always chemical, including toxaemia due to the presence of the tumour, hypercalcaemia, stilboestrol and narcotic analgesics. A phenothiazine antiemetic which acts by decreasing the sensitivity of the chemoreceptor trigger zone in the brain stem

Table 5. Causes of dry mouth in advanced breast cancer.

Local	Moniliasis Mouth breathing		
General	Poor fluid intake		
	Excessive fluid loss	Vomiting Diarrhoea Polyuria Pyrexia	Polyuria: diuretic hypercalcaemia diabetes insipidus
Drugs	(Narcotic analgesics) (Cocaine) Phenothiazines Tricyclic antidepressants Cyclizine		
Psychological	Anxiety Depression		

Table 6. Specific treatment of constipation.

Category	*Treatment*
1. Costive (soft faeces)	Senokot or Dulcolax by mouth on alternate days; adjust dose as necessary
2. Costive (hard faeces)	Dorbanex or Laxoberal by mouth either daily or alternative days
3. Soft impaction	Dulcolax suppositories; manual removal or enema if not effective
4. Hard impaction	Glycerine suppositories or olive oil instillation followed by Dulcolax suppositories. If manual removal necessary, patient may need premedication with ntravenous diazepam and small dose of diamorphine or other narcotic
5. Impaction + spurious diarrhoea	After initial evacuation (see 3 and 4), Dulcolax suppositories daily until poor or no result obtained, then oral preparation according to need

Senokot – proprietary preparation of sennosides A & B, (tablets, granules, syrup)
Dulcolax – proprietary preparation of bisacodyl (tablets, suppositories)
Dorbanex – proprietary preparation containing danthron and poloxamer '188' (capsules, syrup)
Laxoberal – proprietary preparation of sodium picosulphate (syrup)

(Goodman and Gilman, 1975), generally relieves nausea and vomiting. Prochlorperazine (Stemetil®, Compazine®) 5 mg four-hourly may be effective but suppositories (25 mg) or injections (12.5 mg) may be required initially.

If the patient is hypercalcaemic measures designed to correct this should be instituted (see chapter 18). Should the symptoms persist, the dose of prochlorperazine may be doubled, a more potent anti-emetic such as perphenazine (Fentazin®, Trilafon®) prescribed instead, or cyclizine, which acts on the emetic centre itself, prescribed as well. Dietary modification may also help.

Constipation

Constipation often develops and is made worse by narcotic analgesics, phenothiazines and anti-depressants. Correction of predisposing factors such as dehydration and anorexia may help, but specific treatment with laxatives, suppositories, and/or enemas is usually necessary to counteract drug induced constipation (Table 6).

Anorexia and weight loss

Appetite often improves when a patient is admitted to hospital, or when symptoms such as nausea and pain are controlled. As with other alimentary symptoms in breast cancer, anorexia may be due to hypercalcaemia. In other cases where the anorexia is a manifestation of depression, treatment with an anti-depressant causes a return of appetite. When all else fails, it may be worth trying prednisolone 5-10 mg tds for two weeks and if effective, it can be continued.

Some patients receiving chlorpromazine or a glucocorticosteroid become hyperphagic. This is usually welcomed by the patient although, occasionally, modification of the patient's drug regimen is necessary. Weight loss in association with malignant disease is not solely the result of anorexia. Consequently, a return of appetite does not mean that weight loss will be corrected or even halted. Extreme weight loss (cachexia) is, however, rare in breast cancer.

OTHER SYMPTOMS

Dyspnoea

In many cases, dyspnoea is secondary to a pleural effusion and paracentesis may be necessary (see Chapter 17). If, because of an irreversible compression atelectasis, paracentesis results in little benefit, or the patient is too ill for such treatment, symptomatic measures should be used.

For the anxiety and fear that accompany dyspnoea, phenothiazine and benzodiazepine tranquillizers are of value. Diamorphine and morphine with their direct depressant effect on the respiratory centre, are of particular value when the patient is markedly tachypnoeic.

Ulceration

In the presence of ulcerating tumour, its regular inspection by the physician helps to raise and maintain morale in both the patient and the nursing staff. If offensive, eusol in paraffin (1 part in 4) or hydrogen peroxide should be used to clean the lesion two or three times a day. An antibiotic spray helps to combat local sepsis, and sometimes a systemic antibiotic may be necessary. The area should be covered by a non-adhesive dressing.

Weakness

While this may be caused by paraplegia or hypercalcaemia, increasing weakness generally means that the body has lost the battle against the malignant process. It is at this stage that the patient is faced with the fact that death is inevitable. Equally, it is a time when support and companionship are of paramount importance. Although the doctor may feel powerless in the face of death, his continued attendance, indicating that he will stand by the patient no matter what happens, is of inestimable value to the patient, her family and staff.

Smithers (1973) said that any one who hasn't time for chat knows nothing about terminal care, however brilliant a clinical pharmacologist he may be. And in this context, chat means "patient chat" while the doctor listens. Many patients want to talk about their illness, to share their fears and to seek reassurances that they will not suffocate or die in agony. As the doctor has the means of ensuring that a patient will die peacefully, he alone can give the assurance the patient seeks.

Acknowledgements

The author is in receipt of a research fellowship from the Sir Halley Stewart Trust. He wishes to thank Dr. Cicely Saunders for access to patients' case notes and for permission to publish part of a letter from Mrs. V. N. and also Mrs. Esmé Daly for preparing Table 3.

REFERENCES

Anonymous (1971). Dry Mouth. *British Medical Journal 2,* 646.

Brown, A. S. (1966). Absorption of analgesics from the buccal mucous membrane. *Practitioner 196,* 125.

Brunk, S. F. and Delle, M. (1974). Morphine metabolism in man. *Clinical Pharmacology & Therapeutics 16,* 51.

Comroe, J. H. and Dripps, R. D. (1948). Reactions to morphine in ambulatory and bed patients. *Surgery, Gynecology & Obstetrics 87,* 221.

Editorial (1973). Fractures through metastases. *British Medical Journal 3,* 2.

Fidler, M. (1973). Prophylactic internal fixation of secondary neoplastic deposits in long bones. *British Medical Journal 1,* 341.

Galasko, C. S. B. (1972). Skeletal metastases and mammary cancer. *Annals of the Royal College of Surgeons of England 50,* 3.

Goodman, L. S. and Gilman, A. (1975). The pharmacological basis of therapeutics, 5th edition, p. 161, New York: Macmillan.

Harrington, K. D., Johnston, J. O., Turner, R. H. and Green, D. L. (1972). The use of methylacrylate as an adjunct in the internal fixation of malignant neoplastic fractures. *Journal of Bone & Joint Surgery 54A,* 1665.

Marcove, R. C. and Yang, D. J. (1967). Survival times after treatment of pathologic fractures. *Cancer 20,* 2154.

Parrish, F. F. and Murray, J. A. (1970). Surgical treatment for secondary neoplastic fractures. A retrospective study of 96 patients. *Journal of Bone and Joint Surgery 52A,* 665.

Robbie, D. S. and Samarasinghe, J. (1973). Comparison of Aspirin-Codeine and Paracetamol-Dextropropoxyphene compound tablets with pentazocine in relief of cancer pain. *Journal of International Medical Research 1,* 246.

Special correspondence (1971). Vocational training for general practice. *British Medical Journal 2,* 704.

Smithers, D. (1973). Care of the dying: where to die. *British Medical Journal 1,* 34.

Twycross, R. G. (1974). Clinical experience with diamorphine in advanced malignant disease. *International Journal of Clinical Pharmacology, Therapy & Toxicology 9,* 184.

Verebely, K., Volavka, J., Mule, S. and Resnick, R. (1975). Methadone in man: pharmacokinetic and excretion studies in acute and chronic treatment. *Clinical Pharmacology and Therapeutics 18,* 180.

Way, E. L., Young, J. M. and Kemp, J. W. (1965). Metabolism of heroin and its pharmacologic implications. *Bulletin on Narcotics 17,* No. 1, 25.

Wood, A. J. J., Moir, D. C., Campbell, C., Davidson, J. F., Gallon, S. C., Henney, E. and McAllion, S. (1974). Medicines evaluation & monitoring group: central nervous system effects of pentazocine. *British Medical Journal 1,* 305.

SECTION 3

Special Aspects

Chapter

16

ROBERT W. CRICHLOW

Management of Male Breast Cancer

It must be recognized that the biologic behavior of breast cancer in men may differ considerably from that in women. Lessons which are learned on the management of breast cancer from its natural history in women are not necessarily applicable to men. However a major obstacle in studying the natural history of the disease in men is its rarity. Less than 1.5% of cancer in men occurs in the breast and no more than 1% of breast cancers affects the male. Individual series are therefore small and data from several sources must be combined in order to identify the specific features of male breast cancer. It is difficult to achieve valid conclusions also because of the various methods used in reporting, and the omission of important information in many cases.

In 2217 cases of male breast cancer collected from the literature in 1972 (Crichlow, 1972), it was impossible to assess either the crude five-year survival or the clinical stage at presentation in more than half the cases. Acknowledging these inherent difficulties, this review will attempt to identify significant differences in clinical behavior, affecting management and prognosis, between breast cancer in men and that in women.

CLINICAL BEHAVIOR

The average age of males presenting with breast cancer varies in different series between 60 (Crichlow, 1974) and 65 (Scheike, 1975). This average age is 6 to 11 years older than that found in females with breast cancer, but it must be remembered that the latter has two age peaks—one premenopausal and the other postmenopausal. Although once encountered in a five-year-old boy (Simpson and Barson, 1969), breast cancer is clearly a disease of older men, as only 6% of cases are less than 40 years of age (Holleb et al., 1968), and the risk increases exponentially throughout life.

A mass beneath the areola is the initial complaint in almost all men with breast cancer and changes in the nipple or areola are far more frequent in men than in women. Nipple discharge was reported in 14%

Table 1. Pathologic types of male breast carcinoma in six reported series.

Type	*Number*	*Percentage*
Invasive, ductal	595	85.6%
Medullary	37	5.3%
Papillary	35	5.0%
Paget's Disease	8	1.2%
Mucoid	8	1.2%
Inflammatory	5	0.7%
Other	7	1.0%
Total	695	100.0%

of men with malignant tumours and in 2% of those with benign breast tumours (Treves et al., 1956). Serous discharge was seen more often with benign lesions, but three quarters of men with sanguineous discharge had breast cancer—triple the risk in women (Seltzer et al., 1970).

Early and frequent involvement of the nipple and areola is probably a consequence of the proximity of the tumor to the overlying skin. Ulceration is found in 28% and fixation, inversion, encrustation or edema in an additional 37% (Crichlow, 1972). Scheike (1973) has shown a significant correlation between duration of symptoms on the one hand and the tumor size and skin ulceration on the other. Its effect on prognosis will be discussed later.

All of the clinical and histologic varieties of breast cancer encountered in women are found in men with the exception of lobular carcinoma. This probably reflects the lack of lobules in male breast tissue (Stewart, 1950) unless subjected to abnormal hormonal stimulation (Crichlow, 1972). The relative incidence of the various histologic types is indicated in Table 1, drawn from six series reported since 1927 (Crichlow et al., 1972; Haagensen, 1971; Holleb et al., 1968; Sachs, 1941; Visfeldt and Scheike, 1973; Wainwright, 1927). Inflammatory carcinoma and Paget's disease of the breast are clinicopathologic variants which appear to be expressed similarly in both sexes (Crichlow, 1972). In Denmark, Visfeldt and Scheike (1973) found little difference between the sexes in the relative incidence of infiltrating ductal and other carcinomas, if lobular and squamous cell carcinomas were ignored.

The differential diagnosis of a mass in the male breast almost always involves distinction between gynecomastia and carcinoma. Gynecomastia is a hyperplasia of fibrous and epithelial elements of rudimentary male breast tissue, occasionally associated with acinar formation and degenerative changes in connective tissue. A history of prior estrogen therapy, younger age of the patient, bilaterality, tenderness, or pain in the absence of ulceration would suggest gynecomastia. Both conditions tend to show adherence to the overlying areola, but gynecomastia does not tend to fix to underlying pectoral fascia, or produce ulceration or other changes in the nipple and areola. Hardness, eccentricity and lack of definition usually indicate malignancy as opposed to the firm, well defined, central discoid mass of gynecomastia.

Mammography is an increasingly precise and useful tool in the detection of breast cancer in women. While less experience has been acquired in men, the technique appears to be useful, though subject to the same need for careful interpretation in the light of clinical findings (Forman, 1962).

TREATMENT OF EARLY BREAST CANCER

The choice of optimal treatment for potentially curable carcinoma of the female breast has become increasingly controversial in recent decades. The proponents of radical and conservative surgery and radiation therapy are well represented in earlier chapters. Not enough prospective randomized trials have completed 10 year observations capable of providing clear answers in the female, but there are numerous reports of the results of individual or combined modalities of therapy in well defined patient populations. There are no comparable data available to allow comparison of different therapeutic approaches in men.

By and large, surgeons appear to treat carcinoma of the breast in the male as they would in the female, although reasons for selection of one operation over another are often not stated. The small number of cases available for analysis, and frequent failure to relate stage of the disease to treatment and its result, frustrate attempts to define optimal treatment for carcinoma of the male breast. Although criteria for operability are not always stated, there does not appear to be any evidence of significant improvement in recent decades. In 1941 Sachs found 74% of his 264 patients operable, and in 1976 Scheike reported a rate of 78% in 253 cases. Of 495 men collected from 14 reports in the interval, 81% were judged operable, 68% undergoing radical mastectomy and 13% simple mastectomy (Crichlow, 1972).

While some authors favor radical mastectomy (Corwin et al., 1967; Crichlow et al., 1972; Holleb et al., 1968; Somerville, 1952; Wolloch and Dintsman, 1973), others advocate simple mastectomy, particularly in the elderly patient (Greening and Aichroth,

1965; Liechty et al., 1967; Scheike, 1976). Criteria used for choice of the simple as against the radical procedure are rarely defined and it appears that selection of patients for simple mastectomy may be either because of apparently good prognosis (Liechty et al., 1967) or poor prognosis (Crichlow et al., 1972). In those reports in which groups of men and women were treated concurrently, radical mastectomy was generally used with lower frequency in the male (Crichlow et al., 1972; Donegan and Perez-Mesa, 1973).

The comparisons are further obscured by the inconsistent use of adjuvant radiation therapy. Although often combined with simple mastectomy (Greening and Aichroth, 1965; Scheike, 1976), or used in the presence of lymph node metastases (Corwin et al., 1967; Guthorn, 1951; Robinson and Farha, 1967; Somerville, 1952; Stephenson and Gordon, 1969), no consistent pattern has emerged.

Until sufficient useful information about the results of various therapeutic approaches to men with breast cancer can be accumulated, one has no alternative but to proceed on the basis of what is learned from treatment of the disease in women. However, it must be recognized that the common presentation for the male (a central tumor in close proximity to pectoral muscle and epidermis), is rare in the female. Moreover the biologic behavior of the tumor in the male may be quite different because of obvious differences in hormonal environments. Translation of treatment policy from the female patient must therefore be cautious.

Postoperative adjuvant use of single agent or combined chemotherapy has not been reported in males with breast cancer. The experience in females suggests the possibility that postoperative cytotoxic chemotherapy may lead to prolongation of the recurrence-free period (see Chapter 6). Whether or not this will eventually prove to be accompanied by prolongation of survival, it may provide an important gain in the quality of life for the patient with a high risk of recurrence. This consideration may be particularly important in the male, in view of the lower survival rate in general and more especially in the presence of lymph node metastases.

TREATMENT OF ADVANCED BREAST CANCER

There are no obvious differences in patterns of recurrence or metastasis between the sexes (Crichlow, 1972), and radiotherapy and surgery should be applied for symptomatic relief in the same way as in the female. So little experience is reported with cytotoxic chemotherapy in male breast cancer that no specific comment is warranted. However, there is nothing about the observed biologic behavior of male breast cancer to suggest that a difference in response to cytotoxic agents would be likely.

Interesting differences in response to additive and ablative hormonal therapy exist between the sexes. Additive hormonal therapy, a mainstay in the female, has proved of very little value in the male. There have been a few documented responses to estrogens (Donegan and Perez-Mesa, 1973; Haagensen, 1971; Kennedy and Kiang, 1972; Ogilvie, 1961; Treves, 1959), one to androgens (Donegan and Perez-Mesa, 1973) and one to progestogens (Geller et al., 1961). Short term and poorly documented remissions with corticosteroids are reported (Treves, 1959), but this agent is, in the writer's opinion, more useful in improving the patient's sense of well-being and controlling hypercalcemia.

On the other hand, ablative hormonal therapy has been more frequently effective in men than in women. Orchiectomy has produced much higher response rates and longer durations of remission than oophorectomy, and the effect of orchiectomy does not appear to be age-limited. Treves (1959) was uuable to relate the probability of response either to age or to the histologic appearance of the testes in a group of 41 patients aged 39-85 years; 28 (68%) had objective regressions. A subsequent report from the same institution, employing more rigid and objective criteria, documented response in 17 of 38 men (45%), and in nine the duration was in excess of a year (Holleb et al., 1968).

Objective remissions have been observed in 22 of 38 men following castration (58%) in other reports, but the criteria and duration of remissions were not uniformly stated (Crichlow, 1972; Donegan and Perez-Mesa, 1973; Kennedy and Kiang, 1972; Li et al., 1970; Stephens and Muggia, 1974). Because of the high response rate and low morbidity, orchiectomy is often enthusiastically recommended by physicians in the treatment of advanced male breast cancer, only to be rejected by patients. In Treves' (1959) words, "The acquiescence to orchiectomy seems to us to be a triumph of medical persuasion".

Bilateral adrenalectomy has been reported in 26 men with metastatic carcinoma of the breast, but evaluation is limited in many by lack of precise information, short follow-up periods, and associated hormonal therapy (Crichlow, 1972; Hanson et al., 1971; Stephens and Muggia, 1974). In all but one instance, adrenalectomy was preceded or accompanied by orchiectomy. In a review of adrenalec-

tomy in 17 males with metastatic breast carcinoma, Li et al. (1970) found objective evidence of regression in ten of 14 evaluable cases. In two of the responders prior orchiectomy had been unsuccessful, while one of the adrenalectomy failures had previously responded to orchiectomy. In general, orchiectomy and adrenalectomy have been performed sequentially, but response to the combined operation occurred in three of four reported instances (Hanson et al., 1971; Li et al., 1970).

The use of hypophysectomy in male breast cancer has recently been reviewed by Kennedy and Kiang (1972). Of 12 reported attempts, eight cases were evaluable and led to three complete and two partial remissions with an average duration of 20 months. The choice between adrenalectomy and hypophysectomy in women with metastatic breast carcinoma is based on local option, for the results of these two ablative procedures are similar (see Chapter 14). Although protracted remissions appear to be more evident following hypophysectomy in men, the numbers are far too small to allow any firm conclusions, and the choice between adrenalectomy and hypophysectomy is best made on the local availability of appropriate surgical skills.

The selection of men for major ablative procedures has not been evaluated in terms of disease-free interval or dominant site of metastases, two useful predictors of response in women. The need for clinical criteria in selecting patients for endocrine ablation may in the future be obviated by the availability of hormone receptor assays on tumor tissue. Specific estrogen receptors have been demonstrated in a male breast cancer (Wittliff, 1974), and in one instance a positive estrogen receptor assay was associated with response to both orchiectomy and adrenalectomy performed sequentially (Moseley et al., 1974).

RESULTS OF TREATMENT

Continuing disagreement about the relative prognosis of males and females with breast cancer results from conclusions made on inadequate data. Comparative survival rates between the sexes have been variously reported as equivalent (Donegan and Perez-Mesa, 1973; Mausner et al., 1969) and less favorable for men (Moss, 1964; Peltokallio and Kalima, 1969), after correction of data for the greater age and age-related mortality of men. Prognosis has been variously described as equivalent (Holleb et al., 1968) and much inferior (Crichlow, 1974; Haagensen, 1971), for men than women at equivalent stages of breast cancer.

Comparison must be based upon groups defined by common pathologic parameters and treated in similar fashion. The use of pathologic staging allows far more precise identification of relative risk. *Clinical staging* is of value in deciding *pre-operatively* what sort of *therapy* is appropriate for a given patient but *pathologic staging* is more useful in predicting *prognosis.* Estimation of lymph node involvement is the single most important prognostic factor for patients with potentially curable carcinoma of the breast and error is common in the clinical assessment of axillary lymph node involvement. Cutler and Connelly (1969) quote the clinical error as 48% false negative and 37% false positive, based on subsequent pathologic findings. Furthermore, 5 year survival data are inadequate to define the effects of breast cancer treatment in women, and there is no reason to suppose they will serve better in men.

Table 2 lists data based on similarly treated and pathologically staged groups of men from eight reports reviewed by the writer in 1974, (Cortese and Cornell, 1971; Corwin et al., 1967; Crichlow et al., 1972; Haagensen, 1971; Holleb et al., 1968; Liechty et al., 1967; Robinson and Farha, 1967; Somerville, 1952). The 61% operability rate (radical mastectomy) is lower than that usually reported for women and cannot be explained by a different proportion of advanced disease, because the 53% incidence of histologically proven axillary lymph node metastases approximates that reported in women (Haagensen, 1971; Handley, 1972). Five year survival data are available from all but Haagensen's (1971) series, but

Table 2. Collected experience with radical mastectomy in males with breast cancer.

Frequency of radical mastectomy	234/367	(61%)
Incidence of proven axillary lymph node metastases	102/191	(53%)
Survival after radical mastectomy	5 Years	10 Years
Overall	70/143 (49%)	17/49 (35%)
Node Negative	46/58 (79%)	16/26 (62%)
Node Positive	24/85 (28%)	1/23 (4.3%)

10 year data from only three reports (Crichlow et al., 1972; Haagensen, 1971; Liechty et al., 1967).

Without age correction, overall survival is noticeably poorer at both the 5 and 10 year levels than is usually seen among women. For example, Haagensen (1971) reported ten year survivals of 74% among 324 node negative women, and 39% among 298 with axillary metastases. In comparison, the very poor 10 year survival among men with axillary lymph node metastases is marked, and it is doubtful that age correction would significantly change this striking mortality rate.

Of all prognostic factors operating in resectable carcinoma of the male breast, the presence or absence of regional lymph node metastases seems to be the most important. Norris and Taylor (1969) and Scheike (1976) both demonstrated a direct relationship between tumor size and the frequency of palpable axillary lymph nodes. Scheike (1976) also noted that 5 year survival was halved in those men with either axillary adenopathy, skin ulceration or attachment of tumor to underlying structures.

POSSIBLE CAUSES OF POOR PROGNOSIS

Specific factors, both tumor-related and non-tumor-related, may conspire to deny men as good a prognosis for breast cancer as women. They include the effect of their older age group, the tendency for longer delay in seeking treatment by men, and the effect of the location of the tumor and its tendency to early ulceration.

Cancer of the breast in males is a disease of elderly men, and when mortality rates are adjusted for the expected deaths from natural causes, there is an 8-13% improvement in 5 year survival rates in four out of five studies (Scheike, 1976). When this is allowed for, a survival advantage in older men over younger men with breast carcinoma has been found in some series (McDivitt and Stewart, 1966; Peltokallio and Kalima, 1969) although not in others (Scheike, 1976; Vanderbilt and Warren, 1971).

Men tend to delay longer than women in seeking treatment for breast cancer. The duration of time elapsing between onset of symptoms and diagnosis of breast cancer averaged 18 months in 1228 male patients collected since 1900, but was 10 months in those reports since 1951 (Crichlow, 1972). In a study of breast cancer in Philadelphia, Mausner et al. (1969) found delays of more than a year in almost one-third of males compared to one-fifth of women.

While Scheike (1976) observed an increasing frequency of bad prognostic features (such as increasing tumor size and skin ulceration) with increasing duration of symptoms, there was not a direct correlation between delay in treatment as such and prognosis. In fact, in those patients with a duration of symptoms greater than one year the prognosis proved to be as good or better than those with shorter delays in treatment. He believes that this reflects either a naturally slower growing tumor or confusion engendered by preceding benign breast disease upon which carcinoma is later superimposed.

Skin ulceration affects 28% of males with breast cancer (Crichlow, 1972) and in the absence of any other grave sign of locally advanced disease, the presence of skin ulceration in women has been shown to reduce 5 year clinical cure rates from 45% to 36% (Haagensen, 1971). Spatial relationships may be of consequence in male breast cancer, for even a small carcinoma finds itself adjacent to skin and pectoral fascia and there is not the protection offered by the greater bulk of intervening mammary tissue in the female.

Another important prognostic factor is the almost constant central location of breast cancer in men. In women a poorer prognosis is associated with central than with lateral tumors. For example, Handley (1972) achieved a 10 year survival of only 38% in women with central lesions, compared to 52% in women with medial, and 53% in those with lateral tumors. He encountered internal mammary lymph node metastases in centrally placed tumors twice as frequently as in lateral breast lesions. whether with or without axillary lymph node metastases. Such an unfavorable pattern of regional metastasis may contribute significantly to the inferior survival seen in men with relatively small tumors (Norris and Taylor, 1969).

On the other hand, certain histologic features of breast cancer in the male may be associated with a better prognosis. It is well established that there is a direct relationship between histologic grade and prognosis (Greening and Aichroth, 1965; Liechty et al., 1967; Scheike, 1976), and Scheike's analysis (1976) of 150 cases of male breast cancer shows a relatively smaller proportion of Grade III (anaplastic) tumors than among women. Moreover, 19 of the 170 cancers reported by Holleb et al. (1968) and three out of 40 reported by Vanderbilt and Warren (1971) were of the papillary type and this has a relatively good prognosis. The medullary type also has a good prognosis in the female, but in one report on 40 males, the four with medullary type cancer fared no better than those with the other histopathologic types (Vanderbilt and Warren, 1971).

Of all the prognostic factors, involvement of regional lymph nodes seems the most important. In the male with histologically proven axillary node metastasis, survival is significantly worse than in women.

SUMMARY

One of every 100 cancers of the breast occurs in a male. A man with breast cancer will be 6 to 11 years older than his female counterpart, and will probably delay somewhat longer in obtaining treatment, and will present more frequently signs of advanced local disease, such as skin ulceration or tumor fixation. There is nothing to suggest that the primary treatment of cancer in men should differ from that in women, if one bears in mind that tumors in men are necessarily central and close to the pectoral fascia.

Decisions about systemic therapy for metastatic breast cancer should be influenced by the likelihood that response to cytotoxic therapy is alike in the sexes, but that men respond more frequently (and longer and without relation to age) to ablative hormonal therapy and less frequently to additive hormonal therapy than do women. Prognosis is generally regarded as poorer for men than for women with cancer of the breast, and although explained in part by a man's greater age and age-related mortality, the relative disadvantage of men with axillary lymph node metastases is striking.

REFERENCES

Cortese, A. F. and Cornell, G. N. (1971). Carcinoma of the male breast. *Annals of Surgery 173,* 275.

Corwin, J. H., Ferguson, E. F., Moseley, T. and Willey, E. N. (1967). Carcinoma of the male breast. *Southern Medical Journal 60,* 777.

Crichlow, R. W. (1972). Carcinoma of the male breast. *Surgery, Gynecology & Obstetrics 134,* 1011.

Crichlow, R. W. (1974). Breast cancer in men. *Seminars in Oncology 1,* 145.

Crichlow, R. W., Kaplan, E. L. and Kearney, W. H. (1972). Male mammary cancer, an analysis of 32 cases. *Annals of Surgery 175,* 489.

Cutler, S. J. and Connelly, R. R. (1969). Mammary cancer trends. *Cancer 23,* 767.

Dao, T. L., Morreal, C. and Nemoto, T. (1973). Urinary estrogen excretion in men with breast cancer. *New England Journal of Medicine 289,* 138.

Donegan, W. L. and Perez-Mesa, C. M. (1973). Carcinoma of the male breast, a 30 year review of 28 cases. *Archives of Surgery 106,* 273.

Forman, M. (1962). Roentgenography of the male breast. *American Journal of Roentgenology, Radium Therapy and Nuclear Medicine 88,* 1126.

Geller, J., Wol, H. and Lewin, M. (1961). Objective remission of metastatic breast carcinoma in a male who received 17-alpha hydroxy progesterone caproate (delalutin). *Cancer Chemotherapy Reports 14,* 77.

Greening, W. P. and Aichroth, P. M. (1965). Cancer of the male breast. *British Journal of Cancer 19,* 92.

Guthorn, P. J. (1951). Carcinoma of the male breast; a report of 15 cases. *Military Surgeon 109,* 110.

Haagensen, C. D. (1971). *Diseases of the Breast,* (2 nd) Ed. W. B. Saunders Company, Philadelphia.

Haagensen, C. D. (1971). *Diseases of the Breast,* (2nd ed.) W. B. Saunders Company, Philadelphia.

Handley, R. S. (1972). Observations and thoughts on carcinoma of the breast. *Proceedings of the Royal Society of Medicine 65,* 437.

Hanson, E. L., Abramson, S. F., Sage, H. H. and Grier, W. R. N. (1971). Complete remission of metastatic carcinoma of male breast following simultaneous adrenalectomy and orchiectomy. *New York State Journal of Medicine 71,* 670.

Holleb, A. I., Freeman, H. P. and Farrow, J. H. (1968). Cancer of the male breast. *New York State Journal of Medicine 68,* 544 and 656.

Kennedy, B. J. and Kiang, D. T. (1972). Hypophysectomy in the treatment of advanced cancer of the male breast. *Cancer 29,* 1606.

Li, M. C., Janelli, D. E., Kelly, E. J., Kashiwabara, H. and Kim, R. H. (1970). Metastatic carcinoma of the male breast treated with bilateral adrenalectomy and chemotherapy. *Cancer 25,* 678.

Liechty, R. D., Davis, J. and Gleysteen, J. (1967). Cancer of the male breast, forty cases. *Cancer 20,* 1617.

Mausner, J. S., Shimkin, M. B. and Moss, N. H. (1969). Cancer of the breast in Philadelphia hospitals, 1951-1964. *Cancer 23,* 260.

McDivitt, R. W. and Stewart, F. W. (1966). Breast carcinoma in children. *Journal of the American Medical Association 195,* 144.

Moseley, H. S., Fletcher, W. S., Leung, B. S. and Krippaehne, W. W. (1974). Predictive criteria for the selection of breast cancer patients for adrenalectomy. *The American Journal of Surgery 128,* 143.

Moss, N. H. (1964). Cancer of the male breast. *Annals of the New York Academy of Sciences 114,* 937.

Norris, H. J. and Taylor, H. B. (1969). Carcinoma of the male breast. *Cancer 23,* 1428.

Ogilvie, T. A. (1961). Carcinoma of the breast in a male. *Proceedings of the Royal Society of Medicine 54,* 24.

Peltokallio, P. and Kalima, T. V. (1969). Malignant tumors of the male breast in Finland; a report of 51 cases. *British Journal of Cancer 23,* 480.

Robinson, F. W. and Farha, G. C. (1967). Carcinoma of the male breast. *American Journal of Surgery 113,* 394.

Sachs, M. D. (1941). Carcinoma of the male breast. *Radiology 37,* 458.

Scheike, O. (1973). Male breast cancer; 5. clinical manifestations in 257 cases in Denmark. *British Journal of Cancer 28,* 552.

Scheike, O. (1976). Factors provoking male breast cancer. In

Risk Factors in Breast Cancer, p. 173 (Ed. B. A. Stoll). London: Heinemann Medical.

Seltzer, M. H., Perloff, L. J., Kelley, R. I. and Fitts, W. T. (1970). The significance of age in patients with nipple discharge. *Surgery, Gynecology & Obstetrics 131,* 519.

Simpson, J. S. and Barson, A. J. (1969). Breast tumors in infants and children, a 40 year review of cases at a children's hospital. *Canadian Medical Association Journal 101,* 100.

Somerville, P. (1952). Carcinoma of the male breast, a report of 19 cases and a review of the literature. *British Journal of Surgery 39,* 296.

Stephens, R. L. and Muggia, F. M. (1974). Breast cancer in men, report illustrating the values of endocrine ablation. *American Journal of Medicine 57,* 679.

Stephenson, T. R. and Gordon, H. E. (1969). Primary carcinoma of the male breast. *Archives of Surgery 99,* 529.

Stewart, F. W. (1950). Tumors of the breast. In *Atlas of Tumor Pathology,* p. 7 Section IX, Fasicle 34, Armed Forces Institute of Pathology, Washington, D.C.

Treves, N. (1959). The treatment of cancer, especially inoperable cancer, of the male breast by ablative surgery (orchiectomy, adrenalectomy and hypophysectomy) and hormone therapy (estrogens and corticosteroids); an analysis of 42 patients. *Cancer 12,* 820.

Treves, N., Robbins, G. F. and Amoroso, W. L. (1956). Serous and serosanguineous discharge from the male nipple. *Archives of Surgery 73,* 319.

Vanderbilt, P. C. and Warren, S. E. (1971). Forty year experience with carcinoma of the male breast. *Surgery, Gynecology & Obstetrics 133,* 629.

Visfeldt, J. and Scheike, O. (1973). Male breast cancer; I. Histologic typing and grading of 187 Danish cases. *Cancer 32,* 985.

Wainwright, J. M. (1927). Carcinoma of the male breast, clinical and pathologic study. *Archives of Surgery 14,* 836.

Wittliff, J. L. (1974). Specific receptors of the steroid hormones in breast cancer. *Seminars in Oncology 1,* 109.

Wolloch, Y. and Dintsman, M. (1973). Primary carcinoma of the male breast. *American Journal of Surgery 125,* 628.

Chapter

17

CHARLES B. ANDERSON, CHARLES L. ROPER AND THOMAS B. FERGUSON

Management of Pleural Metastases

Pleural effusions in patients with a past history of carcinoma of the breast should be considered malignant until proven otherwise. Pleural effusion is a common complication in patients with carcinoma of the breast and is said to occur in up to 50% of all cases with uncontrolled disease (Fracchia et al., 1970; Ultmann, 1962). The presence of a large effusion will cause severe dyspnea and inevitably death from respiratory failure, but it is important to stress that if the patient's general condition is good, it may be possible to control the effusion and to prolong life for many months or even years. This applies especially in the case of carcinoma of the breast (Ariel et al., 1966).

While in the moribund patient aspiration of the fluid may be adequate, in the patient with more than a short life expectancy, an attempt must be made at pleurodesis-sealing of the pleural space after complete evacuation of the fluid. Dyspnea from pleural effusion will continue as long as the pleural space persists, because the lung is compressed and the mediastinal shift compromises the opposite lung. Multiple attempts at needle aspiration result in loss of protein and electrolytes and run the risk of infection and pneumothorax.

Why is it then that repeated needle aspiration with the occasional introduction of cytotoxic agents, is the therapeutic method practised in over 95% of patients suffering the misery of pleural effusion complicating carcinoma of the breast? It is probably because the variety in the methods of treatment recommended in recent years has left the non-expert confused. Moreover, the various ways in which results are reported, and the different parameters used to measure response, make it difficult to compare the efficacy of the treatment methods advocated.

A thorough understanding of the various methods of treatment and a practical approach in managing these patients is essential for effective palliation. This chapter reviews the pathogenesis and diagnosis of malignant pleural effusion due to carcinoma of the breast and critically evaluates the various modalities now available to treat this entity.

PATHOGENESIS OF MALIGNANT EFFUSIONS

Black (1972) has reviewed in detail the normal physiologic mechanisms of pleural fluid formation

and absorption, as well as the pathophysiologic processes involved in the disease states causing pleural effusion. A variety of factors contribute to the formation of malignant pleural effusion (Dollinger, 1972; Lambert et al., 1967; Leininger et al., 1969; O'Bryan et al., 1968). Altered water metabolism along with changes in lymphatic and capillary permeability have all been implicated. Sodium retention, however, is not a significant factor, and diuretic programs are usually unsuccessful in controlling effusions. Although a detailed review of lymphatic and capillary permeability changes are beyond the scope of this discussion, it is essential that certain basic principles be appreciated.

Factors which result in abnormal pleural fluid formation are those contributing either to increased production or to decreased outflow. Factors which increase fluid production include:

1. Increased permeability of capillaries supplying tumor implants.
2. Increased pleural capillary permeability from pleuritis associated with obstructive pneumonitis.
3. Direct erosion of blood and lymphatic vessels by tumor.
4. Mechanical trauma to the opposing pleural surfaces by tumor implants.
5. Production of fluid by free growing tumor cells in the pleural effusion.

Mechanisms which impede pleural fluid outflow include:

1. Venous and/or lymphatic blockage by tumor cells, primarily in the mediastinum.
2. Pleural thickening.
3. Hypoproteinemia.
4. Depressed respiratory motion which alters intrathoracic pressure and thus hampers the pumping mechanisms.

Pleural fluid protein concentration in patients with malignant serous effusions is usually greater than 3 gm per 100 ml (Leuallen et al., 1955). The high protein concentration is the result of either lymphatic obstruction or increased pleural capillary permeability.

Although the pathogenesis of malignant pleural effusion is poorly understood, this does not detract from the effective treatment of malignant effusions. In our opinion the prime objective of local therapy is obliteration of the pleural space rather than selective modification of production or absorption of fluid. On the other hand, Dollinger (1972) has recently proposed the classification of malignant pleural effusions into three types and suggested appropriate therapy in each circumstance.

In the most common type, tumor implants irritate the serous membranes and cause an effusion containing 50 to 1,000 cells/mm^3 which are differentiated and pleomorphic. Local treatment with radioactive or chemotherapeutic agents is advocated in this situation. In the second type, there is a transudation of fluid as a result of obstruction in the small vessels and lymphatics, and no tumor cells are found in the effusion. Because this type is always associated with large tumor masses, systemic treatment is suggested. In the third type, an effusion similar to the ascitic cell tumor in animals is seen, with large numbers of uniform viable malignant cells present. This type of effusion also responds well to local treatment.

Dollinger (1972) believes therefore that the best response to local chemotherapy is obtained when large numbers of cancer cells are present in the effusion. O'Bryan et al. (1968) on the other hand, could find no correlation between the cytology of the effusion and the effectiveness of radioactive gold or phosphorus therapy. Anderson et al. (1974) have also been unable to correlate effectiveness of treatment with either the number or the characteristics of the cells.

CHARACTERISTICS OF MALIGNANT EFFUSIONS

Malignant pleural effusion is the initial sign of recrudesence in 6.5% of all operated patients with recurrent carcinoma of the breast The effusion is unilateral in a majority of cases but 5 to 20% of patients have bilateral involvement (Fracchia et al, 1970; Anderson et al., 1974; Spratt and Donegan, 1967). Bloody effusions are said to occur in less than 2% of patients (Fracchia et al., 1970). Anaplastic forms of mammary carcinoma have a greater tendency toward pleural metastases and subsequent effusion.

Meyer (1966), in an autopsy study, examined 52 patients with pleural metastases from a variety of tumors. The pleural metastases were confined to the visceral pleura alone in 15 cases, parietal pleura only in one case and both pleural surfaces in 36 cases. Of the 31 patients in whom pleural effusion was present, it was hemorrhagic in nine cases. The presence of pleural effusion was closely related to neoplastic infiltration of the mediastinum but was not related to the extent of pleural involvement by nodular metastatic implants.

With malignant pleural effusion originating in

carcinoma of the breast, cytology is positive in 71 to 75% of cases (Anderson et al., 1974; Jarvi et al., 1972). An even higher recovery of positive cells can be obtained by submitting the sediment from the chest bottle for examination after complete drainage of the effusion by tube thoracostomy. Effusion occurs on the side of the involved or amputated breast in approximately 80% of cases (Stoll and Ellis, 1953). Porter (1965) and Spratt and Donegan, (1967) have interpreted this to be evidence for permeation through the chest wall rather than blood borne metastasis.

Malignant pleural effusions are typically exudates and the distinction between an exudate and transudate is therefore important. Exudates are defined as fluid collections with protein concentrations greater than 3 gm per 100 ml. Since 19% of malignant effusions have a protein concentration less than 3 gm per 100 ml. two other characteristics of exudates are important—the protein and lactic dehydrogenase concentrations (Light et al., 1972). Exudates are characterized by a pleural fluid to serum protein difference greater than 200 u/ml. Also by a higher LDH level than a simultaneous serum specimen (Wroblewski and Wroblewski, 1958; Light et al., 1972). When any two of these three characteristics are present in pleural fluid, the likelihood of its being a transudate are less than 10%.

When the pleural fluid is shown to be an exudate, additional diagnostic maneuvers, such as cytology, cell block or pleural biopsy (needle or open), are needed to make a definitive diagnosis of a malignant effusion before specific therapy is instituted. On the other hand, when the fluid is shown to be a transudate, further local diagnostic and therapeutic maneuvers are not necessary, since etiologic possibilities are limited to congestive heart failure, nephrosis, renal failure, liver cirrhosis or hypoproteinemia.

The finding of malignant cells in the fluid when a pleural effusion is due to carcinoma of the breast connotes a poor prognosis. According to Konikov et al. (1966) 37% of these patients die within one month and another 34% die between one and six months. Nevertheless, the fact that 29% survive for six months or longer emphasizes the importance of controlling the symptoms in these individuals.

DIAGNOSIS

The presenting symptoms of pleural effusion include pleuritic chest pain, dyspnea, fatigue, cough and fever. However, in the early stages, the patient is often asymptomatic and even with large malignant effusions, symptoms may be minimal. If severe symptoms are present, pulmonary metastasis with lymphangitic dissemination should be suspected but this can only be determined after the effusion is removed. Hemothorax occurs rarely with carcinoma of the breast but if other findings of disseminated carcinoma are present, it is evidence of the malignant nature of the effusion. A chest X-ray will identify the effusion and indicate whether it is ipsilateral or bilateral. A lateral decubitus film is helpful in determining that the fluid collection is free within the pleural cavity.

Further differential diagnosis requires that a portion of the fluid should be removed and submitted for protein analysis, LDH content, bacteriological cultures, gram stain, amylase test, occult blood testing and cytologic examination. Fat staining will verify the presence of free fat in the case of chylothorax. A past history of carcinoma of the breast indicates that the effusion is malignant until proven otherwise and in such cases only an amount of fluid adequate to perform the above tests should be aspirated. This is because extensive thoracentesis may interfere with later definitive treatment by tube thoracotomy and the instillation of irritating agents to cause pleural symphysis.

The possibility of other causes of pleural effusion must be eliminated. Abdominal causes include cirrhosis of the liver, Meig's syndrome, renal failure, pancreatitis and subphrenic abscess. Systemic causes include lupus erythematosus, rheumatoid arthritis and congestive heart failure, while thoracic causes include infections of the lung or pleural cavity, pulmonary infarction or embolus, bronchial carcinoma and previous mediastinal irradiation.

A Cope needle biopsy of the pleura may be necessary when the etiology still remains in doubt but rarely is open biopsy indicated. In most patients, it is not necessary to delay treatment while waiting for a final diagnosis. The presumption of malignant effusion can be made in most circumstances and the thoracostomy tube treatment carried out without delay.

MEASUREMENT OF RESPONSE

Although a number of methods have been used to treat malignant pleural effusions, no mode of therapy has emerged as being of paramount advantage. The evaluation and comparison of each type of treatment is complicated by the various ways of reporting results. Some investigators assess the interval before reaccumulation of pleural fluid, but the amount of

fluid which they regard as significant may vary widely. Others measure the time until retreatment is instituted, ignoring the fact that some patients might not obtain therapy as soon as they need it. We have concentrated on the length of time that the patient remains asymptomatic. Since the main objective in therapy is palliation, delay in recurrence of symptoms is probably more important in determining effectiveness of treatment than is recurrence of an effusion, which often may be small and asymptomatic.

Reporting short term improvement from a particular form of therapy, without clearly defining the proportion still under control at varying times subsequently, can result in erroneously favorable statistics. Actuarial analysis of results (see page 180) gives the most accurate assessment of treatment but unfortunately, few reports are expressed in this manner. Other types of therapy used before or after the reported treatment must also be specified because responses in patients who have had or are undergoing external radiation or systemic cytotoxic therapy may be due to either of these methods.

It is clear that standardized methods of reporting data are essential if meaningful information is to be obtained to compare the different treatments of malignant pleural effusion secondary to carcinoma of the breast.

METHODS OF TREATMENT

Techniques used to treat malignant pleural effusions include:

- Systemic chemotherapy
- Thoracentesis
- Thoracentesis and chemotherapeutic agents
- Radioactive isotopes
  - gold (^{198}Au)
  - phosphorus (^{32}P)
  - yttrium (^{90}Y)
- Tube thoracostomy
- Tube thoracostomy and chemotherapeutic agents
  - nitrogen mustard
  - thio-TEPA
  - quinacrine
  - tetracycline
- Talc poudrage
- Radiotherapy
- Pleurectomy

Tube thoracostomy with nitrogen mustard instillation is our preferred method of treating all malignant effusions, especially those due to carcinoma of the breast. In order to justify this strong preference in the management of malignant effusion, it is necessary to review the important aspects of each treatment modality.

Systemic Chemotherapy

Marked improvement in malignant effusions can occur as a result of systemic chemotherapy or hormonal therapy for disseminated carcinoma of the breast. Many patients with effusions also have other evidence of disseminated disease and will have been treated with systemic agents for these additional sites of distant metastases; in some of the patients, the effusion remains intractable and it is necessary to utilize local therapy to give symptomatic relief. Treatment of the effusion should aim at coaptation and symphysis of the pleural surfaces rather than resolution of the malignant process per se.

Thoracentesis

Thoracentesis is inferior to other forms of therapy in this respect (Lambert et al., 1967). We have noted (Anderson et al., 1974) that in 94 unilateral effusions treated only by complete aspiration of pleural fluid, the average time until recurrence of the effusion was 4.2 days. The majority of effusions recurred within 1 to 3 days and 97% recurred within one month. Therefore, repeated thoracenteses are necessary to maintain evacuation of the pleural space. This not only requires frequent visits to the physician but also causes protein depletion, increases the risk of infection and pneumothorax, and often leads to loculation of fluid and trapping of the lung by pleural adhesions which makes subsequent therapy more difficult. Simple thoracentesis is however, the preferred method of managing moribund patients with severe dyspnea just prior to their death.

Thoracentesis and Sclerosing Agents

Thoracentesis in conjunction with the instillation of chemotherapeutic agents is claimed to cause benefit in 59 to 100% of patients, depending upon the series and length of follow up (Dollinger et al., 1967; Hickman and Jones, 1970; Kinsey et al., 1964; Mark et al., 1964; Ultmann et al., 1963; Weisberger et al., 1955). These favorable claims are mainly the result of a liberal interpretation of improvement in relation to subjective change and duration of observation. Improvement of even one month's duration is often classified as a good result. Our experience (Anderson et al., 1974) with local instillation of nitrogen

mustard and thoracentesis has been extremely disappointing. The effusions recurred on the average less than three days after treatment, were all symptomatic and required retreatment.

The technique of thoracentesis with injection of sclerosing agents involves needle aspiration of most of the pleural fluid and subsequent injection of the selected chemical. The patient then changes position frequently to ensure uniform distribution over all pleural surfaces. This will induce a sterile pleuritis which, if the visceral and parietal surfaces are coapted, will result in pleural symphysis and obliteration of the pleural space. A temporary increase in the effusion may be seen because of irritation of the pleural surface and this may require additional thoracenteses over several days or weeks.

Nitrogen mustard is instilled into the pleural space at a dose of 0.4 mg/kg but the dose should be reduced by one half in patients with a history of previous radiotherapy or chemotherapy or in those with depressed marrow function, in order to prevent severe leukopenia or thrombocytopenia. Nausea and vomiting are common but pain is rarely observed. Three weeks later the injection may be repeated if the effusion persists.

Incomplete or partial expansion of the lung can lead to "trapped" lung and loculated collections of pleural fluid. The advantages of nitrogen mustard include its easy availablity, low cost and ease of administration. Weisberger et al. (1955) reported 88 patients with various types of malignant effusion in whom 65% improved after treatment with nitrogen mustard. Kinsey et al. (1964) in 62 patients, and Mark et al. (1964) in 32 patients, noted control in 87 and 92% of patients respectively, when using thoracentesis combined with nitrogen mustard.

The use of quinacrine (Atabrine) involves the injection of 200 mg on alternate days at the conclusion of each thoracentesis. Two-thirds of the fluid is removed and the quinacrine, dissolved in 10 ml of saline, is then instilled. The injections are repeated, usually for 4 to 5 doses, until a mild pleuritis occurs. This is associated with pain and fever in most patients. Resolution of the effusion may be seen in 2 to 3 weeks but may take as long as three months in some cases. Since quinacrine does not result in hematopoietic depression, it is useful in patients with impaired bone marrow function, but the acute toxicity of this drug and the need for repeated injections often requires hospitalization of the patient.

Although quinacrine is cytotoxic for neoplastic cells, it is the inflammatory reaction and subsequent adhesions in the pleural space which are mainly responsible for obliteration of the serous space and resolution of the effusion. Response rates of 64 to 100% have been reported by investigators using this drug (Ultmann et al., 1963; Rochlin et al., 1964; Dollinger et al., 1967; Hickman and Jones, 1970).

Thio-TEPA has given results similar to those of nitrogen mustard but with considerably less risk of nausea and vomiting. Bateman et al. (1955) reported remissions lasting 1 to 9 months in 10 of 17 patients with pleural effusions. Effusions due to breast and ovarian carcinoma are said to respond most favorably and the usual dose is 0.8 mg/kg body weight. 5-Fluorouracil, actinomycin D, hydroxyurea and daunorubicin are additional chemotherapeutic agents which have occasionally been used to treat malignant pleural effusions (Dollinger, 1972).

Thoracentesis and Radioactive Agents

Although radioactive gold (^{198}Au) is frequently mentioned in connection with the intrapleural therapy of malignant effusions, its use has declined within the past decade (O'Bryan et al., 1968; Ariel et al., 1966). The usual dosage varies from 50 to 100 mc. This isotope with a half-life of 2.7 days produces both beta and gamma emission but its therapeutic effect on the tumor appears to be derived from the beta emission which has a tissue penetration of 3.8 mm. Subsequent obliteration of the pleural space occurs by mesothelial fibrosis. The major disadvantages of radioactive gold are its short half-life, expense and radiation hazard.

Radioactive colloidal chromic phosphate ($Cr^{32}PO_4$) has been used by some. Its advantage over ^{198}Au is that ^{32}P emits only beta radiation and this offers a greater degree of radiation safety for both the physician and the patient (O'Bryan et al., 1968; El-Mahdi et al., 1973). This isotope has a half-life of 14.3 days. A dose of 5 to 10 mc can be instilled into the pleural space on an outpatient basis, whereas, the gamma emission from ^{198}Au requires hospitalization of the patient.

Other isotopes such as yttrium (^{90}Y) have had limited usage for pleural instillation therapy (Card et al., 1960; Siegel et al., 1956). All radioactive isotopes are instilled by thoracentesis, and tube thoracostomy should of course be avoided. Open or draining fistulas are additional contraindications to the use of radioactive isotopes. Instillation of radioactive isotopes into the pleural cavity has been reported to give improvement in 30 to 90% of cases (Card et al., 1960; Jacobs, 1958; O'Bryan et al., 1968; Siegel et al., 1956).

Tube Thoracostomy

The treatment of malignant effusions by drainage via a tube thoracostomy alone, without instillation of chemotherapeutic or radioactive agents, has been advocated by Lambert et al., (1967). Although they reported recurrence of effusion in only 14 to 17% of cases, our experience with seven patients treated in this manner indicated that all patients developed recurrent effusions within one month. The concept of complete evacuation of the pleural space to permit pleural symphysis is an important one but it is the addition of sclerosing agents which achieves this objective.

Tube Thoracostomy and Chemotherapeutic Agents

The use of chemotherapeutic agents in conjunction with tube thoracostomy for complete and efficient evacuation of a malignant pleural effusion is a relatively new approach. All authors agree that complete removal of the pleural fluid before and after instillation of chemotherapy is an important factor that improves objective results. Whether the intrapleural agent is tumoricidal or not is seemingly unimportant. One strives for the production of a sterile adhesive pleuritis (pleurodesis) which results in the obliteration of the pleural space.

For a successful result the underlying lung must be re-expanded and there must be almost complete removal of the fluid before the agent is introduced. There must be apposition of the parietal and visceral surfaces during the period of induced pleural inflammation. Although some clinicians feel that asymptomatic effusions do not require treatment even if large, we are of the opinion that the pleural space should be emptied completely as soon as any significant effusion is found. This may prevent the deposition of tumor implants and fibrin, and entrapment of the lung.

Leininger et al., (1969) first reported on this method in 1969, and noted good results in 18 patients with 20 effusions, with only one recurrence several months after chest tube drainage and nitrogen mustard instillation. Malignant pleural effusion from carcinoma of the breast has been treated by tube thoracostomy with nitrogen mustard or thio-TEPA instillation, and objective response rates of 66% at 2 months and 50% at 6 months have been reported (Fracchia et al., 1970; Spratt and Donegan, 1967).

Actuarial analysis of 22 patients with pleural effusion due to breast cancer who were treated with nitrogen mustard and tube thoracostomy demonstrated that the proportion of asymptomatic patients at 1, 2 and 6 months were 77%, 66% and 50% respectively (Anderson et al., 1974). The dosage of nitrogen mustard is 20 mg and for thio-TEPA, 30 mg. Nausea and vomiting occur in approximately 50% of patients after nitrogen mustard but less than 4% develop evidence of bone marrow depression.

Borja and Pugh (1973) reported the use of quinacrine instillation in conjunction with tube thoracostomy. Quinacrine was given in a single dose of 800 mg and a response rate of 70% was reported in their series. Fever, pain and nausea were the most frequent signs of quinacrine toxicity. Hickman and Jones (1970) have advocated administration of quinacrine in daily doses of 180 mg to 360 mg for 2 to 3 days. There was no reported differences between the groups as to the type of toxicity exhibited but the intensity and duration of symptoms in the single dose group was greater.

Rubinson and Bolooki, (1972) reported the use of intrapleural tetracycline for malignant effusion. Tetracycline 500 mg diluted in 30 ml of saline was injected into the pleural space through the thoracostomy tube. Satisfactory results were obtained in 10 of their 12 patients. Advantages claimed for this agent over other intrapleural chemotherapeutic agents include the absence of interference with systemic chemotherapy and a minimal amount of pleuritic pain and fever. However, we have found greater pleuritic pain with the use of tetracycline than with any other intrapleural agent and this is not surprising when one considers that tetracycline solution has a pH of 2.4. Our experience over the past two years with tetracycline as a scarifying agent indicates that it has not given the consistently good results obtained with the use of nitrogen mustard.

Technique: Over the past 15 years at Barnes Hospital, we have preferred the combined use of nitrogen mustard and tube thoracostomy drainage. One hour before the procedure, the patient is premedicated with 100 mg pentobarbital for sedation and 100 mg trimethobenzamide to prevent nausea and vomiting. The procedure is performed using 1% lidocaine local anesthesia. After thoracentesis has demonstrated free egress of fluid at the proposed site of tube insertion, a 2 cm skin incision is made and a #30F to #32F thoracostomy tube with at least two side holes 2 cm from the tip is introduced slightly posterior to the mid-axillary line in the 8th or 9th intercostal space. The tube may be inserted either through a trocar or by means of a curved clamp. The tube is sutured to the skin and then connected to water-sealed drainage. With the patient in the supine position, the pleural fluid is allowed to drain completely into a chest bottle. A chest roentgeno-

gram must confirm full expansion of the lung since a trapped lung is a contraindication to local chemotherapy.

Nitrogen mustard in a dose of 0.4 mg per kilogram of body weight (maximum dose 20 mg), is diluted with 30 ml of saline and injected into the pleural space through the thoracostomy tube which is clamped off approximately 4 cm from the skin surface. Nitrogen mustard solution must be mixed immediately before use. Five to ten minutes are available after injection of the solution to ensure its distribution throughout the pleural space, since the drug rapidly alkylates proteins with which it comes in contact. As soon as the solution is injected, the patient is placed in the prone position, on the right side, in the supine position and on the left side before resuming a semi-recumbent position.

After one hour, the thoracostomy tube is reconnected to underwater seal drainage and 25 cm of constant water suction is applied to facilitate complete evacuation of the pleural space. When the chest tube drainage abates, and the chest roentgenogram indicates full expansion of the lung (usually at 48 hours), the thoracostomy tube is removed. If post-thoracostomy roentgenograms are satisfactory the patient is discharged within the next 24 hours. Thus, the patient hospitalized for thoracostomy is in for only 2 to 3 days.

Nausea and pleuritic chest pain are common following this treatment but these symptoms can be well controlled with antiemetics and analgesics. Slight temperature elevations resolve spontaneously and require no special treatment. Hematopoietic depression is rare provided the patient is not receiving concomitant systemic chemotherapy.

Proper technique in performing tube thoracostomy and nitrogen mustard instillation is important. Technical failures can result from the following: inadequate drainage of the pleural effusion prior to nitrogen mustard instillation: insufficient dosage of nitrogen mustard, inadequate positioning of the patient to ensure thorough distribution of the drug, and incomplete re-expansion of the lung before removal of the thoracostomy tube.

Talc Poudrage

Talc poudrage performed during thoracostomy has yielded excellent results in some series, but is suitable only for those individuals who can withstand a major surgical procedure and have a relatively long life expectancy, or those who require thoracostomy for diagnosis (Camishion et al., 1962; Starkey, 1964). A modification of the talc poudrage method which involves insufflation of talc over the pleural surfaces through a tube thoracostomy has been described as giving satisfactory results (Adler and Rappole, 1967; Jones, 1969).

Radiotherapy

Irradiation to the hemithorax is not a popular method for treating malignant pleural effusion because of the complication of pulmonary fibrosis. Its most effective use may be in cases of bloody effusions, where a 55% response rate has been noted (Chu, 1970). Improvement occurs most commonly with lymphomas, but the benefit from local radiotherapy *per se* is difficult to evaluate because the majority of these patients also receive systemic chemotherapy (Weick et al., 1973). Moving-strip irradiation is said to have resulted in the control of 80% of malignant pleural effusions from non-lymphomatous disease also, without incurring radiation pneumonitis or bone marrow depression (Strober et al., 1973). This technique should probably be reserved for those cases failing response to more standard treatment methods.

Pleurectomy

Pleurectomy with or without decortication has been used to treat malignant effusion, with a high degree of success in properly selected patients. Jensik et al. (1963) reported on 50 patients in whom 52 pleurectomies were performed with a 6% mortality rate. Eighteen of the patients had carcinoma of the breast as the primary lesion. Fifteen of the patients had associated decortication to permit full expansion of the lung, thus facilitating pleural symphysis. Only two patients developed recurrent effusions.

Because of the high mortality and morbidity associated with pleurectomy, lesser procedures should be tried first. This procedure is too radical for the majority of patients with malignant effusion and only those individuals in relatively good condition who are expected to live for at least six months are candidates for stripping of the parietal pleura. Subjective improvement from temporary removal of the effusion by thoracentesis, and the absence of other conditions which might cause pulmonary symptoms must also be established before pleurectomy is planned.

In our experience with pleural effusion secondary to breast carcinoma there is rarely a need for such operative intervention. In the past 15 years, only three patients have required pleurectomy to control recurrent effusions. In two individuals, extensive diagnostic procedures failed to reveal the etiology of

the effusion and pleurectomy was performed during a limited thoractomy carried out primarily for diagnosis. Only with a trapped lung, and therefore the impossibility of pleural symphysis by the method of tube drainage and nitrogen mustard instillation, will pleurectomy be required.

PERICARDIAL EFFUSION

Occasionally, pericardial effusion secondary to breast cancer can occur as an isolated finding but it occurs more often in combination with pleural effusion due to metastatic disease. Radiotherapy is sometimes recommended (see Chapter 10) but if the patient demonstrates any evidence of tamponade, pericardiocentesis is performed immediately. If symptoms recur, the pericardial effusion should be managed by surgical intervention.

Some physicians advocate total pericardectomy for this problem but we have for the past eight years preferred the creation of a "pericardial window". This operation is performed through a limited left anterior intercostal incision in the 4th intercostal space. Large flaps of pericardium are excised anterior and posterior to the phrenic nerve, leaving behind an adequate bridge of pericardium. This prevents herniation of the ventricle through the pericardial opening. Following drainage, chemotherapy or radiation therapy can be directed to the mediastinum without danger of recurrent cardiac tamponade.

SUMMARY

The prime objective in managing patients with malignant pleural effusion secondary to carcinoma of the breast is early diagnosis and rapid alleviation of symptoms. We prefer the use of simple, readily available methods with low mortality and morbidity to effect symptomatic improvement. The choice of treatment for a particular case must be determined by the exigencies of the situation. Some patients are moribund so that no treatment is necessary, while others may require only thoracentesis to bring temporary relief during their last few remaining days. All other individuals are in our opinion best managed by tube thoracostomy and nitrogen mustard instillation. Those rare individuals not responding to this treatment may be considered for pleurectomy or open talc poudrage.

REFERENCES

Adler, R. H. and Rappole, B. W. (1967). Recurrent malignant pleural effusion and talc powder aerosol treatment. *Surgery 62*, 1000.

Anderson, C. B., Philpott, G. W. and Ferguson, T. B. (1974). The treatment of malignant pleural effusions. *Cancer 33*, 916.

Ariel, I. M., Oropeza, R. and Pack, T. G. (1966). Intracavitary administration of radioactive isotopes in the control of effusions due to cancer. *Cancer 19*, 1096.

Bateman, J. C., Moulton, B. and Larson, N. J. (1955). Control of neoplastic effusion by phosphoramide chemotherapy. *Archives of Internal Medicine 95*, 713.

Black, L. F. (1972). The pleural space and pleural fluid. *Mayo Clinic Proceedings 47*, 493.

Borja, E. R. and Pugh, R. P. (1973). Single-dose quinacrine (Atabrine) and thoracostomy in the control of pleural effusions in patients with neoplastic diseases. *Cancer 31*, 899.

Camishion, R. C., Gibbon, J. H., Jr. and Nealon, T. F. (1962). Talc poudrage in the treatment of pleural effusion due to cancer. *Surgical Clinics of North America 42*, 1521.

Card, R. Y., Cole, D. R. and Henschke, U. L. K. (1960). Summary of ten years of the use of radioactive colloids in intracavitary therapy. *Journal of Nuclear Medicine 1*, 195.

Chu, F. C. (1970). Personal communication. Cited in Fracchia, A. A., Knapper, W. H., Carey, J. T. and Farrow, J. H.: Intrapleural chemotherapy for effusion from metastatic breast carcinoma. *Cancer 26*, 626.

Dollinger, M. R., Krakoff, I. H. and Karnofsky, D. A. (1967). Quinacrine (Atabrine) in the treatment of neoplastic effusions. *Annals of Internal Medicine 66*, 249.

Dollinger, M. R. (1972). Management of recurrent malignant effusions. *CA 22*, 138.

El-Mahdi, An, Levene, A. and Lott, S. (1973). Observations and management of malignant pleural effusions in breast carcinoma. *Johns Hopkins Medicine Journal 132*, 4.

Fracchia, A. A., Knapper, W. H., Carey, J. T. and Farrow, J. H. (1970). Intra-pleural chemotherapy for effusion from metastatic breast carcinoma. *Cancer 26*, 626.

Hickman, J. A. and Jones, M. C. (1970). Treatment of neoplastic pleural effusions with local instillation of quinacrine (Mepacrine) hydrochloride. *Thorax 25*, 226.

Jacobs, M. L. (1958). Radioactive colloidal chromic phosphate to control pleural effusions and ascites. *Journal of American Medical Association 166*, 597.

Jarvi, O. H., Kunnas, R. J., Laitio, M. T. and Tyrkko, J. E. S. (1972). The accuracy and significance of cytologic cancer diagnosis of pleural effusions. *Acta Cytologia 16*, 152.

Jensik, R., Cagle, J. E., Jr., Milloy, F., Perlia, C., Taylor, S., Kofman, S. and Beattie, E. J., Jr. (1963). Pleurectomy in the treatment of pleural effusion due to metastatic malignancy. *Journal of Thoracic and Cardiovascular Surgery 46*, 322.

Jones, G. R. (1969). Treatment of recurrent malignant pleural effusion by iodized talc pleurodesis. *Thorax 24*, 69.

Kinsey, D. L., Carter, D. and Klassen, K. P. (1964).

Simplified management of malignant pleural effusion. *Archives of Surgery 89*, 389.

Konikov, N., Bleisch, V. and Piskie, V. (1966). Prognostic significance of cytologic diagnoses of effusions. *Acta Cytologica 10*, 335.

Lambert, C. J., Urschel, H. C., Jr. and Paulson, D. L. (1967). The treatment of malignant pleural effusion by closed trocar tube drainage. *Annals of Thoracic Surgery 3*, 1.

Leininger, B. J., Barker, W. L. and Langston, H. T. (1969). A simplified method for management of malignant pleural effusion. *Journal of Thoracic and Cardiovascular Surgery 58*, 758.

Leuallen, E. C. and Carr, D. T. (1955). Pleural effusion: A statistical study of 436 patients. *New England Journal of Medicine 252*, 79.

Light, R. W., Macgregor, M. I., Luchsinger, P. C. and Ball, W. C., Jr., (1972). Pleural effusions: The diagnostic separation of transudates and exudates. *Annals of Internal Medicine 77*, 507.

Mark, J. B. D., Goldenberg, I. S. and Montague, A. C. W. (1964). Intrapleural mechlorethamine hydrochloride therapy for malignant pleural effusion. *Journal of American Medical Association 187*, 858.

Meyer, P. C. (1966). Metastatic carcinoma of the pleura. *Thorax 21*, 437.

O'Bryan, P. M., Talley, R. W., Brennan, M. J. and San Diego, E. (1968). Critical analysis of the control of malignant effusions with radioisotopes. *Henry Ford Hospital Medicine Journal 16*, 3.

Porter, E. H. (1965). Pleural effusion and breast cancer. *British Medical Journal 1*, 251.

Rochlin, D. B., Smart, C. R., Wagner, D. E. and Silva, A. R. M. (1964). The control of recurrent malignant effusions using quinacrine hydrochloride. *Surgery, Gynecology and Obstetrics 118*, 991.

Rubinson, Richard M. and Bolooki, Hooshang. (1972). Intrapleural tetracycline for control of malignant pleural effusion: A preliminary report. *Southern Medical Journal 65*, 847.

Siegel, E. P., Hart, H. E., Brothers, M., Spencer, H. and Laszlo, D. (1956). Radioyttrium (Y^{90}) for the palliative treatment of effusions due to malignancy. *Journal of American Medical Association 161*, 499.

Spratt, J. S., Jr. and Donegan, W. L. (1967). *Cancer of the Breast*, p. 235, W. B. Saunders Company, Philadelphia.

Starkey, W. B. (1964). Recurrent malignant pleural effusions. *New England Journal of Medicine 270*, 436.

Stoll, B. A. and Ellis, F. (1953). Treatment by oestrogens of pulmonary metastases for breast cancer. *British Medical Journal 2*, 796.

Strober, S. J., Klotz, E., Kuperman, A. and Ghossein, N. A. (1973). Malignant pleural disease. A radiotherapeutic approach to the problem. *Journal of American Medical Association 226*, 296.

Ultmann, J. E. (1962). Diagnosis and treatment of neoplastic effusions. *CA 12*, 42.

Ultmann, J. E., Gellhorn, A., Osnos, M. and Hirschberg, E. (1963). The effect of quinacrine on neoplastic effusions and certain of their enzymes. *Cancer 16*, 283.

Weick, J. K., Kiely, J. M., Harrison, E. G., Carr, D. T. and Scanlon, P. W. (1973). Pleural effusion in lymphoma. *Cancer 31*, 848.

Weisberger, A. S., Levine, B. and Storasli, J. P. (1955). Use of nitrogen mustard in the treatment of serous effusions of neoplastic origin. *Journal of American Medical Association 159*, 1704.

Wroblewski, F. and Wroblewski, R. (1958). The clinical significance of lactic dehydrogenase activity of serous effusions. *Annals of Internal Medicine 48*, 813.

Chapter

18

HUGH L. DAVIS, JR.

Management of Hypercalcemia

Hypercalcemia is a major medical complication of disseminated breast cancer. An episode of hypercalcemia may result in premature death if unrecognized or unsuccessfully managed; thus, awareness of this syndrome is vital to the successful palliation of disseminated breast cancer.

Transient elevations of serum calcium may be seen in 40% of patients with osseous metastases (Thomas et al., 1960; Graham et al., 1963). Symptomatic hypercalcemia is estimated to occur in 5-15% of such patients (Swyer et al., 1950; Myers, 1960; Graham et al., 1963; Jessiman et al., 1963; Davis et al., 1973). The precise etiology of hypercalcemia in breast cancer has not been established, but for practical purposes, the hypercalcemia of breast cancer is almost always associated with osseous metastases whether or not they are demonstrable by X-ray (Kennedy et al., 1955; Jessiman et al., 1963; Galasko and Burn, 1971).

The majority of the episodes of hypercalcemia are spontaneous; that is, they are unassociated with recent hormonal manipulations. The exact proportion of spontaneous to induced hypercalcemia is difficult to estimate, as the numbers vary with the type of treatment and the length of observation. Patients with spontaneous hypercalcemia tend to cluster in the younger age groups and the incidence declines after age 60 (Mannheimer, 1965).

The induction of hypercalcemia immediately after hormonal manipulation was recognised as soon as steroid hormones received their initial trial in metastatic breast cancer. A feature of hormonally-induced hypercalcemia is its rapid onset, generally within 2 weeks of the beginning of a hormone trial, but at times within 24-48 hours (Swaroop and Krant, 1973). In cases where metastatic disease cannot be demonstrated, a search for the other major causes of hypercalcemia is appropriate.

CLINICAL FEATURES OF HYPERCALCEMIA IN BREAST CANCER

The principal symptoms of hypercalcemia are listed in Table 1. The severity and acuteness of these

Table 1. Symptoms of Hypercalcemia.

Gastrointestinal	Anorexia, nausea, vomiting, constipation, abdominal distension, ileus, dysphagia
Renal	Polyuria with accompanying thirst and dry mouth, dehydration and finally oliguria
CNS	Personality changes, depression, somnolence, coma, bulbar palsies, diplopia
Muscular	Variable degrees of muscle weakness
Miscellaneous	Conjunctivitis, pruritus
Bone pain	In great majority of patients there is increased bone pain

symptoms are generally related to the level of the serum calcium and to the rapidity of its rise as well as to other fluid and electrolyte imbalance.

There is nothing specific to be found in the examination of these patients. Dehydration may be prominent due to vomiting, and abdominal distension and hypoactive peristalsis reflect the intestinal hypomotility. Neurological examination may be normal but cranial neuropathies and an organic brain syndrome varying from emotional lability to stupor may occur (Warwick et al., 1961; Petersen, 1968). Electroencephalography reveals the diffuse slow waves of metabolic encephalopathy (Jessiman et al., 1963).

The electrocardiogram may be normal, but with calcium levels above 15 mg% the QT interval is frequently shortened. Arrhythmias are uncommon in the usual clinical presentation. Of special concern is the synergistic effect of elevated calcium and digitalis, and toxic arrhythmias become a serious problem in this setting (Bronsky et al., 1961). Progressive hypercalcemia rapidly leads to renal failure which is not always reversible (Gerbrandy and Hellendoorn, 1958; Frei et al., 1963).

The physiologic consequences of hypercalcemia result in a vicious downhill spiral unless corrected, but the management varies with the individual patient. The course of any degree of hypercalcemia is unpredictable. Persistent levels over 12 mg% may result in varying degrees of permanent renal damage and should be promptly reversed. Mild transient hypercalcemia may spontaneously abate and require no active intervention. Some patients may have hypercalcemia in the course of truly terminal disease, after all specific measures for palliation have been exhausted. This section, therefore, is concerned with the management of significant hypercalcemia where possibilities of active treatment of the disseminated breast cancer still exist.

BASELINE EVALUATION

Stage and extent of disease:

The workup for metastatic breast cancer should include an evaluation to document current progression of the disease but, in acute severe hypercalcemia, valuable time should not be lost in a detailed workup; treatment should have first priority.

Precipitating factors associated with hypercalcemia:

a. The recent initiation of a hormone trial.
b. Pathologic fracture.
c. Other reasons for immobilization.
d. Calcium preparations, excessive milk intake, vitamin D.
e. Thiazide diuretics or spironolactones especially associated with sodium restriction.

History and physical examination:

a. Evidence of an organic brain syndrome.
b. Gastro-intestinal dysfunction—dysphagia, vomiting, constipation, evidence of ileus.
c. Evidence of dehydration and history of thirst and polyuria.
d. A survey for associated illnesses; cardiac disease (potential or actual heart failure), state of renal function, and presence of hypertension.

The current or recent use of digitalis is extremely important.

Laboratory evaluations of importance:

a. Level of serum calcium: although absolute levels differ with methodology, levels <12 mg% are *mild*; levels of 12-15 mg% are *serious*, and levels >15 mg% constitute a medical emergency.
b. Level of serum proteins: the level of the serum albumin is relevant as is that of the total protein. Hypoproteinemia may result in a spuriously low calcium value due to reduction in the protein bound fraction (Myers, 1962), and should be corrected upward by approximately 0.8 mg for each decrease of 1.0 g% of serum albumin.
c. Baseline level of serum phosphorus.
d. BUN, creatinine and urinalysis.
e. Sodium, potassium, chloride, CO_2 in serum.
f. Serum magnesium.
g. Baseline electrocardiogram.

An initial set of orders (modified as appropriate):

These should include:

a. Monitoring of vital signs at suitable intervals.
b. Intake and output from all sources at least daily.
c. Daily weights.

MANAGEMENT OF HYPERCALCEMIA

Table 2 classifies the measures that have been used to manage hypercalcemia according to their postulated mechanism of action.

The restriction of dietary calcium is generally of minor importance unless the patient is receiving calcium supplements. The gastrointestinal symptoms generally result in this restriction occurring spontaneously.

The problem of concurrent hormone therapy is much more controversial. If a patient develops hypercalcemia well into a hormone trial, the likely reason is progression of cancer, not "tumor stimulation" or "acceleration". Even so, discontinuing the hormone would usually be logical at this point, at least while general treatment measures are undertaken. The hypercalcemia occurring early in a trial of additive hormone therapy is often fulminant (Kennedy et al., 1953, 1955) and the utmost caution should be observed here. Usually the hormone should be stopped immediately (Myers, 1973), although it is claimed that ultimate response to the same hormone may be obtained (Hall et al., 1963). I believe the hormone should be stopped, the hypercalcemia corrected, and then the situation re-evaluated: this is surely the most prudent course and in the best interests of the patient.

Ambulatory patients should remain so and movement in bed ordered for those patients who are bedfast to minimize the effects of immobilization.

MEASURES TO INCREASE THE EXCRETION OF CALCIUM

Calcium excretion is closely coupled to sodium excretion (Kleeman et al., 1964; Massry et al., 1973) and, in mild hypercalcemic states a high sodium diet may suffice. Usually the patient will require intravenous administration of normal saline (154 meq sodium/liter) to restore the approximated volume deficit. This is the initial key step in management; with correction of volume deficit, the stage is set for

Table 2. Measures used to treat hypercalcemia.

Reduction of calcium intake and withdrawal of precipitating factors
Eliminate dietary calcium
Stop additive hormone therapy
Increase activity of the patient
Increase excretion of calcium
Increase sodium intake orally or intravenously—volume expansion
Intravenous saline and calciuretic diuretics
Sodium sulfate infusions
Excretion of complexed calcium by sodium citrate or EDTA
Dialysis
Sequestration of calcium
Oral or intravenous phosphate
Reduction of bone resorption
Corticosteroids
Mithramycin, actinomycin D
Calcitonin
Ambulation
Specific treatment of breast cancer
Hormonal manipulation (additive) including corticosteroids
Ablative surgery
Palliative radiation
Single agent or combination chemotherapy

diuresis and perfusion of the kidneys is ensured (Walser, 1970; Suki et al., 1970).

Volume overload remains a constant threat and requires careful monitoring. Following restoration of volume, diuresis is started. Usually this can be accomplished with Furosemide—20 to 40 mg intravenously as necessary to maintain a urine output of 3-5 liters daily. Losses are replaced with 5% dextrose in 0.5 N saline (77 meq sodium/liter), with added potassium as necessary (usually 20-40 meq/KC1 liter). Urinary volumes are best measured hourly and urinary sodium and potassium estimated frequently to ensure accurate replacement of losses (Davis, 1973; Newmark and Himathongkam, 1974).

A more vigorous application of this therapy involves using 80-100 mg of furosemide hourly to maintain an hourly urine volume of approximately 500 ml, with an average hourly calcium excretion of 82 mg (Suki et al., 1970). As might be expected, meticulous attention to volume, potassium and magnesium balance is necessary and the reader would be well advised to review the original publication for details.

Infusions of sodium sulfate markedly increase calcium excretion through natruresis and also excretion of calcium complexed with sulfate (Walser and Browder, 1959). Clinical trials were performed using an 0.12 M solution compounded by adding 38.9 g of sodium sulfate decahydrate to 1 liter of distilled water or 5% dextrose in distilled water (Chakmakjian and Bethune, 1966; Fulmer et al., 1972). The first study used 3 liters of this solution per 24 hours and compared it to 1.45% NaCl given in the same amount per day. This resulted in similar amounts of sodium infused. The sulfate solution was decidedly superior to sodium chloride in terms of both calcium excretion, lowering of serum calcium, and more rapid excretion; sodium chloride frequently resulted in weight gain and edema.

The second study used only one liter of sulfate solution as a single infusion. The decrease in serum calcium averaged 1.9 mg% and lasted 18-24 hours. Neither of these studies used supplemental diuretics. Only a small number of patients with breast cancer are reported with either the intensive diuresis or the sodium sulfate regimens.

Another method of enhancing urinary calcium excretion is as a complex with citrate through the use of intravenous infusion of sodium citrate (Kennedy et al., 1953). Lowering of serum calcium by this method is very transient and moreover, the citrate is metabolized to bicarbonate promoting metabolic alkalosis (Lenhard, 1971).

Disodium ethylenediaminetetraacetate (EDTA) has been utilized with mixed results because of its potential nephrotoxicity (Dudley et al., 1955). Current recommendations restrict its use to situations of urgency where other intravenous therapy is contraindicted. The dose should not exceed 100 mg/kg/day (maximum adult dose 6.0 g in 500 ml of 5% dextrose in water) over 4 hours with constant attendance to monitor the patient for hypotension and symptomatic hypocalcemia (Myers, 1973).

Dialysis has been used for short term control of hypercalcemia and, of course, could provide control of hypercalcemia while controlling renal failure (Myers, 1973; Miach et al., 1975).

MEASURES TO SEQUESTER CALCIUM

The use of oral or intravenous phosphate will predictably lower the serum calcium dependent on the dose administered. It has proved effective in managing the hypercalcemia of primary hyperparathyroidism, as well as that of malignancy (Goldsmith and Ingbar, 1966; Hebert et al., 1966; Massry et al., 1968; Thalassinos and Joplin, 1968; Fulmer et al., 1972). An increased concentration of phosphate has been shown to reduce bone resorption *in vitro* (Raisz and Niemann, 1969). An alternative explanation involves the sequestration of calcium phosphate into a metabolic pool with slow release back into the circulation (Eisenberg, 1970). Since phosphate infusion was often found to elevate the solubility product of calcium X phosphate above accepted safe levels, another explantion was intravascular or extravascular precipitation (Hebert et al., 1966). Renal calcium excretion is reduced.

The sodium and potassium salts used to compound the various formulas contain 31 mg elemental phosphorus/mM. The usual intravenous doses have been studied as single slow infusions (4-8 hrs) of 25, 33, 50 and 100 mM total dose. An abbreviated description of the principal studies of intravenous phosphate is presented in Table 3.

In these studies an inappropriate rise in serum phosphate was noted only occasionally and was associated with preexisting renal insufficiency. Extraskeletal calcification was noted sporadically and a single case of pulmonary edema in a patient receiving 100 mM with the accompanying 162 meq of sodium. More rapid administration (1-3 h) has resulted in fatal hypotension, hypocalcemia and acute renal failure (Shackney and Hasson, 1967). A safe and suitably effective range would be 33-50 mM over 6-8 hours.

Oral phosphate is preferred when possible and provides the opportunity for prolonged control

Table 3. Intravenous Phosphate Therapy.

Authors	*Preparation*	*Phosphorus (g/mM)*	*Results*
Goldsmith and Ingbar (1966)	.081 M Na_2HPO_4 .019 M KH_2PO_4	3g/100 mM	max fall 1-5 days from single infusion
Thalassinos and Joplin (1968)	*same*	1g/33 mM	max effect in 3 days; little rise in serum phosphorus
Massry et al. (1968)	*Inphos®* .081 M Na_2HPO_4 .019 M KH_2PO_4	1-3 g/33-100 mM	similar to above
Fulmer et al. (1972)	*same*	25,50,75 & 100 mM	dose dependent; fall in serum calcium 25mM decrease of 1.1 mg% 50mM decrease of 2.4 mg% 75mM decrease of 4.13 mg% 100mM decrease of 6.08 mg%

Note: These intravenous preparations contain 162 meq/L of sodium, 19 meq potassium and 100 mM (3.1 g) phosphorus/liter.

(Thalassinos and Joplin, 1968). The daily dose is from 1-3 g phosphorus/day and the smallest effective dose should be used as maintenance. Although extraskeletal calcification can occur with prolonged usage, the most frequent adverse reaction is diarrhea.

MEASURES WHICH DECREASE BONE RESORPTION

Corticosteroids

Corticosteroids have been the most frequently used treatment for cancer hypercalcemia. The long term effect of corticosteroids is to promote bone resorption and hypercalciuria (Massry et al., 1973), but this is usually not the case in acute treatment. Further, when calcium balance studies have been done in *hypercalcemic* breast cancer patients, urinary calcium was usually decreased along with the serum calcium (Myers, 1958; Jessiman, 1963; Mannheimer, 1965). Although steroids are a valuable measure because of the high ultimate response rate (60-90%), the maximum response usually takes 5-14 days (Davis, 1973; Goldsmith, 1972). Typical response rates are 48/59 episodes in Jessiman's series and 46/59 successfully treated episodes of *spontaneous* hypercalcemia in Mannheimer's series.

The minimum starting daily dosages advocated are either 200-300 mg of cortisone or hydrocortisone orally or parenterally; at least 80 mg methylprednisolone parenterally; or 60-80 mg oral prednisone. Following restoration of serum calcium to normal levels, steroids are gradually tapered off but at times, maintenance levels of 15-20 mg of prednisone or its equivalent are necessary for prolonged periods.

Antitumor Antibiotics and Cytotoxic Drugs

In 1956, the antitumor antibiotic 6-diazo-5-oxo-L-norleucine (DON) was shown to reverse hypercalcemia and reduce urinary calcium excretion without noticeable antitumor effect in 8/13 patients (Myers and Magill, 1956). Subsequently methotrexate was reported to prevent recurrent hormone-induced hypercalcemia in a small series and to arrest spontaneous hypercalcemia in a single case (Nevinny and Hall, 1962). Since this drug is active in breast cancer, it is difficult to ascribe specificity to this effect.

Actinomycin D has been shown to reverse hypercalcemia for periods up to 1 week after a single 2 mg dose (Muggia and Heinemann, 1970), but the most widely studied agent of this class is mithramycin. This antitumor antibiotic is rarely effective in tumors other than germ cell testicular neoplasms (Kennedy, 1970), but is effective in a wide variety of hypercalcemic states in a broad spectrum of malignant disease (Parsons et al., 1967; Perlia et al., 1970; Slayton et al., 1971; Fillastre et al., 1974; Lenhard, 1971).

The usual dose which is required to lower serum calcium is 25 μg/kg by direct intravenous injection. It may be repeated daily or every 3-4 days for several doses. Toxicity generally has been mild, but several instances of thrombocytopenia were noted in a small series of breast cancer patients with extensive bone disease (Davis et al., 1973).

Mithramycin appears to temporarily interfere with osteoclastic function and rapidly reduces the serum calcium, with maximum effect being seen in 2-3 days (Perlia et al., 1970; Slayton et al., 1971). It is associated with marked decrease in urinary calcium (Parsons et al., 1967; Fillastre et al., 1974) and urinary hydroxyproline (Parsons et al., 1967) which is indicative of marked reduction of active bone resorption. Fairly extensive experience has accrued in the hypercalcemia of breast cancer. Perlia observed a fall to normal levels with a single injection of 25 μg/kg in 18 of 25 episodes and hypercalcemia was corrected in five additional episodes by further injections. Slayton found 23 cases of breast cancer "the most responsive" in his series of 89 patients with a variety of tumors.

Calcitonin

Porcine or synthetic salmon calcitonin has recently been studied in the hypercalcemia of malignancy (Silva and Becker, 1973; Vaughn and Vaitkevicius, 1974). In both these reports no major adverse reactions were reported and the cases reported included patients with cardiac disease or renal failure. Moderate falls in serum calcium level were obtained in 17/23 and 9/10 trials, respectively. The two breast cancer patients both responded to short courses of intramuscular calcitonin given at 6 hour intervals and further studies are awaited with interest. Long term control of hypercalcemia of parathyroid carcinoma has been achieved with calcitonin and steroids (Au, 1975).

SPECIFIC ANTICANCER TREATMENT

Measures of importance here include: trial of appropriate hormonal manipulation in spontaneous hypercalcemia: resumption of hormone that has previously induced hypercalcemia: ablative surgery in the hypercalcemic patient: the role of cytotoxic chemotherapy.

Hormonal trial

It would seem logical to offer appropriate hormonal manipulations to the as yet untested patient with spontaneous hypercalcemia, and this has indeed been recommended (Muirhead, 1967). The selected therapy is that most appropriate for the age, menopausal status, extent of disease, the "free interval", and presence of estrogen receptors—all features reported to influence the response to the various hormonal manipulations (Rozencweig and Heuson, 1975). It is mandatory to carefully manage the hypercalcemia with appropriate methods during this trial, with a plan to promptly discontinue the administered hormone if the hypercalcemia worsens or does not remit to safe levels (<12 mg%).

Resumption of previous hormonal therapy

Resumption of a hormone previously demonstrated to induce hypercalcemia has been advised by some authorities, but there are conflicting opinions mostly based on anecdotal observations. With perseverance, 6 of 13 estrogen trials associated with hypercalcemia were continued and three patients responded to the estrogen (Hall et al., 1963). This was distinctly higher than the total response rate in 259 estrogen treated patients. Six of 11 testosterone treated patients likewise could be continued with two objective regressions. These authors futher showed some patients could tolerate estrogens a second time if they were pretreated with 2.5 mg methotrexate to the point of mild leucopenia (Nevinny and Hall, 1962).

It has also been demonstrated that estrogen could be continued in the face of induced hypercalcemia when mithramycin was used to control the hypercalcemia (Perlia et al., 1970). Long term observations on most of these patients are lacking and clinicians electing to rechallenge patients with the previously inciting hormone are, in my opinion, taking a risk.

Ablative Surgery

More justification appears to be available when ablative surgery is considered, even though there are occasional instances of severe hypercalcemia occurring soon after ablative procedures (Galasko and Burn, 1971). Major evidence in this area comes from observations of estrogen-induced hypercalcemia and subsequent response to ablative surgery (Muirhead, 1967; Jessiman et al., 1963; Galasko and Burn, 1971; Emerson and Jessiman, 1956). The numerous case reports suggest that an appropriate course of action should include consideration of major endocrine ablative surgery (Beckett, 1969). The spontaneously occurring hypercalcemia patient presents no special clues as to responsiveness to endocrine ablative surgery; after correction of hypercalcemia, each patient should be evaluated individually.

Cytotoxic chemotherapy

The "protective" effect of methotrexate was alluded to previously, as was the effect on osteolysis of selected antitumor agents. Hypercalcemia has abated

after 5FU therapy (Davis et al., 1973). Antitumor response is now so frequent with combination chemotherapy, it would indeed be surprising if remission of hypercalcemia was not observed, but no specific attempts have been made to document this. On the negative side, a recent trial of combined stilbestrol and cyclophosphamide therapy failed to abolish early hypercalcemia presumed to be induced by estrogens (Kennedy and Kiang, 1975).

CONCLUSIONS

Hypercalcemia remains a serious complication of breast cancer with 10-30% mortality (Jessiman et al., 1963, Davis et al., 1973). However, by observing the proper priorities the mortality rate from this complication should be minimized.

1. The expert use of volume expansion and forced diuresis, and the early recognition of hypercalcemia are probably the two most vital factors in management. It has been stated that 50% of episodes can be successfully managed by volume expansion and diuresis alone (Gordan, 1974).

2. The use of corticosteroids in large divided doses (60-80 mg prednisone or equivalent daily) when added to supportive therapy, remains the single most valuable pharmacologic measure in breast cancer. The mechanism of action remains unknown. It may well be a direct antitumor action, or inhibition of the unknown humoral factors thought to be locally released from the tumor.

3. If these measures fail to reverse the hypercalcemia in 7-10 days, *or* the levels remain critically high with progressive threat of renal insufficiency or cerebral dysfunction, the clinician has two excellent modalities to consider—phosphate and mithramycin. Mithramycin is very effective in short term control and appropriate phosphate preparations may result in both short term and prolonged control.

Two cautions are appropriate:

a. Mithramycin can be very toxic in patients with pre-existing marrow depression and might best be avoided if aggressive chemotherapy is being considered.

b. The tendency of hypercalcemia of breast cancer to cause renal dysfunction means that phosphate preparations must be used with extra care. A total of 15 breast cancer patients are reported in the articles surveyed; they represented failures of conventional therapy and generally manifested an unfavorable clinical course even though responding to phosphate.

We have used intravenous phosphate (Inphos®-50 mM/6-8 h) and oral phosphate as Neutra Phos® or Fleets Phospho Soda® in a few patients who were steroid unresponsive and had bone marrow depression: Two patients with compromised renal function developed hyperphosphatemia of 9-10 mg% while control of the serum calcium was temporarily achieved. Autopsy study revealed extensive metastatic calcifications in both. Thus, our preference is to use mithramycin whenever possible.

4. Long term control can only be achieved by successful specific treatment. Since hormonal manipulations usually result in longer remissions than chemotherapy, initial efforts should lean in this direction and estrogen receptor data appear to be excellent in predicting response to hormonal methods. A combined approach might be considered for rapidly progressive disease, utilizing both hormonal and chemotherapeutic measures to ensure the maximum response. Radiation therapy for osteolytic lesions may provide the additional control necessary to relieve the hypercalcemia.

Further developments in therapy seem imminent. The demonstration of osteolytic prostaglandins in a variety of other tumors, if extended to breast cancer, might provide further rationale for the use of steroids, indomethacin and aspirin. There is no clinical evidence at present to recommend the last two agents in hypercalcemia of breast cancer.

Perhaps calcitonin might be useful as an adjunct to reduce osteolysis. Diphosphonate (sodium etidronate) is under preliminary investigation also as an additive to the treatment of osteolytic metastases. Results of this study are pending, but published results in Paget's disease indicate a marked decrease in bone resorption and clinical improvement (Altman et al., 1973). Thus considerable progress continues with promise of further therapeutic benefit in this distressingly common malignancy.

Acknowledgements

Support is acknowledged from Center Grant CA 14520, COG Grant CA 13290 and Breast Grant CA 04594.

REFERENCES

Altman, R. D., Johnston, C. C., Khairi, M. R. A., Wellman, H., Serafini, A. N. and Sankey, R. R. (1973). Influence of disodium etidronate on clinical and laboratory manifestations of Paget's disease of bone (Osteitis Deformans). *New England Journal of Medicine 289*, 1379.

Au, W. Y. W. (1975). Calcitonin treatment of hypercalcemia

due to parathyroid carcinoma. *Archives of Internal Medicine 135,* 1594.

Beckett, V. L. (1969). Hypercalcemia associated with estrogen administration in patients with breast carcinoma. *Cancer 24,* 610.

Bronsky, D., Dubin, A., Waldstein, S. S. and Kuschner, D. S. (1961). Review: Calcium and the electrocardiogram (3 parts). *American Journal of Cardiology 7,* 823, 833, 840.

Chakmakjian, Z. H. and Bethune, J. E. (1966). Sodium sulfate treatment of hypercalcemia. *New England Journal of Medicine 275,* 862.

Davis, H. L. Jr., Wiseley, A. N., Ramirez, G. and Ansfield, F. J. (1973). Hypercalcemia complicating breast cancer. *Oncology 28,* 126.

Dudley, H. R., Ritchie, A. C., Schilling, A. and Baker, W. H. (1955). Pathologic changes associated with the use of sodium ethylene diamine tetra-acetate in the treatment of hypercalcemia. *New England Journal of Medicine 252,* 331.

Eisenberg, E. (1970). Effect of intravenous phosphate on serum strontium and calcium. *New England Journal of Medicine 282,* 889.

Emerson, K. Jr. and Jessiman, A. G. (1956). Hormonal influences on the growth and progression of cancer. Tests for hormone dependency in mammary and prostatic cancer. *New England Journal of Medicine 254,* 252.

Fillastre, J. P., Maitrot, J., Canonne, M. A., Gray, H., Jeanne, C., Bastit, P. and Bourgeois, T. (1974). Renal function and alterations in plasma electrolyte levels in normocalcaemic and hypercalcaemic patients with malignant diseases, given an intravenous infusion of mithramycin. *Chemotherapy 20,* 280.

Frei, E. III, Bentzel, C. J., Rieselbach, R. and Block, J. B. (1963). Renal complications of neoplastic disease. *Journal of Chronic Diseases 16,* 757.

Fulmer, D. H., Dimich, A. B., Rothschild, E. O. and Myers, W. P. L. (1972). Treatment of hypercalcemia. Comparison of intravenously administered phosphate, sulfate, and hydrocortisone. *Archives of Internal Medicine 129,* 923.

Galasko, C. S. B. and Burn, J. I. (1971). Hypercalcemia in patients with advanced mammary cancer. *British Medical Journal 3,* 573.

Gerbrandy, J. and Hellendoorn, H. B. A. (1958). Renal failure during acute hypercalcaemia in patients with metastasized mammary carcinoma. *Clinica Chimica Acta 3,* 435.

Goldsmith, R. S. (1972). Treatment of hypercalcemia. *Medical Clinics of North America 56,* 951.

Goldsmith, R. S. and Ingbar, S. H. (1966). Inorganic phosphate treatment of hypercalcemia of diverse etiologies. *New England* Journal of Medicine 274, 1.

Gordan, G. S. (1974). Hyper- and hypocalcemia: Pathogenesis and treatments. *Annals of the New York Academy of Sciences 230,* 181.

Graham, W. P. III, Gardner, B., Thomas, A. N., Gordan, G. S., Loken, H. F. and Goldman, L. (1963). Hypercalcemia in carcinoma of the female breast. *Surgery, Gynecology and Obstetrics 117,* 709.

Hall, T. C., Dederick, M. M. and Nevinny, H. B. (1963). Prognostic value of hormonally induced hypercalcemia in breast cancer. *Cancer Chemotherapy Reports 30,* 21.

Hebert, L. A., Lemann, J. Jr., Petersen, J. R. and Lennon, E. J. (1966). Studies of the mechanism by which phosphate infusion lowers serum calcium concentration. *Journal of Clinical Investigation 45,* 1886.

Jessiman, A. G., Emerson, K. Jr., Shah, R. C. and Moore, F. D. (1963). Hypercalcemia in carcinoma of the breast. *Annals of Surgery 157,* 377.

Kennedy, B. J. (1970). Mithramycin therapy in advanced testicular neoplasms. *Cancer 26,* 755.

Kennedy, B. J. and Kiang, D. T. (1975). The effect of short-term cyclophosphamide on estrogen therapy in metastatic breast cancer. *Medical and Pediatric Oncology 1,* 265.

Kennedy, B. J., Nathanson, I. T., Tibbetts, D. M. and Aub, J. C. (1955). Biochemical alterations during steroid hormone therapy of advanced breast cancer. *American Journal of Medicine 19,* 337.

Kennedy, B. J., Tibbetts, D. M., Nathanson, I. T. and Aub, J. C. (1953). Hypercalcemia, a complication of hormone therapy of advanced breast cancer. *Cancer Research 13,* 445.

Kleeman, C. R., Bohannan, J., Bernstein, D., Ling, S. and Maxwell, M. H. (1964). Effect of variations in sodium intake on calcium excretion in normal humans. *Proceedings of the Society of Experimental Biology and Medicine 115,* 29.

Lenhard, R. E. Jr. (Moderator) (1971). Clinical Case Records in Chemotherapy: The management of hypercalcemia complicating cancer. *Cancer Chemotherapy Reports 55,* 509.

Mannheimer, I. H. (1965). Hypercalcemia of breast cancer. Management with corticosteroids. *Cancer 18,* 679.

Massry, S. G., Friedler, R. M. and Coburn, J. W. (1973). Excretion of phosphate and calcium. Physiology of their renal handling and relation to clinical medicine. *Archives of Internal Medicine 131,* 828.

Massry, S. G., Mueller, E., Silverman, A. G. and Kleeman, C. R. (1968). Inorganic phosphate treatment of hypercalcemia. *Archives of Internal Medicine 121,* 307.

Miach, P. J., Dawborn, J. K., Martin, T. J. and Moon, W. J. (1975). Management of the hypercalcaemia of malignancy by peritoneal dialysis. *Medical Journal of Australia 1,* 782.

Muggia, F. M. and Heinemann, H. O. (1970). Hypercalcemia associated with neoplastic disease. *Annals of Internal Medicine 73,* 281.

Muirhead, W. (1967). Hormonal treatment of hypercalcemia caused by bone metastases. *Canadian Medical Association Journal 97,* 569.

Myers, W. P. L. (1958). Cortisone in the treatment of hypercalcemia in neoplastic disease. *Cancer 11,* 83.

Myers, W. P. L. (1960). Hypercalcemia in neoplastic disease. *A. M. A. Archives of Surgery 80,* 308.

Myers, W. P. L. (1973). Hypercalcemia associated with malignant diseases. *In Endocrine and Nonendocrine Hormone-Producing Tumors,* p. 147. Proceedings of the Annual Clinical Conference on Cancer, University of Texas, M. D. Anderson Hospita and Tumor Institute. Year Book Medical Publishers, Chicago.

Myers, W. P. L. and Magill, G. B. (1956). Alterations in calcium metabolism in cancer patients treated with 6-diazo-5-oxo-L-norleucine (22741). *Proceedings of the Society for Experimental Biology and Medicine 93,* 314.

Newmark, S. R. and Himathongkam, T. (1974). Hypercalcemic and hypocalcemic crises. *The Journal of the American Medical Association 230,* 1438.

Nevinny, H. B. and Hall, T. C. (1962). Prevention of hormone-induced hypercalcemia by the use of methotrexate. *Cancer Chemotherapy Reports 16,* 305.

Parsons, V.. Baum, M. and Self, M. (1967). Effect of

mithramycin on calcium and hydroxyproline metabolism in patients with malignant disease. *British Medical Journal 1,* 474.

Perlia, C. P., Gubisch, N. J., Wolter, J., Edelberg, D., Dederick, M. M. and Taylor, S. G. III (1970). Mithramycin treatment of hypercalcemia. *Cancer 25,* 389.

Petersen, P. (1968). Psychiatric disorders in primary hyperparathyroidism. *Journal of Clinical Endocrinology and Metabolism 28,* 1491.

Raisz, L. G. and Niemann, I. (1969). Effect of phosphate, calcium and magnesium in bone resorption and hormonal responses in tissue culture. *Endocrinology 85,* 446.

Rozencweig, M. and Heuson, J.-C. (1975). Breast cancer: Prognostic factors and clinical evaluation. In *Cancer Therapy: Prognostic Factors and Critieria of Response,* p. 167 (Ed. M. J. Staquet). New York: Raven Press.

Silva, O. L. and Becker, K. L. (1973). Salmon calcitonin in the treatment of hypercalcemia. *Archives of Internal Medicine 132,* 337.

Slayton, R. E., Shnider, B. I., Elias, E., Horton, J. and Perlia, C. P. (1971). New approaches to the treatment of hypercalcemia. The effect of short term treatment with mithramycin. *Clinical Pharmacology and Therapeutics 12,* 833.

Suki, W. N., Yium, J. J., Von Minden, M., Saller-Hebert, C., Eknoyan, G., and Martinez-Maldonado, M. (1970). Acute treatment of hypercalcemia with furosemide. *The New England Journal of Medicine 283,* 836.

Swaroop, S. and Krant, M. J. (1973). Rapid estrogen-induced hypercalcemia. *The Journal of the American Medical Association 223,* 913.

Swyer, A. J., Berger, J. S., Gordon, H. M. and Laszlo, D. (1950). Hypercalcemia in osteolytic metastatic cancer of the breast. *American Journal of Medicine 8,* 724.

Thalassinos, N. and Joplin, G. F. (1968). Phosphate treatment of hypercalcaemia due to carcinoma. *British Medical Journal 4,* 14.

Thomas, A. N., Loken, H. F., Gordan, G. S. and Goldman, L. (1960). Hypercalcemia of metastatic breast cancer. *Surgical Forum XI,* 70.

Vaughn, C. B. and Vaitkevicius, V. K. (1974). The effects of calcitonin in hypercalcemia in patients with malignancy. *Cancer 34,* 1268.

Walser, M. (1970). Treatment of hypercalcemias. *Modern Treatment 7,* 662.

Walser, M. and Browder, A. A. (1959). Ion association. III. Effect of sulfate infusion on calcium excretion. *The Journal of Clinical Investigation 38,* 1404.

Warwick, O. H., Yendt, E. R. and Olin, J. S. (1961). The clinical features of hypercalcemia associated with malignant disease. *Canadian Medical Association Journal 85,* 719.

Chapter

19

WILLIAM L. DONEGAN

Management of Pregnancy and Lactation

INTRODUCTION

Since 17% of breast cancers occur in women of reproductive age, pregnancy will sometimes coincide with the malignancy or follow its treatment (Donegan, 1972). Breast cancers discovered during pregnancy or in the postpartum period, i.e. during "lactation", are presumed to have been potentially influenced by these conditions, while any occult residual tumor after mastectomy is subject to the influence of a subsequent conception. The association of pregnancy with breast cancer is a special situation inasmuch as the physician is confronted with the responsibility for two lives, that of the future mother and that of the fetus. Effective treatment for the former can victimize the unborn child and judgements and priorities made in this regard may at times encompass problems beyond those of medical science.

The suspicion that pregnancy has an unfavorable influence upon cancer of the breast is based firstly on the physiologic changes which occur during pregnancy and secondly on clinical observations reported in the past. In 1880 Samuel Gross noted that when breast cancer appeared during pregnancy or during lactation, "its growth is wonderfully rapid and its course excessively malignant" (Treves and Holleb, 1958). The physiologic changes which accompany pregnancy appear ideally suited to promote the growth and spread of this neoplasm. The enlarging breasts tend to hide its appearance, their unusual density hinders radiographic detection and the associated vascular congestion provides ample opportunity for dissemination.

The hormonal changes of pregnancy also have been suspected of favoring tumor growth. Since 1896 when Beatson reported the beneficial effects of castration on advanced cases, breast cancer has been known to be hormonally dependent in some patients. The original work of Lacassagne and the investigations which followed, demonstrated the stimulating effects of estrogens upon mammary cancer in mice and by implication were thought to incriminate estrogens in the promotion of this tumor in humans.

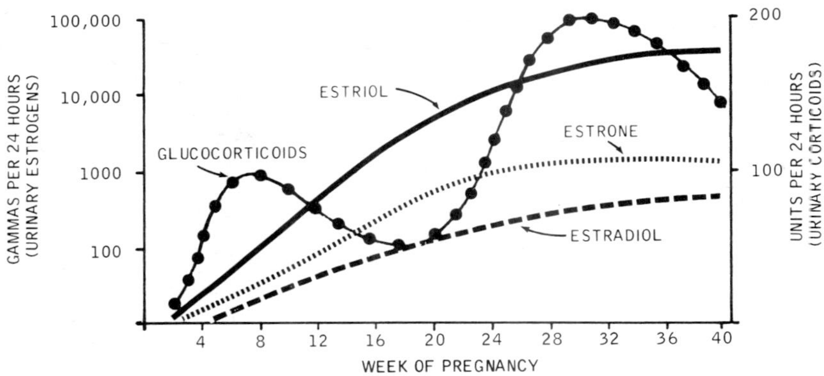

Figure 1. Estrogen and glucocorticoid levels in urine during the course of normal pregnancy (adopted from Davis and Plotz, 1965).

Thus, the striking rise in estrogen production during pregnancy, regularly reaching three hundredfold in the final trimester (Figure 1), has been of sufficient concern that its reversal and subsequent avoidance have been considered by many an important therapeutic objective.

Rises in circulating adrenal corticosteroid levels due to a two to three fold increase in production, are a regular accompaniment of pregnancy (Davis and Plotz, 1965). In animals, adrenal steroids are known to facilitate the implantation and spread of neoplasms. Depressed cellular immune competence is characteristic of pregnancy (Campion and Currey, 1972). It is apparently a mechanism to permit fetal implantation, but is also associated with reduced host resistance to neoplasia (Purtilo et al. 1972). A reduction in the normal proportion of circulating T lymphocytes occurs during early pregnancy and returns to normal only after the twentieth week (Strelkavskos et al., 1975).

Finally, during lactation high levels of prolactin are observed. This hypophyseal hormone, upon which lactation depends, is known to promote the growth of DMBA-induced mammary tumors in mice. In humans, however, its significance is not as yet established: the levels in breast cancer patients are not significantly different from those of controls, and prolactin suppression with ergot compounds or L-dopa has not proved of value therapeutically (Wilson et al., 1974). However, it has been claimed in some reports that women whose bone pain is relieved by L-dopa seem often to be benefited by endocrine ablation (Minton, 1974).

Whatever the reason, patients with breast cancers diagnosed during pregnancy or shortly thereafter have generally presented with advanced neoplasms and have often shown a disappointing clinical course. Early in this century, the results of treatment were so poor that the question was raised whether curative efforts were even justified. The mystique of pregnancy may have contributed to this pessimism, and delays resulting from an overly cautious attitude toward the pregnant patient may, in fact, be the real culprit.

Recurring questions about pregnancy associated with breast cancer include the following: How can the prognosis of these patients be improved? Is standard therapy for the primary appropriate? Is therapeutic abortion indicated? Should prophylactic castration be advised? Are future pregnancies contraindicated? The following sections attempt to reflect current thinking on these subjects.

INCIDENCE AND DIAGNOSIS

Because breast cancer generally affects an older population, obstetricians can expect to find relatively few cases in their routine practice. Finn reported approximately one case per 1,360 patients (Lewison, 1954), while White (1955) found only one per 3,200 pregnancies. The age range in the group is from 21 to 44 years with a modal average of 34 years. The physician examining patients with breast cancer is more likely to find a pregnancy. Among 45,881 cases of breast cancer collected from the literature, White (1955) found 2.8% with a coincident or recent pregnancy, while smaller but more recent series have set the figure for associated pregnancy between 0.75% and 3.1% (Rosemond, 1964: Peters, 1968: Applewhite et al., 1973).

If only women of childbearing age are considered the frequency of coincident pregnancy is considerable. Applewhite et al., (1973) reported that

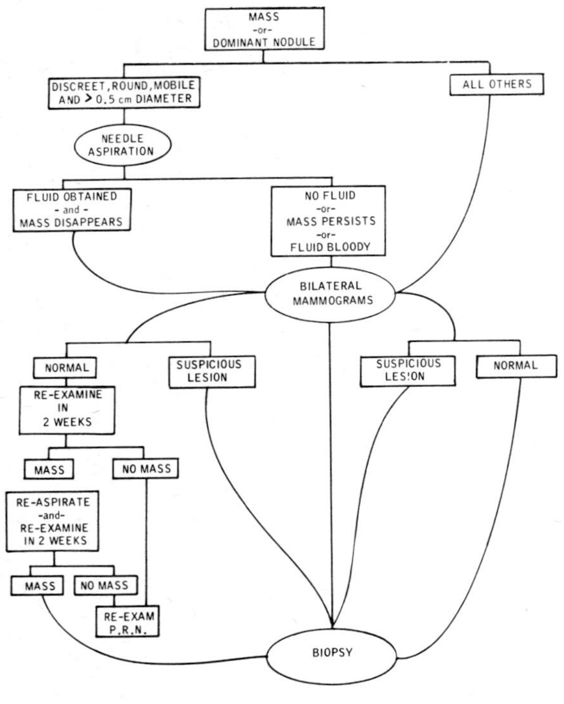

Figure 2. Management diagram used for diagnosis of breast masses at Breast Clinic, Medical College of Wisconsin.

7.3% of 655 women with breast cancer under 45 years of age were found to be pregnant or lactating, while an impressive 14% concurrent pregnancy rate was found by Treves and Holleb (1958) among 549 patients less than 35 years of age.

There tends to be a continuing delay in the diagnosis of breast cancer during pregnancy. The duration of symptoms before treatment in some series averages 11 to 15 months, exceeding the usual duration by 6 or 7 months (Applewhite et al., 1973: White and White, 1956: Rosemond, 1964: Peters 1968). This delay is only partly the patient's fault, and Byrd et al. (1962) attributed 75% of the delay to physician procrastination. Physicians are perhaps too ready to attribute signs of neoplasia to normal physiologic changes in pregnant or lactating women, or to delay action until after delivery.

Although nipple discharge from multiple ducts, sometimes of a thin bloody character, is a normal physiologic accompaniment of late pregnancy, the presence of abnormal masses or other suspicious changes deserves a prompt definitive diagnosis. Obstetricians more than anyone else have the opportunity for detecting breast cancer during pregnancy through regular breast examinations. Simple needle aspiration of masses serves to quickly distinguish cysts or galactoceles from solid tumors; the latter must then be biopsied. Due to the radiographic density of the breast during this time, mammography is seldom useful.

In Byrd's 1925-1960 series at Vanderbilt, 134 breast biopsies under general anesthesia during pregnancy or lactation produced 29 cancers, approximately one cancer per 4.6 biopsies and similar to the 1:5.4 ratio in the non-pregnant population (Byrd et al., 1962). Most of the benign lesions were fibroadenomas, lipomas, and papillomas, followed in frequency by cystic disease, galactoceles, lobular hyperplasia, and inflammatory lesions.

The risk of these surgical procedures to the mother is negligible, and to the fetus it is small. In the series reported by Byrd et al. (1962) one spontaneous abortion occurred among the 86 pregnant patients subjected to biopsy or mastectomy and this followed three weeks after the removal of a benign cyst. This 1.2% risk is minute compared to the fetal loss of 36% which accompanied mastectomy at the Mayo Clinic prior to 1933 (Harrington, 1937) or even the 5% reported in 1964 (Westberg, 1946).

Figure 2 is the management diagram used for diagnosis of breast masses at the Breast Clinic of the Medical College of Wisconsin. It applies equally well during pregnancy or in its absence. Biopsy under local anesthesia would seem best in pregnancy.

EFFECT OF PREGNANCY ON PROGNOSIS

The influence of pregnancy upon the prognosis of breast cancer has been considered increasingly less ominous over the past 40 years. In 1943, Haagensen and Stout found that of 20 such patients at the Columbia-Presbyterian Hospital in New York, all except one presented with axillary metastases and none were cured. As a result, such patients were categorically declared incurable and unsuitable for radical mastectomy (Haagensen, 1967). Not all shared this extreme opinion however. In a review of 92 cases treated by radical mastectomy between 1910 and 1933, Harrington at the Mayo Clinic found most cases to have presented at an advanced stage, but drew attention to the favorable prognosis in patients without axillary metastases, 61.5% of whom had survived for 5 years (Harrington, 1937). However, even as late as 1953, Cheek surveyed 47 authorities on this subject and found little individual experience and even less enthusiasm. Not more than 5.3% of their composite group of patients had survived 5 years.

Since these earlier years the overall results of treatment have improved and since 1953, reported 5

Table 1. Prognosis of patients with breast cancer during pregnancy or in the postpartum period.

Years reviewed	Total patients	Average duration symptoms	Overall 5 yr survival	Percent operable	Percent with AX+	5 yr survival All	AX+	AX−	Reference
1960-1973	33			88%	75%		27%	33%	Cheek (1973)
1948-1967	48	12 mos	25%	69%	50%	36%	18%	56%	Applewhite (1973)
1930-1964	46		39%	83%	50%		28%	68%	Earley et al. (1969)
1921-1962	17			71%	67%	100%	100%	100%	Horsley et al. (1969)
1938-1961	187		33%						Peters (1968)
1925-1960	29		55%	72%		71%	33%	100%	Byrd et al. (1962)
Ante 1956	37	11 mos		Operable only	68%	22%	8%	50%	White & White (1956)
1920-1953	133		31%		72%	30%	17%	65%	Holleb & Farrow (1964)
Ante 1953	20		40%	90%	75%	50%	42%	75%	Hochman & Schreiber (1953)
1910-1933	92			Operable only	85%	15%	6%	62%	Harrington (1937)

year survivals have varied from 25% to 55% (Table 1). Ten year survivals of 8.5% and 15% are reported (Applewhite et al., 1973; White 1955). Operable cases managed by a variety of operations and adjunctive treatments show between 22% and 100% of patients surviving 5 years (Horsley et al., 1969) and 15% surviving 10 years (Applewhite et al., 1973). As no revolution in treatment occurred during this time, it may be speculated that the trend reflects a reduction in the extent of the disease at diagnosis and more incisive management.

Yet the results of treatment usually, although not invariably, are still inferior to those of the non-pregnant population. Many have commented upon the good prognosis when axillary nodes are found to be uninvolved in pregnancy, although Table 1, in which nine reports are summarized, suggests variation in results. At the Ellis Fischel State Cancer Hospital 20 women treated during pregnancy or the puerperium had relative survival rates at 5 years of 52% and at 10 years of 39%. These results are not inferior to the 54% and 40% corresponding rates for 175 non-pregnant premenopausal women treated with radical mastectomy between 1940-1965 (Donegan, 1972). On the other hand, comparing 41 pregnant patients treated with radical mastectomy with a larger series of non-pregnant patients of all ages, Haagensen (1967) found a lower 10 year survival for the former, 29.5% vs 56.7% respectively, and a constant deficit in each clinical stage, e.g. Stage A 62.5% vs 70.2%; Stage B 12.5% vs 40.1%; Stage C 12.5% vs 22.8%, and Stage D 0% vs 18.2%.

Inconsistent results can be attributed to the small size of most series and where deficits do exist, the influence of pregnancy per se is believed by some to be minimal. Rissanen (1969) observed that early cancers were not appreciably less curable in pregnant patients than in women of comparable age, and Peters' review of 187 pregnant patients treated in Toronto supports this view (Peters, 1968). When these patients were matched with a control group for age and stage of disease, Peters found no more than a 10% to 15% deficit in 5 year survival in each clinical stage. Those patients 36-40 years old fared equally as well as their non-pregnant counterparts, and the difference in actuarial survival between the two total groups over a 10 year period was unimpressive. These data justified the conclusion that pregnancy alone had slight, if any, unfavorable effect on prognosis when stage and age were taken into consideration.

Other factors notwithstanding, there is evidence that the stage of pregnancy during which the cancer is treated will affect the prognosis. Women treated in the latter part of pregnancy seem to fare worse than those treated in the first two trimesters or during the postpartum period. White (1955) found 5 year survival rates after treatment during the second and third trimesters of pregnancy (8% and 10%) to be only half those after treatment earlier in pregnancy (16%) or during lactation (16%). He ascribed the adverse effect to a tendency to treat either less promptly or less adequately in late pregnancy. A poorer prognosis in late pregnancy was also observed by Peters (1968) who could not attribute it to a disproportion of advanced clinical stages, and moreover, could not show that those cases treated promptly had a good prognosis.

The grave implications suggested for cancer in the later stage of pregnancy are of interest in view of its concurrence with the peak corticosteroid production displayed in Figure 1. Irrespective of the time of diagnosis, the highest 5 year survival in Peters' series was associated with treatment during the early postpartum period, i.e. 77%, versus 57% and 14% for the first and second halves of pregnancy respectively. However, there is no indication for postponing treatment of patients near term for this reason. It seems likely that the better prognosis in the women

treated in the early postpartum period in the series was due to postponing the treatment of slower growing tumors till after parturition. The more malignant tumors forced an operation in the second half of pregnancy and this probably accounts for their remarkably poor prognosis (Stoll and Dexeus, 1976).

THERAPEUTIC ABORTION

There is no evidence that termination of pregnancy increases the likelihood of cure in the case of early breast cancer associated with pregnancy. Pregnancy was of concern to surgeons of the last century primarily because of the excess hemorrhage and shock which attended mastectomy in the gravid state. Billroth solved this problem with premature induction of labor, but was not convinced that abortion contributed to cure (Peters, 1968). However, the impression that pregnancy had an adverse effect upon breast cancer induced most authorities prior to 1953 to advise interruption of pregnancy. Some still advise therapeutic abortion, but the majority deny its value, and accumulating data substantiate this view (Helman and Bennett, 1963: Rissanen, 1969: Haagensen, 1967: Erwald, 1967: Rosemond, 1964: Holleb, 1965: Byrd et al., 1962).

Four reports, in which the effect of abortion in operable cases was compared with those cases in which pregnancy was allowed to progress to term, are shown in Table 2. The cases are few and comparison by stage is not possible, but within these limitations there is nothing to suggest a beneficial effect from therapeutic abortion. Most authorities at present would probably agree that pregnancy has a minor effect upon prognosis and should be left undisturbed. Rather than concentrate upon terminating the pregnancy, Byrd pointedly advises, the evidence suggests that physicians should terminate the cancer (Byrd et al., 1962).

However, in the case of advanced disease, therapeutic abortion is usually a necessity if effective palliation methods are to be applied successfully. Ordinarily, surgical castration is the first step in the management of the premenopausal woman with disseminated mammary cancer. In the pregnant woman, a therapeutic abortion is required to remove the source of placental hormones also. In the first trimester of pregnancy this is accomplished by dilatation and curettage of the uterus; later in pregnancy a hysterotomy or hysterectomy is required. Recently, intraamniotic instillation of prostaglandin F2 alpha, as well as the occasional use of hypertonic (20%) saline, have been suggested for interruption of second trimester pregnancies.

Table 2. Results of therapeutic abortion for operable breast cancer concurrent with pregnancy.

Reference	*5 year survival* *Abortion*	*No abortion*
Peete et al. (1966)	2/7 (29%)	3/6 (50%)
Helman & Bennett (1963)	4/7 (57%)	3/3 (100%)
Hochman & Schreiber (1953)	4/6 (67%)	4/10 (40%)
Rissanen (1968)	3/4 (75%)	8/10 (80%)
	13/24 (54%)	18/29 (62%)

When the pregnancy is near term the decision to carry out abortion depends mainly upon the patient's attitude and the urgency of palliation. A short wait until term or until a viable fetus can be obtained may not involve significant progress of an advanced neoplasm. Continued gestation represents no threat to the fetus, as the risk of cancer passing the placenta and metastasizing to the fetus is negligible (Rosemond, 1964).

Chemotherapy with cytotoxic agents and radiation therapy are both contra-indicated in the presence of a viable fetus. Normal development is possible, but the risk of anomalies is significant. Pregnancy should be terminated if treatment with radiotherapy or cytotoxic agents is contemplated.

PROPHYLACTIC CASTRATION

There are two arguments for including castration in the management of operable breast cancer in relation to pregnancy, and both are questionable. The first is that castration of the young patient will prevent future pregnancies which might cause recrudesence of the disease through hormonal stimulation. As will be discussed in a subsequent section, there is no convincing evidence that this is so. The second reason is that by eliminating the ovarian source of oestrogen production, any remaining tumor cells not removed by mastectomy will be slowed in their growth and recurrence will thereby be prevented or retarded.

This second expectation is based upon the observation that therapeutic castration in advanced breast cancer leads to temporary tumor regression in approximately one-third of cases. On this premise, only modest results can be anticipated in pregnancy because therapeutic castration is more effective for women approaching the menopause, while the population most likely to be pregnant is under 35 years old, and this age group is said to respond in no

more than 22% of cases (Fracchia et al., 1969: Taylor, 1962). Furthermore, since only the uncured fraction of the operable group could be expected to derive benefit, only 22% of the 50% not cured by mastectomy (or 11%) would perhaps be helped. Almost 90% would have had a needless operation.

The results of randomised trials of prophylactic castration in breast cancer are discussed fully in chapters 6 and 8 and provide no clear evidence of improved 5 year survival rates. Data on trials in pregnant patients are scanty and controlled studies are lacking, but there is no reason to expect that the results would be any more promising. In a small group of pregnant patients in operable stages, Hochman and Schreiber (1953) found 5 year survival rates virtually identical whether or not castration had been performed. Five of 12 castrates (42%) survived 5 years as did three of seven patients (43%) with intact ovaries. Influenced by such unimpressive results and the negative results of controlled trials in non-pregnant patients, clinicians interested in this field have increasingly abandoned prophylactic castration (Rissanen, 1969: Byrd et al., 1962: Peters, 1968: Holleb, 1965).

Witholding castration unless and until recurrence makes its appearance has certain positive advantages. Those who actually need the procedure will be the ones to receive it, and then at a time when it is known to be effective. Furthermore, it is widely accepted that knowing a patient's response to therapeutic castration is a useful predictor of likely response to further endocrine ablation. In view of the fact that subsequent pregnancies do not appear to jeopardize survival, preservation of the ovaries has the final advantage of permitting a life of normal reproductive potential for those whom mastectomy has cured, an act of compassion for these patients.

PREGNANCY SUBSEQUENT TO MASTECTOMY

The incidence of pregnancy subsequent to treatment for breast cancer is influenced by many factors including whether sterilization was a part of therapy, whether recommendations were made against child-bearing and also the duration of patient survival. The literature suggests that as many as 7% of fertile women have one or more pregnancies after mastectomy, most of which can be expected within the first 5 years (Applewhite et al., 1973: Cooper and Butterfield, 1970: Rissanen, 1969).

What should the physician advise the patient who has had a potentially curative mastectomy about future pregnancies? Should they be avoided; should they be terminated if they occur? Two major considerations are involved. The first is whether a future pregnancy will promote recurrence of the cancer; the second is the probability of the patient having been cured.

It is now generally believed that women who become pregnant subsequent to mastectomy have a surprisingly good prognosis, far better than those whose pregnancy coexisted with the primary tumor, and often better than mastectomy patients overall. Eight (67%) of White's 12 patients lived at least 5 years and 58% for 10 years (White and White, 1956). This experience was shared by Rissanen (1969) whose 53 patients had corresponding survivals of 77.4% and 69.5%. On the other hand, Cheek (1973) reported 50% and Applewhite et al. (1973) reported 29% of 5 year survivals in such patients.

To explain the unexpectedly good results in some series, the point is often made that those women who do become pregnant are a selected group. Women with a poor prognosis die early, leaving those who have a better prognosis to become pregnant. Credence was given to this argument by the finding of a lower incidence of axillary nodal metastases in this group when compared to the total mastectomy population. In the large series of Holleb and Farrow (1964) only 46% of patients who became pregnant later, had involved nodes at the time of mastectomy, compared to 72% and 73% of all those treated during pregnancy and lactation respectively.

However, elimination of this bias by case matching suggests that the apparently beneficial effect of pregnancy may not be illusory. Ninety-six patients with a subsequent pregnancy were matched with respect to both age and clinical stage with mastectomy patients who had no subsequent pregnancy (Peters, 1968). The former not only demonstrated better survival rates than the controls, but also had longer recurrence-free intervals when cases with tumor recurrence were compared.

Furthermore, when the factor of selection through early death was minimized by considering only those who became pregnant within six months of mastectomy, as many as 54% were found to survive five years. In an even more exacting analysis, Cooper and Butterfield (1970) examined 40 cases each matched with two controls according to clinical stage, age, status of axillary involvement and length of survival to the time of pregnancy. They found that the survival of the patients who became pregnant was still superior to that of the controls.

While on the basis of these studies it may be presumptuous to conclude that pregnancy subsequent to mastectomy improves the prognosis, it seems

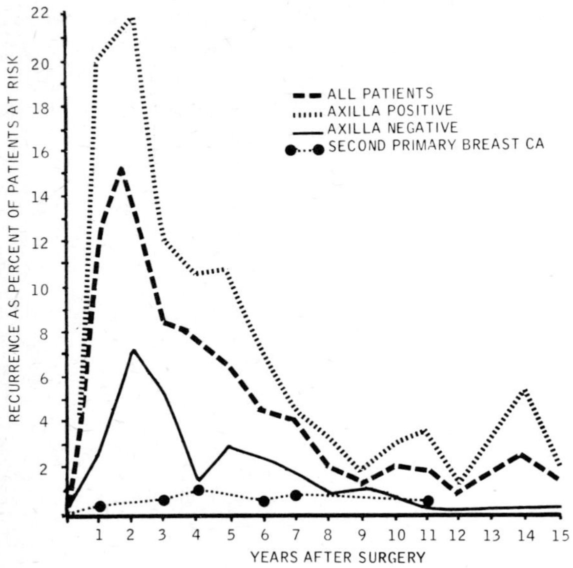

Figure 3. Annual incidence of recurrence and new second primaries after radical mastectomy for unilateral mammary carcinoma. (703 patients—Ellis Fischel Hospital, 1940-1958).

reasonably safe to conclude that it is not detrimental. Consequently, if a pregnancy occurs, there appears to be no justification for recommending its termination in patients apparently cured by mastectomy. The point must however be made that pregnancy in no way guarantees against a subsequent recurrence, and cases are known in which multiple pregnancies have eventually been followed by recurrence (Cooper and Butterfield, 1970: Rissanen, 1969).

A second major consideration in formulating a recommendation on future pregnancies is the normally expected risk of recurrence and death after mastectomy. In Figure 3 is shown the annual incidence of recurrence observed during 15 years among 703 women treated with radical mastectomy at the Ellis Fischel State Cancer Hospital. As would be expected, the annual recurrence rate is constantly higher among patients who had involved axillary nodes than among those who did not. The incidence of recurrence is highest in the first three years after mastectomy and then gradually falls to a low level. Although even up to 15 years the risk never entirely disappears, approximately one third of the population at risk show tumor recurrence during the first 3 years. Contralateral breast cancers, an independent threat, appear at a constant rate of 1% per year.

It is evident from this data that the earlier a pregnancy occurs after mastectomy, the more likely it is to be followed by recurrence and the less likely will the mother be to give continuing care to her child. If a pregnancy is desired therefore, it would seem best to advise deferment until after 3 to 5 years, especially if the axillary nodes were involved. However, as it is the patient who takes the risk, it should be her privilege to weigh the desirability of the pregnancy against her risk of dying prematurely from the disease.

A difficult problem is the management of recurrence during a subsequent pregnancy. There is considerable danger of damage to the fetus from irradiation of a large area of chest wall by cobalt or high voltage beams. Effective systemic treatment of dissemination beyond the local site also generally requires interruption of pregnancy. Whether this can be avoided depends upon the closeness of the pregnancy to term and the urgency of the need for palliation.

SUMMARY

Pertinent information about breast cancer and pregnancy may be summarized as follows: About 3% of breast cancers are accompanied by pregnancy, the peak incidence being among women in the fourth decade of life. The prognosis of these patients, and of those whose cancers are discovered and treated during the postpartum period, is less favorable than that of others, largely because they present with more advanced disease. If age and stage of disease are taken into account, pregnancy alone seems to have a minor influence upon prognosis.

Radical mastectomy can be expected to be almost as curative as for other patients with operable cancers, and with little risk of fetal loss. Therapeutic abortion does not improve the chances for cure, nor does prophylactic castration.

For the patient with inoperable or disseminated disease, effective radiation therapy, endocrine therapy or chemotherapy requires therapeutic abortion, and early pregnancy is best terminated without delay. The management of pregnancy near term depends greatly upon the desire of the patient for a child. Unless palliation is urgent, treatment sometimes can be delayed until after delivery without jeopardy to the infant or significant deterioration in the mother's condition.

Pregnancy subsequent to mastectomy appears neither to promote nor diminish the chances of continued wellbeing. Unless recurrent cancer is evident, or some other consideration is present, there is nothing to be gained therapeutically by interrupting such a pregnancy. A successful pregnancy, however, is no guarantee against a future recurrence, and

as the risk of recurrence diminishes rapidly with time, a prudent course is to defer pregnancy after mastectomy until the period of greatest risk is past and cure seems reasonably certain.

The treatment of patients during pregnancy and lactation is more successful at present than it was four decades ago. Continued progress depends upon a keen awareness that breast cancers do occur during this period, that they are curable, and that pregnancy should neither deter the prompt diagnosis of breast masses nor interfere with definitive treatment.

REFERENCES

Applewhite, R. R., Smith, L. R. and DiVincenti, F. (1973). Carcinoma of the breast associated with pregnancy and lactation. *The American Surgeon 39,* 101.

Beatson, G. T. (1896). On the treatment of inoperable cases of carcinoma of the mamma; suggestions for a new method of treatment with illustrative cases. *Lancet 2,* 104.

Byrd, Jr., B. F., Bayer, D. S., Robertson, J. C. and Stephenson, Jr., S. E. (1962). Treatment of breast tumors associated with pregnancy and lactation. *Annals of Surgery 155,* 940.

Campion, P. D. and Currey, H. L. F. (1972). Cell-mediated immunity in pregnancy. *Lancet 2,* 830.

Cheek, J. H. (1953). Surgery of current opinions concerning carcinoma of the breast occurring during pregnancy. *Archives of Surgery 66,* 664.

Cheek, J. H. (1973). Cancer of the breast in pregnancy and lactation. *American Journal of Surgery 126,* 729.

Cooper, D. R. and Butterfield, J. (1970). Pregnancy subsequent to mastectomy for cancer of the breast. *Annals of Surgery 171,* 429.

Davis, M. E. and Plotz, E. J. (1965). *Obstetrics,* p. 233, 13th ed., W. B. Saunders Company, Philadelphia.

Donegan, W. L. (1972). *Advances in Surgery,* Volume 6, p. 1, Year Book Medical Publishers, Incorporated, Chicago.

Earley, T. K., Gallagher, J. Q. and Chapman, K. E. (1969). Carcinoma of the breast in women under thirty years of age. *American Journal of Surgery 118,* 832.

Erwald, R. (1967). Mammary carcinoma and pregnancy. *Acta Obstetrica et Gynecologica Scandinavica 46,* 316.

Fracchia, A. A., Farrow, J. H., DePalo, A. J., Connolly, D. P. and Huvos, A. G. (1969). Castration for primary inoperable or recurrent breast carcinoma. *Surgery, Gynecology and Obstetrics 128,* 1226.

Haagensen, C. D. (1967). Cancer of the breast in pregnancy and during lactation. *American Journal of Obstetrics and Gynecology 98,* 141.

Harrington, S. W. (1937). Carcinoma of the breast, results of surgical treatment when the carcinoma occurred in the course of pregnancy or lactation and when pregnancy occurred subsequent to operation. *Annals of Surgery 106,* 690.

Helman, P. and Bennett, M. B. (1963). Breast cancer and pregnancy. *South African Medical Journal 37,* 1236.

Hochman, A. and Schreiber, H. (1953). Pregnancy and cancer of the breast. *Obstetrics and Gynecology 2,* 268.

Holleb, A. I. (1965). Breast cancer and pregnancy. *CA—A Cancer Journal for Clinicians 15,* 182.

Holleb, A. I. and Farrow, J. H. (1964). Breast cancer and pregnancy. *Extrait de Acta Union Internationale Contre Le Cancer XX,* No. 6-7.

Horsley, III, J. S., Alrich, E. M. and Wright, C. B. (1969). Carcinoma of the breast in women 35 years of age or younger. *Annals of Surgery 196,* 839.

Lewison, E. F. (1954). Breast cancer and pregnancy or lactation. *Surgery, Gynecology, and Obstetrics 99,* 417.

Minton, J. P. (1974). Proceedings: the response of breast cancer patients with bone pain to L-dopa. *Cancer 33,* 358.

Peete, Jr., C. H., Huneycutt, Jr., H. C. and Cherny, W. B. (1966). Cancer of the breast in pregnancy. *North Carolina Medical Journal 27,* 514.

Peters, M. V. (1968). The effect of pregnancy in breast cancer. In *Prognostic Factors in Breast Cancer,* (Ed. by A. P. M. Forrest and P. B. Kunkler). Baltimore: Williams and Wilkins Company.

Purtilo, D. T., Hallgren, H. M. and Yunis, E. S. (1972). Depressed maternal lymphocyte response to PHA in human pregnancy. *Lancet 1,* 769.

Rissanen, P. M. (1969). Pregnancy following treatment of mammary cancer. *Acta Radiologica 8,* 415.

Rosemond, G. P. (1964). Management of patients with carcinoma of the breast in pregnancy. *Annals of the New York Academy of Science 114,* 851.

Stoll, B. A. and Dexeus, S. (1976). Effect of pregnancy and lactation on prognosis. In *Risk Factors in Breast Cancer,* (Ed. B. A. Stoll). Heinemann Medical and Year Book Publishers, p. 164.

Strelkavskos, A. J., Wilson, B. S., Dray, and Dodson, M. (1975). Inversion of levels of human T & B cells in early pregnancy. *Nature "D",* 331.

Taylor, S. (1962). Endocrine ablation in disseminated mammary carcinoma. *Surgery, Gynecology, and Obstetrics 115,* 443.

Treves, N. and Holleb, A. I. (1958). A report of 549 cases of breast cancer in women 35 years of age or younger. *Surgery, Gynecology, and Obstetrics 107,* 271.

Westberg, S. V. (1946). Prognosis of breast cancer for pregnant and nursing women. *Acta Obstetrica et Gynecologica Scandinavica, Suppl. No. 4.*

White, T. T. (1955). Prognosis of breast cancer for pregnant and nursing women. *Surgery, Gynecology, and Obstetrics 100,* 661.

White, T. T. and White, W. C. (1956). Breast cancer and pregnancy, report of 49 cases followed 5 years. *Annals of Surgery 144,* 384.

Wilson, R. G., Buchan, R., Roberts, M. M. et al. (1974). Plasma prolactin and breast cancer. *Cancer 33,* 1325.

Chapter

20

JOHN A. McCREDIE

Management of the Contralateral Breast

INTRODUCTION

It is sometimes forgotten that the woman with the greatest risk of developing carcinoma of the breast is the one who has had the disease. It is true that these women are generally examined at regular intervals and a biopsy performed of any suspicious lesion in the contralateral breast, but this regime had been challenged because it has not resulted in the second carcinoma being diagnosed at an earlier stage than the first tumour. Three alternative managements have been suggested; regular review with mammography or thermography performed once a year; excision of the mirror image or upper lateral quadrant of the contralateral breast at the time of treating the first carcinoma; or subcutaneous or simple mastectomy with or without insertion of a prosthesis.

It has been suggested that it may be possible to select for mastectomy those patients with an especially high risk of developing contralateral carcinoma of the breast. Factors to be considered are the microscopic findings in the first breast including the histology of the primary tumour, the presence of mammary dysplasia and the presence of multiple independent carcinomas. In addition, the microscopic findings in a biopsy from the opposite breast may influence the decision.

The prognosis from the first carcinoma is also important in selecting cases for contralateral mastectomy. There is less concern about the contralateral breast in women whose primary tumour carries a bad prognosis such as a large infiltrating carcinoma with fibrosis, or those who have metastases in the axillary nodes, since about 80% of the latter will develop recurrence within 10 years. Age is also important in the selection since older women are less likely to survive long enough to develop a second carcinoma than are younger women. Finally, to help in making a decision, a family history of carcinoma of the breast must also be considered.

We define synchronous carcinoma of the two breasts as those diagnosed at the same time or within six months of each other. What then are the criteria suggesting that a consecutive carcinoma of the breast

is a new primary and not a metastasis? The major ones used are that the tumour is an invasive carcinoma within the mammary lobules and that other metastases are not demonstrable at the time of diagnosing the second carcinoma. Only occasionally is it possible to demonstrate that the two breast tumours differ microscopically. Robbins and Berg (1964) stressed thaat in situ changes were almost invariably present adjacent to a second carcinoma of the multifocal type. This does not of course apply in those cases with two primaries of different microscopic types or in those with medullary carcinoma associated with lymphoid infiltration.

INCIDENCE AND PROGNOSIS OF CONSECUTIVE CARCINOMAS

Moertel (1966) found that the incidence of carcinoma of the contralateral breast was highest initially and then decreased exponentially with time. Robbins and Berg (1964) found that the incidence was 0.7% per year for the patients at risk at any one time and that this was five times greater than in the general population. It was ten times the general incidence in women before the age of 50 years but only less than twice that expected after the age of 70 years.

We observed 88 consecutive tumours among 1489 patients with carcinoma of the breast seen between 1953 and 1971 in the London Clinic of the Ontario Cancer Treatment and Research Foundation (McCredie et al., 1975a). The cumulative probability of developing a consecutive nonsynchronous carcinoma of the breast was found to be 1% per year throughout the total period of 20 years. This percentage applied to the total number of patients at risk each year and not to the total number of people who were first entered into the study. However the true value must be over 2% per year since the mortality from carcinoma of the breast is just less than one-half the incidence, and many patients die from other causes before the second carcinoma can become clinically manifest.

In our study of bilateral carcinoma of the breast, survival rates were higher in women aged under 50 years than in older women, and also in those who had a long interval between the first and second tumours. Five year survival rates were similar among women with unilateral tumours as in those with bilateral tumours, about 50%. Survival at 5 years was 40% in those who had synchronous tumours but 70% in those with consecutive tumours.

Contralateral breast cancer is usually discovered late. Axillary metastases were found in 51% of these patients compared with 47% of those with unilateral carcinoma. It should be mentioned that only during the last 3 years of this study (1969, 1970 and 1971) was mammography of the remaining breast performed as a routine once per year. Mammography, perhaps combined with thermography, should lead to earlier detection of non-palpable tumours, an increase in the number of contralateral biopsies and therefore a decreased proportion with axillary metastases in resected specimens.

Wilson and Alberty (1973) found that 80 women with consecutive carcinomas of the breast were on the average 5 years younger than those with unilateral tumours. Also that the most important factor influencing prognosis was the interval between diagnosing the first and second tumours—the longer the interval, the greater the survival rate. Rather remarkably, they found that the prognosis was better in women who developed non-synchronous consecutive carcinomas than in those with unilateral disease. Also that the incidence of axillary metastases, 30%, was about one-half that in women with unilateral carcinomas.

They postulated that women with tumours with a bad prognosis might not live long enough to develop second tumours, or that the second tumour might in some way improve the immune response against the tumour. However, observations by Watson (1966) on the prognosis of these cases are similar to our own. Five year survival rates in women with consecutive tumours are similar to those following unilateral tumours—namely about 50%.

EFFECT OF IMMUNOSUPPRESSION

Recently there has been concern that treatment of cancer by surgery, radiotherapy or chemotherapy may decrease host resistance and increase the incidence of metastases and new primary cancers. It has been suggested that removal of the regional nodes or their destruction by radiotherapy may decrease host resistance and increase distant metastases. In animals the evidence is based mainly on the fact that the cell-mediated immune response to an allograft is initially confined to the regional nodes. This evidence need not necessarily apply to human tumours.

Stjernsward (1974) quoted five controlled clinical trials using prophylactic postoperative radiotherapy in carcinoma of the breast and pointed out that 5-year survival was significantly worse, varying from 1% to 10% in those who were irradiated compared to those who were not. However, in some of these studies inadequate data are presented to show that

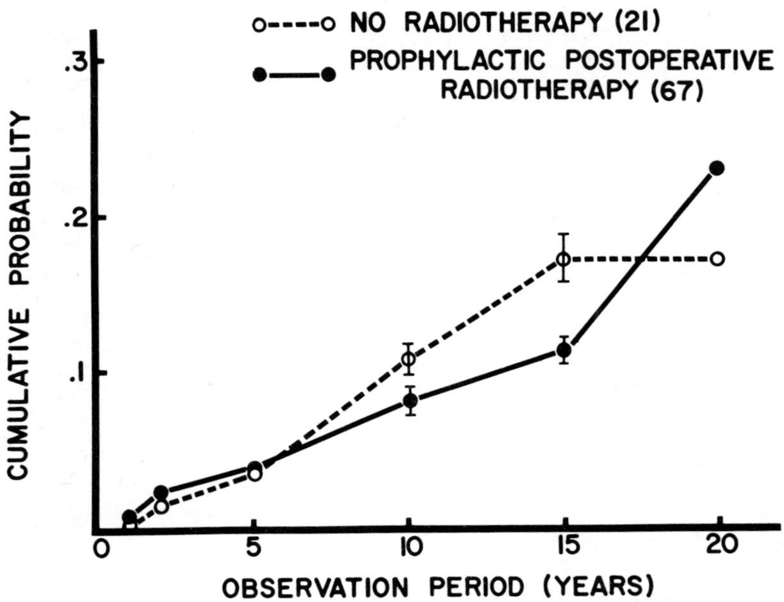

Fig. 1. Cumulative probability of developing a nonsynchronous carcinoma of the contralateral breast in women who were or were not given prophylactic postoperative radiotherapy. (From McCredie et al., 1975a. Reprinted by permission Editor *Cancer).*

the groups were equally matched, especially in the size of the tumours and the presence or absence of metastases in the regional nodes. No prospective controlled clinical trials in carcinoma of the breast have so far shown that radiotherapy is associated with an increase in carcinoma of the contralateral breast or at distant sites.

We made a retrospective study of the effect of prophylactic postoperative radiotherapy on the incidence of carcinoma of the contralateral breast (McCredie et al., 1975b). For 369 women treated by radical mastectomy with or without prophylactic postoperative radiotherapy, a 20-year life table showed no difference at any time between the groups in the incidence of contralateral carcinoma (Fig. 1). Also there was no difference in the incidence of other primary cancers in the two groups. It suggests that the immunosuppression produced by radiotherapy for carcinoma of the breast is not of sufficient severity or prolonged enough to increase carcinogenesis.

However, women given immunosuppressant drugs after renal transplantation show an increase in mesenchymal and epithelial cancers, including carcinoma of the breast (Penn and Starzl, 1973). The agents used most frequently were azathioprine, prednisone and antilymphocytic serum. Arseneau et al. (1972) have reported a three-fold increase in new primary cancers in patients given extended field radiotherapy for Hodgkin's disease and a thirty-fold increase in those treated by extended field radiotherapy and chemotherapy. Nevertheless, in more recent studies, no increase in new primary cancers was observed in patients treated for Hodgkin's disease (Rosenberg and Kaplan, 1975: Sutherland et al., 1976).

EFFECT OF FAMILY HISTORY

Opinions differ on the importance of a family history of carcinoma of the breast but it is possible that there are families with a genetic predilection to develop carcinoma of the breast. Anderson (1973) compared the incidence of carcinoma of the breast in 567 mothers, sisters and daughters of 178 patients who had a history of carcinoma of the breast, with the incidence in 699 mothers, sisters and daughters of 217 patients who had a family history of other types of cancer. He found that there was a two-fold increase in risk in the relatives of patients with a positive history of carcinoma of the breast.

But the daughters of women who had bilateral breast carcinoma before the age of 50 years had a *nine-fold* increase compared with controls who did not have the disease. If the overall incidence is about 5%, about 50% of this group developed the disease. Anderson also noted that the carcinomas developed

at a younger age than in the relatives of women with unilateral tumours. These findings suggest that a women with carcinoma of the breast whose mother had the disease before the age of 50 years may carry a high risk of developing a carcinoma of the contralateral breast. The risks involved when the mother developed the disease after the age of 50 years, and those associated with a history of breast cancer in other relatives, still remain controversial.

EFFECT OF MAMMARY DYSPLASIA

There is considerable controversy on the relationship of mammary dysplasia to carcinoma of the breast, but it needs to be reviewed in relation to the development of bilateral tumours. Warren (1940) found a 4.5-fold increase in the incidence of breast carcinoma in women with mammary dysplasia, and a 12-fold increase in those with marked epithelial proliferation, among 1200 cases observed over a period of 5 years. Haagensen (1971) found a 4-fold increase in carcinoma associated with dysplasia, in 1,700 patients matched for age and for period of observation. McDivitt et al., (1968) in an excellent review of the subject did not agree with Warren's findings and concluded that the relation of mammary dysplasia to carcinoma of the breast is not known.

The practical problem, however, is not whether mammary dysplasia is premalignant but whether a carcinoma is also present. In an autopsy study of 100 women with clinically normal breasts, Ryan and Coady (1962) found that 12% had intraductal epithelial proliferation, while in 100 women with carcinoma of the breast the incidence was four times as great. They concluded that this condition was precancerous. Others, however, consider only the observation of atypicism with dyskaryosis to be premalignant. It may be that the factor responsible for hyperplasia is similar to that for carcinoma but that the one does not progress to the other.

Opinions differ also on the relation of papillomas and papillomatosis to carcinoma of the breast. Conclusions have been based on the incidence of carcinoma among women who have previously had this diagnosis made on excised specimens. Warren (1940) and Haagensen (1971) considered that both conditions were benign and were not associated with an increase in carcinoma. On the other hand, Foote and Stewart (1945) and Buhl-Jorgensen et al. (1968) stated that they were associated with an increase in malignancy.

One agrees with the conclusion of McDivitt et al. (1968) that there is still insufficient evidence that any of the various manifestations of mammary dysplasia is precancerous.

EFFECT OF MULTICENTRICITY

Recently there has been interest in the microscopic changes in normal breast tissue both in the ipsilateral and contralateral breasts of patients with breast carcinoma. In 1931, Cheatle and Cutler recognized the multicentric origin of a number of carcinomas of the breast, and demonstrated extensive involvement of single ducts, but with intervening normal regions within the ducts. They reported one case with three independent primary carcinomas within the same breast. Foote and Stewart (1945) also noted that multicentricity was frequent within a single segment and recognised that other segments might also be involved.

Qualheim and Gall (1957) emphasized the multicentricity of carcinoma of the breast and found more than one cancer in 54% of specimens. They found that only 17% were confined to the same segment while 37% were in other segments. Gallager and Martin (1969) on examination of whole organ section, found multiple carcinomas in the ipsilateral breast in 48% of cases and intraductal hyperplastic changes in all cases.

Fisher et al. (1975) found a significantly greater incidence of multicentricity in those with carcinomas greater than 5 cm than in those with smaller tumours, and noted that twice as many lesions were non-invasive as were invasive. It is interesting to note the number of microscopic carcinomas left in the breast after performing a local excision of the tumour with a 2 to 3 cm margin of normal breast tissue segments. Morgenstern et al. (1975) found that 30% of 500 patients had microscopic evidence of cancer in residual breast tissue.

The upper lateral or mirror image segment of the contralateral breast has been removed at the time of treating the first breast. Urban (1969) found that 16% of 281 women had occult carcinomas in the mirror image biopsy, and of the tumours, 13 were infiltrating and 18 non-infiltrating. Fenig et al. (1975) removed 30% of the mirror image segment of the contralateral breast in 314 patients and found that 7.3% had in situ or invasive carcinomas. Yet these biopsies represent only 25% and 10% respectively of the total breast tissue in these patients. One must conclude therefore that the majority of contralateral breasts must contain invasive or non-invasive occult carcinomas.

Fenig et al. (1975) did not find that the size of the

primary tumour was related to the incidence of occult carcinomas, unlike the report of Fisher et al. (1975) mentioned earlier. It is interesting that only 6 of their 291 patients treated during 1966 and 1972 had developed metachronous tumours up to 1975. This is considerably less than the expected 1% per year and suggests that excision of 30% of the mirror image segment removes the commonest site of consecutive carcinoma.

The natural history of these small carcinomas is not known but many may remain small and not develop into palpable tumours. It has been stated that the finding of multiple carcinomas in the first breast suggests that the patient may be at greater risk of developing a contralateral carcinoma than when a single tumour is found. It now appears that most patients with carcinoma of the breast have occult carcinomas in both breasts.

Other chapters in this book debate the merits of removing a small primary carcinoma with 2 to 3 cm. margin of normal breast tissue compared with removing all the breast tissue. The concern of those advocating mastectomy is that additional tumours may be left on the affected side. Recent studies show that there is the same incidence of independent carcinomas, invasive and non invasive, in the contralateral as in the ipsilateral breast. This suggests that the treatment and methods of observation recommended for the residual ipsilateral breast need to be considered for the contralateral breast.

EFFECT OF TUMOUR TYPE

Intraductal Carcinoma

The diagnosis of in situ intraductal carcinoma is now being made more frequently since the introduction of mammography and the more thorough histological examination of grossly normal breast tissues. About 2% of cancers of the breast are intraductal carcinomas. Westbrook and Gallager (1975) made a particularly valuable study of 64 such cases and found that 12.5% developed bilateral carcinoma. The authors stress the high incidence of bilateral carcinomas in these patients and that, since many of the lesions are located centrally, the nipple and areola should be removed if subcutaneous mastectomy is carried out.

Lobular Carcinoma

At least 5% and possibly as many as 10% of breast cancers, are infiltrating lobular carcinomas (Newman, 1966), and about one-third of patients with in situ or invasive lobular carcinoma in one breast develop a similar tumour in the contralateral breast within 10 years. The diagnosis of in situ lobular carcinomas is often made on tissue that does not contain a palpable tumour and the tissue is often adjacent to a segment showing mammary dysplasia. The extremely high incidence of multicentricity involving the ipsilateral and the contralateral breasts places these patients at extremely high risk of developing further disease.

Medullary Carcinoma with Lymphoid Infiltration

Between 1 and 5% of carcinomas of the breast are medullary or circumscribed tumours. They tend to be large and soft and have a lower incidence of spread to the regional nodes than do infiltrating adenocarcinomas with fibrosis. The five-year survival is excellent, about 90% and few patients die from the tumour after that time. Nevertheless, Haagensen (1971) found that among 140 patients with this tumour a carcinoma of the same or another type developed in 10% of patients.

MANAGEMENT

Regular Review

At present the most frequent management of the contralateral breast is to examine the patient at regular intervals and to perform mammography once per year. The patient is also advised to perform a monthly self examination. In some centres mammography and thermography are performed at the first examination and thermography once per year. Mammography is then performed if an abnormality is noted on clinical examination or changes are observed on thermography. Biopsy is performed if a tumour is palpated or if any change suggestive of malignancy is noted on mammography. While Clark (1973) champions the use of thermography, Burn (1971) considered that the incidence of false positives was too high for the test to be of value.

Supporters of the regime of repeated examination and mammography with or without thermography state that it avoids mutilation of the contralateral breast and that tumours can be detected at a small size, often before they are palpable. On the other hand, a number of women do not attend regularly for follow-up, and patients are often unreliable in carrying out regular monthly self-examination, whatever its value.

There is so far no proof that the addition of

mammography of the opposite breast can improve survival rates in breast carcinoma patients after treatment. Nevertheless, it is possible that with further refinements in mammography, a contralateral carcinoma will be diagnosed at an earlier stage than formerly. The incidence of false positives and false negatives with mammography are each about 10 to 20%. While the false positives lead to unnecessary biopsies, the high incidence of false negatives means that reliance must still be placed on clinical judgement. Finally, since the natural history of non palpable carcinomas detected on mammography is unknown it is uncertain whether this regime will lead to a marked improvement in survival in those patients developing carcinoma of the contralateral breast.

Radiation received by the breast during repeated fluoroscopy of the chest in patients with pulmonary tuberculosis, has been shown to increase the risk of breast carcinoma on the affected side (MacKenzie, 1965). There has, therefore, been concern that radiation given during repeated mammography may also be carcinogenic. With the original technique taking three views of each breast, a high dose, 20 to 25 rads. was delivered to each breast. More recently a dose as low as 6 rads. has been given and even less if xeroradiography is used. Although several doses at this low level are unlikely to be harmful, long term observation is essential.

There has recently been an interest in the presence of cancer specific cell markers which might show up the presence of carcinoma of the breast. Carcinoembryonic antigen (CEA) is increased in many patients with carcinoma and the antibody to CEA can be tagged with an isotope. If taken up by the cancer cells containing CEA (Hoffer et al., 1973), this could possibly be used for the early detection of carcinoma in the contralateral breast.

It can be concluded that regular examination of the contralateral breast (often with mammography) has so far failed to lead to significantly earlier diagnosis of consecutive breast carcinoma although some improvement may be anticipated from the more extensive use of mammography, possibly combined with thermography. This regime is indicated in those patients who have a bad prognosis suggested by the histopathology of the primary tumour and axillary nodes, or if the patient is aged and has other serious diseases (Table 1).

Since 1% of the women at risk each year develop a clinically palpable carcinoma of the contralateral breast, this regime would appear to be inadequate in women with a good prognosis suggested by the histopathology of the primary tumour and nodes, especially if they have the type of tumour which tends to be more often bilateral, and if they have a life expectancy of more than 20 years.

Segmental Excision

It has been suggested that at the time of treating the first carcinoma, the mirror image or upper lateral segment of the opposite clinically normal breast should be removed. If either an in situ or an invasive occult carcinoma is found, it is then recommended that a simple mastectomy be performed on the contralateral side. The axillary nodes are generally not removed since less than 5% contain metastases at that stage.

From the observations of Urban (1969) and Fenig et al. (1975) mentioned earlier, it can be concluded that if all the contralateral breast was examined, using many whole organ sections, a high proportion would be found to contain either non-invasive or invasive occult carcinomas. Since carcinoma of the breast is most often a multicentric disease and the natural history of these microscopic tumours is not known, a mirror image or upper lateral segment excision of clinically normal contralateral breast tissue does not appear to be indicated in the writer's opinion.

Table 1. Management of contralateral breast.

		Tumor type frequently bilateral*	*Carcinoma with fibrosis*	*Axillary nodes*		*Life expectancy (years)*		*Family history***	
				−ve	*+ve*	*>20*	*<20*	*−ve*	*+ve*
Review and Mammography		−	−	−	+	−	+	−	−
Subcutaneous mastectomy	(a) Highly recommended	+	−	+	−	+	−	−	−
	(b) Discussed	−	+	+	−	−	−	−	+

* In situ and infiltrating lobular, medullary and intraductal carcinomas.
** Mother had carcinoma breast at <50 years.

Mastectomy

Bloodgood (1921) suggested that since the incidence of carcinoma of the contralateral breast is 7%, prophylactic mastectomy is indicated as a routine, and thirty years later this view was endorsed by Pack (1951). This approach is too radical because it includes women who would die from metastases or not live long enough to have a high likelihood of developing the disease in the contralateral breast. Leis (1971) has made an important contribution in defining groups at special risk who might benefit from prophylactic mastectomy. He insists that the patient should have a good prognosis from the first carcinoma since it would be wrong to recommend operation if there was a high likelihood of recurrence.

The most important factor determining prognosis is the presence of metastases in the axillary nodes, since 80% of cases with positive nodes develop recurrence within 10 years. Leis (1971) stated that other microscopic findings that place the patient at special risk were lobular carcinoma and the presence of multiple carcinomas in the ipsilateral breast. Other factors were a positive family history of carcinoma of the breast and a patient aged less than 50 years. He recommended that the operation be performed one year after the first operation if extensive investigations, including bone scan, failed to show metastases and he found that less than one in three women met these criteria. In 91 patients treated by delayed prophylactic simple mastectomy he found that the incidence of occult invasive carcinomas was 17%.

The writer suggests that women with medullary carcinomas, or in situ and invasive lobular and intraductal carcinomas, be strongly recommended to have some form of contralateral mastectomy provided that the ipsilateral axillary nodes were free of metastases at the primary operation. Operation should be recommended at one year after the first operation. In those women found to have infiltrating adenocarcinomas with fibrosis, the prognosis is worse and the incidence of bilateral tumours is lower but the possibility of performing mastectomy should still be discussed with these patients. Thorough investigation for metastases is performed in both groups prior to considering mastectomy.

In the writer's opinion, the finding of multiple cancers in the breast is probably not important in making a decision because carcinoma of the breast is generally a multifocal disease. As far as the family history is concerned it is definite that the patient whose mother had a carcinoma of the breast before the age of 50 years has an enormously increased risk of developing carcinoma of the breast. It is therefore advisable to recommend contralateral mastectomy in the daughter. A history of breast cancer in the mother after the age of 50 years or in other relatives, would appear to be insufficient to recommend the operation. The patient should have a life expectation of at least 20 years, this being a more important consideration than that she should be less than 50 years old.

In the operation of subcutaneous mastectomy a curved incision is made in the skin fold below the breast and the mammary lobules are removed with preservation of the subcutaneous fat, the nipple and the areola. Mammary lobular tissue is left below the areola and nipple, in the periphery of the gland, and the axillary tail of Spence may not be removed. An alternative form of subcutaneous mastectomy is to make transverse incisions above and below the areola and to remove the nipple and areola. The ductal tissue deep to the areola is then removed. Mammary carcinoma may still develop in the small amount of residual lobular tissue. Repeated clinical examination and mammography at least once a year are therefore essential.

In total mastectomy all the mammary lobules are removed along with subcutaneous fat superficial and deep to the lobules, and the axillary tail of Spence is excised as it passes through the axillary fascia to make contact with the anterior pectoral nodes. The deep fascia covering the pectoralis major and the serratus anterior muscles may or may not be excised. The less mammary tissue removed the better the cosmetic effect, but the greater the risk of developing a carcinoma in the remaining tissue.

It has often been stated that a prosthesis should not be inserted because it may induce a fibrotic reaction that is difficult to differentiate from a tumour. This is a rapidly advancing field with the introduction of new materials that are relatively inert and well tolerated by the tissues. Consideration should therefore be given to performing a subcutaneous mastectomy and inserting a prosthesis after either 3 days or a longer interval.

SUMMARY

Carcinoma of the breast develops most often in women who have previously had the disease. The incidence is 1% per year for all women at risk at any one time and remains at this level for up to 20 years. There is however a special risk in younger women and in those whose mother developed a breast carcinoma before the age of 50 years. The prognosis depends on

the interval between the first and second tumours. The longer the interval, the better the chance of survival.

In the past, management most often consisted of repeated clinical examination although more recently, mammography, and in some centres, thermography, have been added at yearly intervals. So far, this regime has not been proved to improve survival and it has therefore been suggested that women at special risk should be strongly recommended to undergo some form of prophylactic mastectomy.

The operation is especially recommended in the case of tumours which tend more often to be bilateral such as medullary carcinoma, and in situ and invasive lobular and intraductal carcinomas. Only women with a life expectancy of more than 20 years and those whose axillary nodes did not contain metastases at primary operation should be considered. Subcutaneous mastectomy should be carried out 12 months after the first operation, after careful investigation has made sure that there is no clinical evidence of metastases. The case for operating upon women with infiltrating carcinomas with fibrosis is less strong, but the advisability should nevertheless be discussed with the patient one year after the first operation.

Carcinoma of the breast is most often a multifocal disease involving both breasts. For this reason the presence of multiple carcinomas in the ipsilateral breast is not important in deciding the risk of contralateral breast carcinoma nor is the presence of mammary dysplasia. For the same reason, a mirror image or upper lateral segment biopsy of the contralateral breast is not indicated.

A subcutaneous mastectomy should be performed using an infra-mammary incision with preservation of the nipple, areola and subcutaneous fat but this does not apply to those patients with intraductal carcinomas because of the high incidence of centrally located tumours. Consideration should be given to immediate or delayed insertion of a prosthesis. Following operation, regular clinical examinations are essential, with mammography once a year, since some mammary lobular tissue is almost invariably left behind and could be the site of a second carcinoma.

REFERENCES

Anderson, D. E. (1973). A high-risk group for breast cancer. *Cancer Bulletin 25,* 23.

Arseneau, I. C., Sponzo, R. W., Levin, D. L., Schnipper, L. E., Bonner, H., Young, R. C., Canellos, G. P., Johnson, R. E. and DeVita, V. T. (1972). Nonlymphomatous malignant tumors complicating Hodgkin's disease. *N. Engl. J. Med. 287,* 1119.

Bloodgood, J. C. (1921). The remaining breast after radical removal of the opposite side for carcinoma. *J. Southern Surg. Ass. 34,* 223.

Buhl-Jorgensen, S. E., Fischermann, K., Johansen, H. and Petersen, B. (1968). Cancer risk in intraductal papilloma and papillomatosis. *Surg. Gynec. and Obstet 127,* 1307.

Burn, J. I. (1971). Diagnostic methods in breast cancer. *Proc. Royal Society of Med. 64,* 254.

Cheatle, G. L. and Cutler, M. (1931). *Tumours of the breast.* London: Edward Arnold and Co.

Clark, R. M. (1973). An approach to the detection and management of early breast cancer. *Canad. Med. Assoc. J. 108,* 599.

Fenig, J., Arlen, M., Livingston, S. F. and Levowitz, B. S. (1975). The potential for carcinoma existing synchronously on a microscopic level within the second breast. *Surg. Gynec. and Obstet. 141,* 394.

Fisher, E. R., Gregorio, R., Redmond, C., Vellios, F., Sommers, S. C. and Fisher, B. (1975). Pathologic findings from the national surgical adjuvant breast project (Protocol No. 4) I. Observations concerning the multicentricity of mammary cancer. *Cancer 35,* 247.

Foote, F. W. and Stewart, F. W. (1945). Comparative studies of cancerous versus noncancerous breasts. *Ann. Surg. 121,* 197.

Gallager, H. S. and Martin, J. E. (1969). The study of mammary carcinoma by mammography and whole organ sectioning. Early observations. *Cancer 23,* 855.

Haagensen, C. D. (1971). *Diseases of the Breast,* p. 170. W. B. Saunders Company, Philadelphia, Pa.

Hoffer, P. B., Lathrop, K., Bekerman, C., Fang, V. S. and Refetoff, S. (1973). Use of ^{131}I-CEA antibody as a tumour scanning agent. *J. Nuclear Med. 15,* 323.

Leis, H. P. (1971). Selective, elective, prophylactic contralateral mastectomy. *Cancer 28,* 956.

MacKenzie, I. (1965). Breast cancer following multiple fluoroscopies. *Brit. J. Cancer 19,* 1.

McCredie, J. A., Inch, W. R. and Alderson, M. (1975a). Consecutive primary carcinomas of the breast. *Cancer 35,* 1472.

McCredie, J. A., Inch, W. R. and Alderson, M. (1975b). Effect of local radiotherapy on consecutive primary cancers in patients with carcinoma of the breast. In *Multiple Primary Malignant Tumours.* Proc. Vth Perugia Quadrennial International Conference on Cancer, Perugia.

McDivitt, R. W., Stewart, F. W. and Berg, J. W. (1968). *Tumours of the Breast.* Armed Forces Institute of Pathology, Washington, D. C.

Moertel, C. G. (1966). Multiple primary malignant neoplasms: Their incidence and significance. In *Recent Results in Cancer Research,* p. 82. Springer-Verlag, New York.

Morgenstern, L., Kaufman, P. A. and Friedman, N. B. (1975). The case against tylectomy for carcinoma of the breast. *Amer. J. Surg. 130,* 251.

Newman, W. (1966). Lobular carcinoma of the female breast. Report of 73 cases. *Ann. Surg. 164,* 305.

Pack, G. T. (1951). Argument for bilateral mastectomy. *Surg. 29,* 929.

Penn, I. and Starzl, T. E. (1973). Immunosuppression and cancer transplant. *Proc. 5,* 943.

Qualheim, R. E. and Gall, E. A. (1957). Breast carcinoma with multiple sites of origin. *Cancer 10,* 460.

Robbins, G. F. and Berg, J. W. (1964). Bilateral primary breast cancers. A prospective clinicopathological study. *Cancer 17,* 1501.

Rosenberg, S. A. and Kaplan, H. S. (1975). The management of stages I, II and III Hodgkin's disease with combined radiotherapy and chemotherapy. *Cancer 35,* 55.

Ryan, J. A. and Coady, C. J. (1962). Intraductal epithelial proliferation in the human breast—A comparative study. *Canad. J. Surg. 5,* 12.

Stjernsward, J. (1974). Decreased survival related to irradiation postoperatively in early operable breast cancer. *Lancet 11,* 1285.

Sutherland, R. M., McCredie, J. A. and Inch, W. R. (1975). Effect of splenectomy and radiotherapy on lymphocytes in Hodgkin's disease. *Clin. Oncol. 1,* 275.

Urban, J. A. (1969). Bilaterality of breast cancer—Biopsy of the other breast. *Cancer 24,* 1310.

Warren, S. (1940). The relation of "chronic mastitis" to carcinoma of the breast. *Surg. Gynec. and Obstet. 71,* 257.

Watson, T. A. (1966). Cancer of the breast; The Janeway Lecture—1965. *Amer. J. Roentgenol. 96,* 547.

Westbrook, K. C. and Gallager, H. S. (1975). Intraductal carcinoma of the breast—A comparative study. *Amer. J. Surg. 130,* 667.

Wilson, N. D. and Alberty, R. E. (1973). Bilateral carcinoma of the breast. *Amer. J. Surg. 126,* 244.

Chapter

21 G. KEITH STILLWELL

Management of Arm Edema

A review of the literature on postmastectomy edema (Stillwell, 1959, 1969) revealed that several syndromes were being discussed. One was an acute transient edema occurring immediately after surgery. The second was an acute painful edema beginning 3 to 4 weeks postoperatively, and for which such a diversity of successful treatments was reported (corticosteroids, phenylbutazone, antibiotics and sympathetic block), that it seemed likely to be a self-limited disorder. Leis et al. (1966) listed as another type the edema that accompanies and persists after an attack of lymphangitis, naming it "erysipeloid edema".

The syndrome with which we are principally concerned is a persistent and usually painless edema that may develop weeks, months or years after the operation. Pain is not usually a problem, other than discomfort at the shoulder, which seems associated with the heaviness of the more severe swollen arms.

In severe cases puncture wounds may drain lymph for several hours or even days. Limitation of motion of the elbow and the digits may result from the swelling. Episodes of cellulitis or lymphangitis may complicate the more severe lymphedemas. Resembling erysipelas, the more severe attacks are associated with chills and fever, prostrating malaise, vomiting, and a blotchy erythema in the limb. The patient may be disabled and bedridden for 3 or 4 days with such an event, and they may occur at intervals of a few months to several years.

MEASUREMENT AND INCIDENCE

Many reports on the incidence of postmastectomy lymphedema have been based on measurement of the circumference of the upper limbs at various points. However, measurements can be affected considerably by the softness of the limb, the regularity of its contour, and the snugness with which the measuring tape is applied to the skin. Because edema is by definition an excess amount of interstitial fluid, it is more appropriate to measure the volume of the arm rather than the circumference. This is done relatively easily by determination of the volume of water displaced when the limb is immersed.

Volume measurements must be supplemented by

Table 1. Patients with postmastectomy lymphedema classified according to criteria of Tracy et al. (1961).

Severity of edema		*No.**		*No.†*	
Insignificant	(<150 ml)	56	53%	17	3%
Slight	(150-400 ml)	20	19%	104	16%
Moderate	(400-750 ml)	17	16%	188	30%
Severe	(>750 ml)	13	12%	319	51%
Total		106		628	

* Data from Tracy et al., 1961.
† Data from Tinkham and Stillwell, 1965.

visual observation, determination of the presence of pitting, and circumference measurements in deciding if the patient has edema (Tinkham and Stillwell, 1965). The latter observations will sometimes give an indication that the fluid is distributed differently, even though the volume has not changed (Wakim et al., 1955; Stillwell et al., 1957).

The volume of water displaced can be determined either by measuring the volume of water that spills from a filled container when the limb is immersed, or by measuring the change in water level when the limb is immersed. Kettle et al. (1958) found that in normal women the mean difference in the volumes of the upper extremities was 51 ml, with a standard deviation of 71 ml. Engler and Sweat (1962) reported a mean difference of 41 ml, with a standard deviation of 54 ml.

Tracey et al. (1961), defining edema of the upper limb as a difference of volume of 150 ml or more, found that 47% of 106 consecutive patients with radical mastectomy had edema (Table 1). Using different criteria, Healey (1971) reported that the incidence of lymphedema by volume measurements was 39.9%, and Leclaire and Dupuis (1972) reported it to be 28.5%. After radical mastectomy the average incidence is probably between 40 and 45%, while it is about 5% for patients treated by simple mastectomy and radiotherapy (Tough, 1968).

Classification of the severity of the edema has been based either on its absolute magnitude or on the volume of the edema relative to the volume of the contralateral limb. In Figure 1 a comparison is given of the classification of edema in 67 patients, by absolute volume (Tracy et al., 1961) and as a percentage of the normal limb (Stillwell, 1969). The geometric division of the ordinate gives a classification that more closely reflects the amount of trouble the patients have with the edema.

MECHANISM OF PRODUCTION OF POST-MASTECTOMY LYMPHEDEMA

There has been considerable controversy about the relative roles of lymphatic and venous obstruction, as

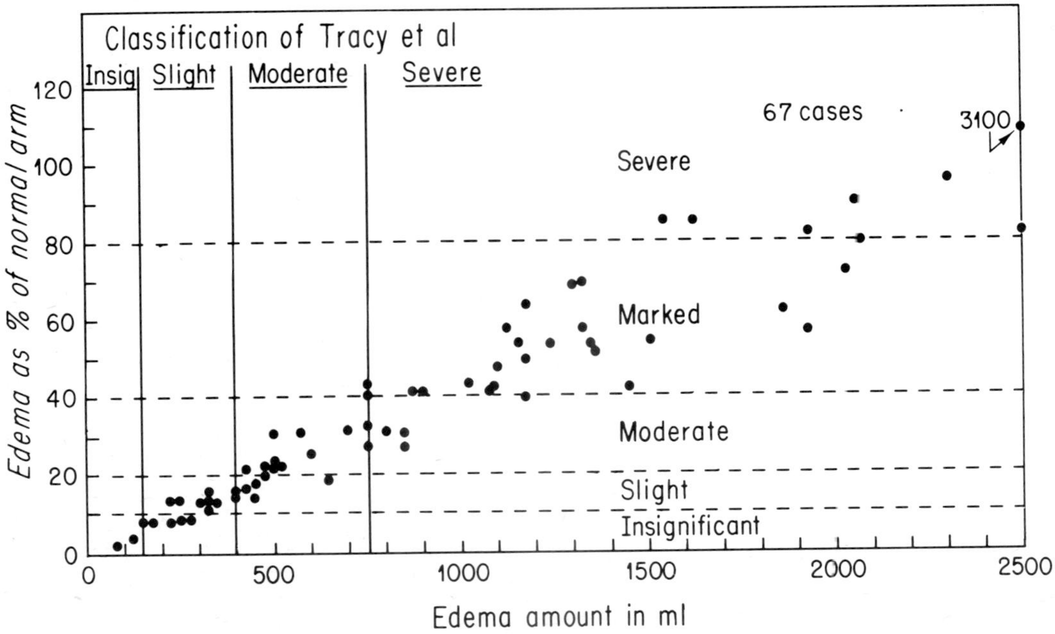

Figure 1. Distribution of volume of edema in 67 patients seen in 1967. Vertical lines subdivide the distribution according to the classification of Tracy et al. (1961). Horizontal lines subdivide it according to the classification proposed by Stillwell(1969).

well as those of other factors, in the causation of postmastectomy lymphedema. The current consensus is that the problem is primarily one of lymphatic insufficiency, which may be aggravated secondarily by factors such as obesity or venous obstruction.

Lymphatic Obstruction

The lymphatic system can be considered as a sump pump that keeps the interstitial system dry of free water by removing proteins and some water in the normal situation, and maintaining a subatmospheric pressure in the interstitial fluid. The work of Taylor et al. is cited by Guyton et al. (1971), showing that as the interstitial fluid pressure increases from −6 to 0 mm Hg, the lymph flow increases 12 to 50 fold. However, as the interstitial fluid pressure increases further *above* atmospheric pressure, there is no further increase in the rate of flow because the increase in pressure both impedes and augments the lymph flow equally, even though more water is available.

As the edema increases, the edematous limb can slowly enlarge without being tense. Acute episodes that temporarily cause tense increase in the size of the limb may be followed by a persistent increase in the size of the limb after the tension has subsided.

Hollander et al. (1961) found that, with lymphatic obstruction, the clearance of ^{131}I-labeled human serum albumin (RIHSA) from a limb was slowed. Ju et al. (1954) also found the rate of clearance of RIHSA to be greatly slowed in lymphedema, as did Emmett et al. (1967) and Harvey (1969).

A major advance in the understanding of lymphatic disorders was the development by Kinmonth and Taylor (1954) of practical lymphangiography. The lymphangiographic characteristics of obstructive lymphopathies include varicosities, delayed emptying, retrograde flow and dermal backflow, discontinuity of the lymph node chain, occasional hypertrophy of other lymph nodes and, infrequently, collateral vessels. Burn (1968) reported that it is the dermal backflow which correlates best with lymphedema, and that some of the other changes may be associated with little swelling of the limb.

Danese et al. (1962) in experiments on dogs, found that transected lymphatic vessels regenerate, regaining continuity and function in about 1 month, but that resected vessels do not. In the latter instance, collateral vessels take over the function but may later enlarger and more tortuous; they tend to develop valvular incompetence or occlusions due to infection, with ensuing edema. They noted that infection may lead to edema as a complication of the mere transection of lymphatic vessels.

Danese and Howard (1965) reported that, in the human upper extremity, three groups of antebrachial lymphatic pathways parallel respectively the radial, median, and ulnar veins. In postmastectomy patients without edema, they found one or two channels which bypassed the axilla, generally along the cephalic vein. The forearm lymphatic vessels were normal apart from some superficial abnormality at the elbow and the distal two-thirds of the arm. However in eight patients with edema, there was marked dilatation of the lymphatic vessels of the forearm and arm which involved the subdermic and occasionally the intradermic plexus. Dermal backflow and reflux were present.

Venous Obstruction

The role of venous obstruction in postmastectomy lymphedema is apparently an infrequent one. Danese et al. (1968a) reported on the production of chronic postsurgical lymphedema in dogs, with no change in the normal phlebograms. Haagensen (1971) cited the work of Kister et al. showing that either the cephalic or the axillary vein can provide adequate venous drainage from the arm. Mustard and Murillo (1961) reported that the preservation of the areolar tissue around the axillary vein lowered the incidence of postmastectomy lymphedema from 53 to 4% and the presumption was that the perivenous lymphatic vessels remained intact and were responsible for this improvement.

However, venous obstruction may play some part in the development of edema. Phlebograms on 35 normal women and 14 with radical mastectomy were compared by Larson and Crampton (1973). In the normal women, when the shoulder was abducted, the axillary vein was normal in all, but when the shoulder was adducted, the vein was normal in only 23%, being obstructed in 34% and narrowed in 43%. In the postmastectomy patients, with the shoulder abducted, the axillary vein was obstructed in 8%, narrowed in 23%, and normal only in 69%; with the shoulder adducted, the vein was obstructed in 50% and narrowed in 21%. In eight lymphedematous patients, they decompressed the axillary and subclavian veins, with much improvement in five.

Hughes and Patel (1966) found the axillary vein ensheathed in scar tissue from which they liberated it, with good results in 12 of 19 patients. Arnulf (1973) found a similar situation in seven patients with severe edema, and Lipshutz (1969) noted good results up to 5 years in four patients. On the other hand, Feijoo

Osorio (1969) noted venous obstruction in only one patient, Conte et al. (1968) in very few of their 29 patients, and Timossi (1969) noted it only in those with severe edema.

Radiation Therapy

Radiation may damage small blood vessels and lymphatic vessels directly and by cicatrization (Tough, 1968; Hirshowitz et al., 1969; Peters, 1970). It is common for the patient to first become aware of lymphedema a few weeks after the completion of postoperative radiation therapy.

Metastasis

Treves (1957) found that metastatic involvement of the axillary lymph nodes at surgery was not related to the incidence or severity of the edema. However, the late onset of edema may signal the development of metastatic involvement in the axilla or supraclavicular area with lymphatic or venous obstruction.

It would appear then that postmastectomy lymphedema is primarily and usually due to lymphatic obstruction and insufficiency. In very severe lymphedema, there also may be obstruction of the axillary vein, usually due to scar formation around the vein, which in turn may relate to the surgical procedure, wound infection, or fibrosis secondary to radiation therapy.

Generally, however, the likelihood of lymphedema developing after radical mastectomy depends on the original endowment with lymphatic vessels, particularly those that bypass the axilla. This should be explained to the patient lest she compare herself with her friends who have had a radical mastectomy and have not developed lymphedema, and then attributes her plight to some defect in her operation.

OTHER FACTORS AND PROPHYLAXIS

Infection

Wound infection when acting alone during the postoperative period was not incriminated by Treves (1957), but it was found to augment the severity and incidence of edema in conjunction with other factors such as obesity. In addition to frank cellulitis or "lymphangitis", many believe that lesser degrees of infection precipitate or aggravate the edema (Britton and Nelson, 1962; Tough, 1968; Haagensen, 1971; Leclaire and Dupuis, 1972; Zeissler et al., 1972; Byrd, 1973; Larson and Crampton, 1973; Robbins and Markel, 1973). All agree on the need for avoiding infection of the lymphedematous limb through any sort of puncture wound lest more lymphatic vessels become occluded (Robbins and Markel, 1973). There is less support for the postulate that every patient is already infected, perhaps subclinically, and should be treated with antibiotics.

Trauma

Trauma to the arm on the same side as the radical mastectomy may often precipitate or aggravate the lymphedema. Open wounds may do this by the admission of infection, but closed injuries such as fractures or severe sprains or bruises also may upset the delicate balance. As stated by Treves (1957):

> "It is well to remember that the onset of swelling in patients previously free from this complication may be initiated by any minor infection or trauma. Friction from clothing, trauma to the arm, a scratch or a mosquito bite, sunburn or a minor thermal injury, paronychia or ringworm of the nail, a cut at the time of manicure, any of these may induce lymphedema, which often persists. The circulatory balance is so fine that seemingly trivial incidents may produce this distressing complication and, once produced, the process is rarely reversible."

Robbins and Markel (1973) listed some things that the patient should do to avoid precipitation or aggravation of lymphedema. These included avoidance of cutting cuticles during care of the nails; protection with garden gloves, kitchen gloves, oven mitts, and thimbles; shaving the arm with an electric razor, if at all; avoidance of sunburn and of cigarette burns; avoidance of venipuncture and other needle punctures; avoidance of blood pressure measurement on that limb; and avoidance of heavy lifting and of constricting garments and jewelry. Foley (1968) has cautioned about the constricting action of brassiere straps.

Obesity

This has been incriminated as an etiologic factor (Treves, 1957; Hughes and Patel, 1966; Haagensen, 1971). The skin of an arm already large because of obesity may be less able to resist further enlargement than would that of a small arm because of the physical relationship expressed in the law of Laplace (see p. 219). Haagensen (1971) commented on the difficulty in avoiding infection in the obese patient.

Excessive Limb Use

Excessive use of the limb can precipitate or aggravate the edema (Stillwell, 1969; Zeissler et al., 1972). The work need not be heavy and the duration of the work may be the key factor. If an elastic support is worn during the work and for an hour or so afterward, the patient may be able to perform more work with impunity. Patients are often encouraged to try to use the arm "normally" or "as much as possible," with the result that they may use it too much. They should be encouraged to change a task after 20 or 30 minutes to one that will rest the arm awhile. Sports activities that use the arm more or less continuously, such as tennis, may be less well tolerated than those in which the use of the arm is periodic, such as golf.

Local Application of Heat

Application of heat has as one of its principal side effects the tendency to edema formation (Stillwell, 1971). Heat should be avoided in patients with postmastectomy lymphedema unless it is strongly indicated for the management of other problems such as cellulitis or pain. Damage to the cutaneous circulation by prior radiation therapy decreases the tolerance to local heating and is an additional contraindication to its use (Stillwell, 1969).

Generalized Heating

Immersion in hot tub baths or whirlpool baths or exposure to hot weather can cause vasodilatation in the extremities, which tends to generate edema. Patients with mastectomy should avoid prolonged hot baths and should be less active in hot weather (Stillwell, 1969).

TREATMENT

Physical Measures

Treatment used at the Mayo Clinic consists of procedures to promote the removal of fluid from the limb and measures to impede the accumulation of new fluid in it. In essence, the former consists of elevation, massage, and exercise to activate the "muscular pump," and the latter consists of external elastic support. Treatments are usually given twice daily for a period of 3 or 4 days, and the patient then continues on a program of home treatment. Patients who have insignificant or slight edema may merely be followed, and the treatment withheld until and if the edema becomes worse. Periodic measurements of the volume and circumference of the limb help to assess the progress and elicit the cooperation of the patient.

The treatment plan is explained in some detail to the patient, along with a discussion about the results that can be expected. The long-term nature of the program is stressed. The patient then decides whether to undertake the program and when she wants to start.

Elevation. The arm is elevated with the help of the supporting device (Figure 2) during the massage and exercise parts of the treatment, which last 60 to 90 minutes. The arm should be elevated comfortably with the shoulder abducted about 20° to 45° from the side and the limb subtending an angle of about 45° to 60° from the horizontal. The hand should be higher than the elbow and the elbow higher than the shoulder. Elevation so that the limb is vertical may be difficult or uncomfortable, unless supported by a device such as that of Foley (1958). Elevation of the limb with the arm alongside the head may be self-defeating as some patients who try this at night awaken with more rather than less swelling, presumably due to some obstruction at the costoclavicular space.

In the home program, the patient is encouraged to elevate the limb for as much of the time at night as she can, and still get adequate sleep. During the day, periodic elevation for half an hour or longer is encouraged, as is resting the limb in the horizontal position when convenient. Repeated volume measurements on a series of patients (Stillwell, 1969) showed that the greatest reduction in edema usually occurred overnight with prolonged elevation rather than with other components of the treatment program. We believe that periods of elevation as short as 10 minutes are of little value.

Massage. Massage may be administered by pneumatically operated compression devices or by hand, and we generally use both. After 1 hour with the pneumatic device, some areas in the arm may be more firm than others, and it is to these areas that the physical therapist directs most attention during the 10-minute period of manual massage. The latter is a gentle kneading and friction type of massage rather than light stroking.

During the past 25 years, we have used three different types of pneumatic pumping devices. A study by Tinkham and Stillwell (1965) compared the relative efficacy of these devices with each other, and with a 45-minute period of elevation alone instead of the 60-minute period of elevation with the device. The results during the initial 3 or 4 days of treatment were slightly better with the pumping devices in that about half of the patients so treated obtained a

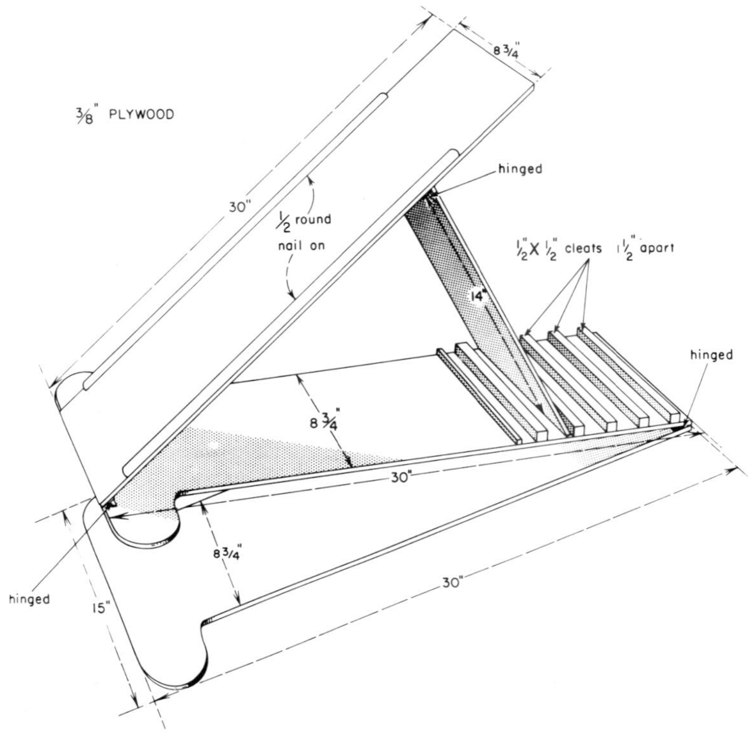

Figure 2. Arm support board. Lowermost board can be swung down to act as a leg, supporting the right-hand end of the board. Degree of elevation of the arm is easily varied. (From Stillwell (1962) by permission of W. B. Saunders Company.)

reduction of 30% or more of their edema, while only one-third of those treated without a device accomplished this. Successful treatment of the problem is, therefore, not dependent on the use of the pneumatic pumping devices, but they are of some value. They also motivate patients to have enough treatment sessions in the beginning to learn how to carry out the home program properly.

Exercise. A relatively small amount of active exercise of the muscles of the forearm and arm is used to activate the muscular pump in the hope that this may increase lymphatic and venous emptying. Exercise is best done with minimal motion of the extremity so that the patient can do it unobtrusively whenever she wishes. Five to 10 repetitions performed every 5 minutes or so will suffice. The exercise may be more effective if done with elastic support on, rather than off. Excessive repetition of the exercise may lead to a sufficient increase of blood flow into the limb to increase edema formation. In my experience, the remainder of the program is not of much help in patients who have a flaccid paralysis of the lymphedematous limb and therefore are unable to carry out any exercise.

The type of exercise to regain or retain the range of motion of the shoulder is different from that employed for the muscular pumping activity. The vast majority of our patients regain shoulder motion fairly early in the postoperative period under the guidance of the surgeons and the nurses, and do not require the services of the physical therapist for this.

External Elastic Support. Except for patients with minimal lymphedema, adequate external elastic support is the sine qua non of the entire program. The accumulation of new water and protein in the interstitial space must be prevented. During the initial 6 to 8 weeks of our program, we prefer the use of double-length elasticized bandages (3-inch width). As the size of the limb decreases in the early period, the elastic support will continue to conform to it. After the limb has stabilized at a smaller size, the improvement is more easily maintained with an elasticized sleeve.

Initially, the bandage is applied from the level of the metacarpophalangeal joints up to about the level of the insertion of the deltoid muscle. A simple spiral technique, even if the bandage stays in place poorly around the elbow, seems preferable to the figure-of-

eight technique at the elbow. The latter method may result in a tightened up bandage at the elbow with movement and lead to increased swelling of the forearm and hand. Patients with more marked edema may develop deep creases under the bandage at the wrist or occasionally on the flexor aspect of the elbow. These creases may be prevented or corrected by the use of thin felt cuffs under the bandage until the edema is adequately relieved and the crease formation ceases. Frequently, after about 4 weeks of the program, if the edema of the hand has disappeared, the hand can be excluded from the bandage without recurrence of swelling there.

The patient is taught to apply the bandage by herself. This is difficult but not impossible. Because the bandage must be removed and reapplied about every 2 hours during the day and the patient is the only person who will invariably be available to perform the task, she must be able to do it well. If the bandage is not reapplied frequently the limb becomes ridged and lumpy and uncomfortable. With frequent changes, the limb becomes smoother since the bandage is never reapplied identically on consecutive wrappings. Elastic support is not worn at night, and its use is optional when the limb is elevated during the day.

Elasticized sleeves are easier to put on, and they stay in place properly at the elbow. They maintain the limb at a specific size, although when first put into use they also may help to further reduce the edema, particularly around the elbow. Foley (1954) described a method of manufacture of a sleeve. Various commercial sleeves are available. We have made use of supports fabricated by the Jobst Institute of Toledo, OH (Brush et al., 1959).

After the lymphedema has been held at its minimal size for about 3 months and the interstitial space and skin have regained some of their elasticity, the patient is encouraged to leave the elastic support off for progressively longer periods at the end of each day. In this way, she can ascertain how long she can be without the elastic support and still not have noticeable recurrence of the swelling. Since the basic cause for the lymphedema is still present, the elastic support usually cannot be abandoned permanently. The patient must decide whether to accept a recurrence of the lymphedema or permanent part-time use of the support. Most decide in favor of the latter. It is believed to be more important to wear the sleeve while using the arm and for an hour or so afterwards.

An important consideration in the use of elastic support is the relationship between limb radius (R), the circumferential tension (T) in the support, and the transmural pressure (P) engendered by the support. This is expressed in the law of Laplace (Stillwell, 1973) which is that $P = T/R$. To exert any given amount of transmural pressure, the tension must be greater if the radius is greater. In effect, the greater the size of the limb, the less effective will be the external elastic support.

This treatment results in the patients losing an average of about one-third of their edema during the initial 3 to 5 days of treatment in the department (Figure 3) (Stillwell et al., 1957; Stillwell and Redford, 1958; Stillwell, 1959, 1962, 1969; Tinkham and Stillwell, 1965). About an additional one-third of the edema may be lost during the first 4 to 6 weeks of the home program prior to fitting of the sleeve, but we do not have accurate data on this. Nor do we have accurate long-term data on later events such as continued use of the elastic support in the control of the edema.

Wilhelm et al. (1974) reported on a similar method of treatment but without the use of elastic support until the end of the 4th week. Of 17 patients followed, three-fourths initially had moderate or marked edema (as measured volumetrically) but only one-third had such edema 3 months later. Leclaire and Dupuis (1972) compared results in 12 patients treated by pneumatic pumping with results in 14 patients treated by a wrapping technique using cord 1 cm in diameter (ficelage). The pneumatic pumping group averaged a reduction of 29% in edema (or 8 ml per treatment). Those with the "ficelage" averaged a reduction of 12% (or about 6 ml per treatment). Another report from Canada (Godfrey, 1969) on the use of elevation, pneumatic pumping, exercise, and bandaging in a group of 242 patients noted that 65% lost some of the swelling and 34% lost half of it.

Brush and Wylie (1964) reported on the use of pneumatic pumping for 5 to 10 days, followed by fitting with a sleeve, and noted good results in 138 of 166 patients during a 10-year period. A similar approach has been reported from the Cleveland Clinic (Nelson, 1966; Zeissler et al., 1972); there, all patients with postmastectomy lymphedema are treated for 1 week on oral antibiotic medication, then treated for 6 hours with a pneumatic pump, and then measured for a sleeve. After 2 to 3 months, the patient is treated again with the pump for 3 hours and then measured for a new sleeve. Figure 4 shows changes occurring with repeated sleeve measurements. Zeissler et al. (1972) had follow-up data ranging from 1 to 12 years on 339 patients and found that 184 had been helped by the program. Having been alerted to the hazards of infection, 41% took better care of their arms. Of 183 who were still alive, 96 used the sleeve daily and 25 used it occasionally.

Foley (1968) emphasized that the major or sole

lymphatic drainage from the upper limb after radical mastectomy is over the top of the shoulder and that this pathway is often occluded by the pressure of a brassiere strap. In addition to causing or aggravating lymphedema, the pressure of the strap also may be responsible for causing costoclavicular compression, occasional occlusion of the subclavian vein or stenosis of the subclavian artery, and at times brachial plexopathy.

Surgical Measures

Obstruction to the flow in the axillary vein may be a contributing factor in severe lymphedema, particularly if the cephalic vein is not fully patent, and decompression of the axillary vein may therefore be helpful. Various attempts have been made to restore lymph flow but the only operation to stand the test of time is the buried skin flap procedure of Thompson (1962, 1970) described fully in Chapter 11.

If the dermal lymphatic plexus has been destroyed by infection or severe fibrosis, the procedure is less likely to be beneficial. It is also more difficult to do in grossly obese patients. The usual indications are frequent attacks of cellulitis which cannot be prevented by prophylactic antibiotic medication, or occasionally the excessive weight of the limb. It is not done primarily for cosmetic purposes. Thompson classified his results as "good" when the swelling was reduced by 75% or more and the main complaint was completely relieved and normal function restored; "satisfactory" when the swelling was reduced appreciably, the main complaint was alleviated, and function was improved, with complete arrest of progress of the disease; and "bad" when there was no improvement.

In 1970, Thompson reported his results in 23 cases of operation on upper extremities, with the primary complaint being recurrent severe cellulitis in 5 and excessive weight in 18. In five of the latter group, there had been associated minor attacks of cellulitis. Of the 23 patients with upper extremity lymphedema, 2 had had radiotherapy alone, 17 patients had had radical mastectomy and radiotherapy, and 4 had had radical mastectomy only. Two patients had satisfactory results after the first stage of the procedure, and two had metastatic cancer that became apparent before the second stage could be carried out; the other 19 patients had the two-stage procedure.

In patients followed up 5 to 8 years, the results were "good" in three and "satisfactory" in one. In those followed 3 to 5 years, the results were "good"

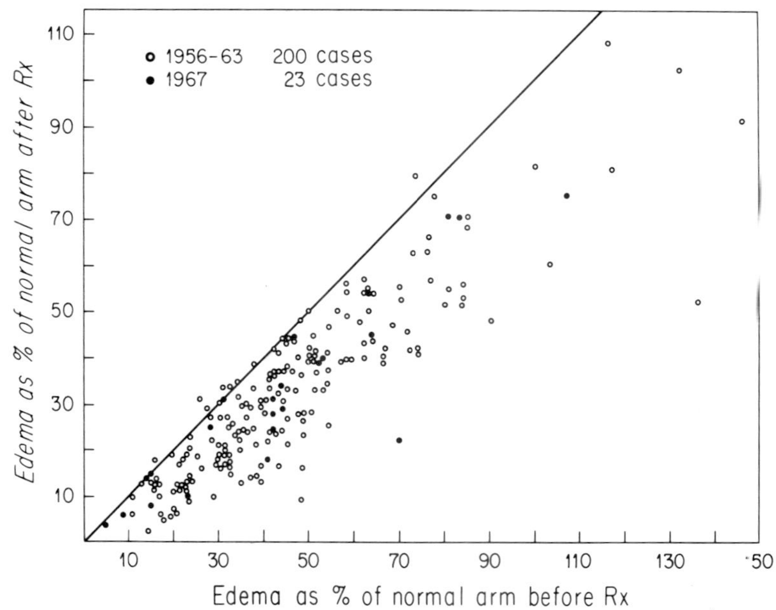

Figure 3. Scatter diagram showing results of initial series of treatments in the Department of Physical Medicine and Rehabilitation at the Mayo Clinic. Open circles represent 200 patients reported by Tinkham and Stillwell (1965); solid circles represent 23 patients treated in 1967; diagonal line indicates no change. Circles below the line represent patients with reduction in the volume of the edematous limb; circles above the line represent patients whose condition worsened.

in nine, "satisfactory" in one, and "bad" in one (the patient with a bad result had lymphedema secondary to radiation and an infective arthritis of the shoulder). Of patients followed 1 to 2 years, the results were "good" in two and "satisfactory" in six. Of the 10 patients with recurrent attacks of cellulitis, 8 had the attacks abolished and 2 had them alleviated. The use of the buried dermal flap has also been reported by Rigas et al. (1970) and Hugo (1971).

Danese et al. (1968b) expressed some pessimism about the efficacy of the buried dermal flap procedure, whereas Harvey (1969) reported an improved clearance of radioiodinated human serum albumin in all of the eight patients he studied. When the time required for clearance of one-half the injected dose was measured, the preoperative observations ranged from 9 to 200 hours, with a mean of 90 hours, while the postoperative range was 9 to 112 hours, with a mean of 50 hours. There was usually some irregularity in the rate of clearance during the first few hours, but the mean percentage that was cleared during the first 24 hours was 16.9 preoperatively (range 10 to 88) and 30.2 postoperatively (range 10 to 51).

Miscellaneous Methods

Cytotoxic Drugs. Nielsen (1967) administered cyclophosphamide intralymphatically into three patients who had metastatic involvement of the axillary glands and noted a reduction in pain and swelling and an increase in mobility in all three. Kitchen and Garrett (1971) tried the same procedure for four patients with metastases in axillary or supraclavicular nodes. Two had good relief of symptoms and measurable reduction of the edema, one had a little reduction of the edema, while the fourth felt better, with a softer limb but no change in the circumference.

Enzymes. Schwartz (1955) reported on the use of hyaluronidase by iontophoresis in one case of postmastectomy lymphedema. With a treatment of 20 to 30 minutes, the volume of the arm decreased an average of almost 230 ml, the greatest amount being 510 ml. Mufson et al. (1956) used subcutaneous injection of hyaluronidase not directly into the edematous area and believed that it was more helpful when the edema was due to venous obstruction than to other causes. However, Foley (1955) found that such subcutaneous injection was not helpful in reducing the edema.

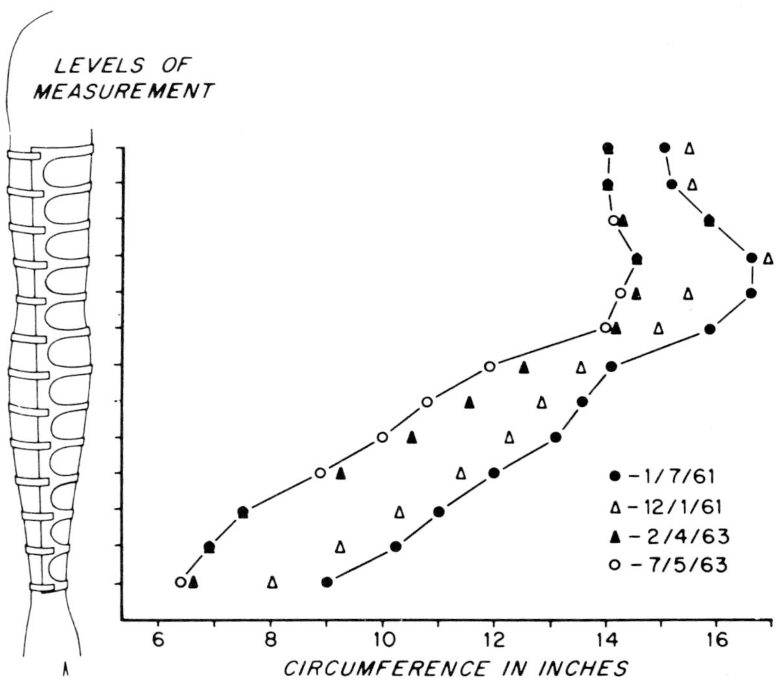

Figure 4. Series of circumferential measurements of lymphedematous arm showing progressive decrease in size with treatment program from 1-7-61 (solid circles) to 7-5-63 (open circles). (From Zeissler et al. (1972), by permission of American Congress of Rehabilitation Medicine.)

Gros and Haehnel (1974) reported on the prophylactic use of oral amylase in 25 patients and its therapeutic use (with associated physical therapy) in 45 patients with post-mastectomy lymphedema and in 8 with lymphedema after irradiation. An analgesic effect was noted in all patients in the therapeutic group and the authors believed that the enzyme helped reduce the edema. The prophylactic group included 20 patients who underwent mastectomy and 5 who had radiation therapy. Only four developed edema, and three of the four had not had a mastectomy.

Antibiotic Therapy. The general medical management of lymphedema at our institution has been outlined by Schirger (1962) and includes antibiotics if necessary. We do not routinely treat patients with antibiotics unless there appears to be infection or inflammation, since the nonspecific use of antibiotics may eventually promote the development of resistant organisms. However, patients with recurrent attacks of lymphangitis may be controlled with prophylactic antibiotic therapy (Babb et al., 1966). Others report a more frequent use of antibiotic therapy, sometimes noting that the edema may improve considerably with this treatment alone or with minimal concurrent treatment (Nelson, 1966; Haagensen, 1971; Leclaire and Dupuis, 1972; Zeissler et al., 1972; Byrd, 1973; Wilhelm et al., 1974; Golematis et al., 1975).

Diuretic Therapy. Facilitation of removal of water from the blood by diuretic medications should theoretically promote the transudation of water from the interstitial space into the blood. Many include this as part of their program for postmastectomy lymphedema in some patients (Schirger, 1962; Nelson, 1966; Haagensen, 1971; Zeissler et al., 1972). We do not use diuretics routinely or even frequently. Diuresis presumably will not influence the removal of protein from the interstitial space, and this removal must be considered to be as important as the removal of water. However, in the presence of cardiac failure, diuretics may be indicated in some patients with massive edema of the upper extremity or more particularly, the lower extremity.

COMPLICATIONS

The most frequent complication of postmastectomy lymphedema is infection of the stagnant lymph, variously referred to as lymphangitis or cellulitis. Usually preceded by a puncture wound or similar penetrating injury, the onset is abrupt, with the development of blotchy areas of inflammation in the subcutaneous tissues and skin. It is associated with chills and fever and malaise and an increase in the tension of the edema. Since additional lymphatic channels may be closed off by such episodes, the edema may be permanently worse afterward.

Generally, the incidence of such attacks is less if the volume of the edema is less, but there are few precise data to support this. When it is not otherwise controllable, the use of periodic antibiotic therapy may prevent the recurrent attacks (Babb et al., 1966).

A less frequent but usually fatal late complication of postmastectomy lymphedema is lymphangiosarcoma, described more fully in Chapter 11. Gruffaz (1971) described 26 patients who had post-radiation brachial plexopathy associated with the presence of painful inflammatory edema.

REFERENCES

Arnulf, G. (1973). Lymphoedema of the upper limb after Halsted's operation of radical mastectomy: lymphography and phlebography therapeutic consequences. *Vascular Surgery 7,* 36.

Babb, R. R., Spittell, J. A., Jr., Martin, W. J. and Schirger, A. (1966). Prophylaxis of recurrent lymphangitis complicating lymphedema. *Journal of the American Medical Association 195,* 871.

Britton, R. C. and Nelson, P. A. (1962). Causes and treatment of postmastectomy lymphedema of the arm: report of 114 cases. *Journal of the American Medical Association 180,* 95.

Brush, B. E. and Wylie, J. H., Jr. (1964). The management of the swollen arm following mastectomy. *Pacific Medicine and Surgery, 72,* 64.

Brush, B. E., Wylie, J. H., Jr. and Beninson, J. (1959). Some devices for the management of lymphedema of the extremities. *Surgical Clinics of North America 39,* 1493.

Burn, J. I. (1968). Obstructive lymphopathy. *Annals of the Royal College of Surgeons of England 42,* 93.

Byrd, B. F., Jr. (1973). Rehabilitation of the patient with breast cancer. *Proceedings of the National Cancer Conference 7,* 309.

Conte, G., Bevilaqua, L., Vangelista, R., Grigoletto, E. and Pizzi, G. (1968). Studio radiologico delle alterazioni del deflusso linfo-venoso nell'edema post-chirurgico dell'arto superiore. *Acta Chirurgica Italica* (Supplement), *24,* 571.

Danese, C. and Howard, J. M. (1965). Postmastectomy lymphedema. *Surgery, Gynecology and Obstetrics 120,* 797.

Danese, C., Howard, J. M. and Bower, R. (1962). Regeneration of lymphatic vessels: a radiographic study. *Annals of Surgery 156,* 61.

Danese, C. A., Georgalas-Bertakis, M. and Morales, L. E. (1968a). A model of chronic postsurgical lymphedema in dogs' limbs. *Surgery 64,* 814.

Danese, C. A., Papaioannou, A. N., Morales, L. E. and

Mitsuda, S. (1968b). Surgical approaches to lymphatic blocks. *Surgery 64,* 821.

Emmett, A. J. J., Barron, J. N. and Veall, N. (1967). The use of I^{131} albumin tissue clearance measurements and other physiological tests for the clinical assessment of patients with lymphoedema. *British Journal of Plastic Surgery 20,* 1.

Engler, H. S. and Sweat, R. D. (1962). Volumetric arm measurements: technique and results. *American Surgeon 28,* 465.

Feijoo Osorio, J. J. (1969). Linfedema gigante del brazo postmastectomia: relato de un caso de interés. *Angiologia 21,* 16.

Foley, W. T. (1954). An elastic sleeve for edema of the arm (letter to the editor). *New York State Journal of Medicine 54,* 1082.

Foley, W. T. (1955). The treatment of lymphedema. *Surgery, Gynecology and Obstetrics 101,* 25.

Foley, W. T. (1958). The treatment of lymphedema of the arms and legs. *GP 17,* 83.

Foley, W. T. (1968). "El sindrome del sostén": linfedema del brazo. *Angiologia 20,* 283.

Godfrey, C. M. (1969). Postmastectomy lymphedema. *Applied Therapeutics 11,* 440.

Golematis, B. C., Delikaris, P. G., Balarutsos, C. and Karamanakos, P. P. (1975). Lymphedema of the upper limb after surgery for breast cancer. *American Journal of Surgery 129,* 286.

Gros, M. and Haehnel, P. (1974). Intérêt de l'Oramyl-Salvoxyl-Wander dans les "gros bras" après mastectomie. *Therapeutique 50* 467.

Gruffaz, J. (1971). Le syndrome neurologique des "gros bras" après mammectomie et télécobaltothérapie pour cancer du sein. *Presse Medicale 79,* 755.

Guyton, A. C., Granger, H. J. and Taylor, A. E. (1971). Interstitial fluid pressure. *Physiological Reviews 51,* 527.

Haagensen, C. D. (1971). *Diseases of the Breast,* 2nd edition, p. 718, W. B. Saunders Company, Philadelphia.

Harvey, R. F. (1969). The use of ^{131}I labelled human serum albumin in the assessment of improved lymph flow following the buried dermis flap operation in cases of post-mastectomy lymphoedema of the arm. *British Journal of Radiology 42,* 260.

Healey, J. E., Jr. (1971). Role of rehabilitation medicine in the care of the patient with breast cancer. *Cancer 28,* 1666.

Hirshowitz, B., Mahler, D. and Goldan, S. (1969). Surgical treatment of chronic radiation injuries of axilla and shoulder. *Plastic and Reconstructive Surgery 44,* 261.

Hollander, W., Reilly, P. and Burrows, B. A. (1961). Lymphatic flow in human subjects as indicated by the disappearance of I^{131}-labeled albumin from the subcutaneous tissue. *Journal of Clinical Investigation 40,* 222.

Hughes, J. H. and Patel, A. R. (1966). Swelling of the arm following radical mastectomy. *British Journal of Surgery 53,* 4.

Hugo, N. E. (1971). Recent advances in the treatment of lymphedema. *Surgical Clinics of North America 51,* 111.

Ju, D. M. C., Blakemore, A. and Stevenson, T. W. (1954). A lymphatic function test. *Surgical Forum 5,* 607.

Kettle, J. H., Rundle, F. F. and Oddie, T. H. (1958). Measurement of upper limb volumes: a clinical method. *Australian and New Zealand Journal of Surgery 27,* 263.

Kinmonth, J. B. and Taylor, G. W. (1954). The lymphatic circulation in lymphedema. *Annals of Surgery 139,* 129.

Kitchen, G. and Garrett, M. J. (1971). A trial of intralymphatic cyclophosphamide in patients with arm lymphoedema due to metastatic breast carcinoma. *Clinical Radiology 22,* 379.

Larson, N. E. and Crampton, A. R. (1973). A surgical procedure for postmastectomy edema. *Archives of Surgery 106,* 475.

Leclaire, R. and Dupuis, M. (1972). Traitement physiatrique du lymphoedème post-mastectomie. *Union Medicale du Canada 101,* 2702.

Leis, H. P., Jr., Bowers, W. F. and Dursi, J. (1966). Post-mastectomy edema of arm. *New York State Journal of Medicine 66,* 618.

Lipshutz, H. (1969). Decompression, an adjunct to the treatment of lymphedema of the arm. *Panminerva Medica 11,* 205.

Mufson, I., Goldman, L., Radle, L. and Sheiman, M. (1956). Treatment of edema caused by chronic phlebothrombosis and other peripheral vascular diseases with hyaluronidase. *New York State Journal of Medicine 56,* 2093.

Mustard, R. L. and Murillo, C. (1961). Prevention of arm lymphedema following radical mastectomy. *Annals of Surgery* (Supplement), *154,* 282.

Nelson, P. A. (1966). Recent advances in treatment of lymphedema of the extremities. *Geriatrics 21,* 162.

Nielsen, R. (1967). Injection intra-lymphatique de cyclophosphamide: un cancer du sein avec gros bras. *Presse Medicale 75,* 2117.

Peters, M. V. (1970). Radiation therapy in the management of breast cancer. *Proceedings of the National Cancer Conference 6,* 163.

Rigas, A., Chrysanthakopoulos, S. and Tsardakas, E. (1970). Diagnostic and therapeutic applications of lymphangiography in clinical medicine. *American Journal of Surgery 120,* 66.

Robbins, G. F. and Markel, W. M. (1973). The postmastectomy lymphedematous arm. *Medical Annals of the District of Columbia 42,* 495.

Schirger, A. (1962). Postoperative lymphedema: etiologic and diagnostic factors. *Medical Clinics of North America 46,* 1045.

Schwartz, M. S. (1955). Use of hyaluronidase by iontophoresis in treatment of lymphedema. *Archives of Internal Medicine 95,* 662.

Stillwell, G. K. (1959). Physical medicine in management of patients with postmastectomy lymphedema. *Journal of the American Medical Association 171,* 2285.

Stillwell, G. K. (1962). The physiatric management of postoperative lymphedema. *Medical Clinics of North America 46,* 1051.

Stillwell, G. K. (1969). Treatment of postmastectomy lymphedema. *Modern Treatment 6,* 396.

Stillwell, G. K. (1971). *Handbook of Physical Medicine and Rehabilitation,* 2nd edition, p. 261, W. B. Saunders Company, Philadelphia.

Stillwell, G. K. (1973). The law of Laplace: some clinical applications. *Mayo Clinic Proceedings 48,* 863.

Stillwell, G. K. and Redford, J. W. B. (1958). Physical treatment of postmastectomy lymphedema. *Proceedings of the Staff Meetings of the Mayo Clinic 33,* 1.

Stillwell. G. K., Redford, J. W. B. and Krusen, F. H. (1957). Further studies on the treatment of lymphedema. *Archives of Physical Medicine and Rehabilitation 38,* 435.

Thompson, N. (1962). Surgical treatment of chronic lymphoedema of the lower limb: with preliminary report of new operation. *British Medical Journal 2,* 1566.

Thompson, N. (1970). Buried dermal flap operation for chronic lymphedema of the extremities: ten-year survey of results in 79 cases. *Plastic and Reconstructive Surgery 45,* 541.

Timossi, G. (1969). L'edema del braccio conseguente ad intervento di mastectomia radicale: quadri flebografici e considerazioni etio-patogenetiche. *Minerva Chirurgica 24,* 377.

Tinkham, R. G. and Stillwell, G. K. (1965). The role of pneumatic pumping devices in the treatment of post-mastectomy lymphedema. *Archives of Physical Medicine and Rehabilitation 46,* 193.

Tough, I. C. K. (1968). Oedema of the arm after simple mastectomy and radiotherapy for breast cancer. *Journal of the Royal College of Surgeons of Edinburgh 13,* 312.

Tracy, G. D., Reeve, T. S., FitzSimons, E. and Rundle, F. F. (1961). Observations on the swollen arm after radical mastectomy. *Australian and New Zealand Journal of Surgery 30,* 204.

Treves, N. (1957). An evaluation of the etiological factors of lymphedema following radical mastectomy: an analysis of 1,007 cases. *Cancer 10,* 444.

Wakim, K. G., Martin, G. M. and Krusen, F. H. (1955). Influence of centripetal rhythmic compression on localized edema of an extremity. *Archives of Physical Medicine and Rehabilitation 36,* 98.

Wilhelm, M. C., Saul, P. B. and Morgan, J. A. (1974). Post-mastectomy lymphedema. *Virginia Medical Monthly 101,* 465.

Zeissler, R. H., Rose, G. B. and Nelson, P. A. (1972). Post-mastectomy lymphedema: late results of treatment in 385 patients. *Archives of Physical Medicine and Rehabilitation 53,* 159.

Chapter

22

J. S. LYON

Management of Psychological Problems in Breast Cancer

The discovery of a lump in the breast carries for most women the implication of probable cancer and possible death. This usually occurs in an otherwise fit person and therefore its impact is correspondingly greater. Such a reaction is normal but it may have more serious implications requiring the help of the physician.

It is remarkable how little scientific investigation has been undertaken in this field. Most clinicians have their own ideas and experience but they show a very wide variety in awareness and acceptance of these reactions in patients. For this reason, I propose to discuss the basis and management of the psychological reactions to a diagnosis, or feared diagnosis, of cancer; also the basis and management of the psychological and psychiatric reactions associated with surgery or radiotherapy in the breast cancer patient.

Psychological reactions to physical illness tend to follow a pattern (Holland and Ward, 1966). The pattern is an initial denial of illness or of its seriousness ("Oh, it's nothing"), followed by a period of anxiety. Defences against this anxiety may lead to regression ("She's such a baby when she's sick"), dependency on family or therapists, or sometimes a paranoid reaction against either. This may in turn be followed by a depression leading ultimately to the goal of a realistic adaptation to the illness. Many will achieve this but some may remain arrested at any of the stages, depending on their own personality make-up and the attitude they have to cancer as such. This may in turn be affected by their own experience of relatives or acquaintances with a similar diagnosis.

STAGE OF DENIAL

Denial of illness is a major factor in the delay so commonly encountered in seeking treatment for carcinoma of the breast. Henderson (1966) discussed the various reasons for a delay of over three months in 38 of his sample of 50 patients suffering from cancer of the breast, cervix or large bowel. He found the mechanisms of denial to be a prominent factor. Those who delayed tended to be people who had

previous experience of friends or relatives with a fatal cancer, who did not have a confident relationship with their family physician, or who had a previous history of psychiatric treatment. On the other hand, exposure to a "cancer education programme" did not appear to influence whether or not any delay occurred. Cameron and Hinton (1968) found that 20% of their sample of 83 patients with mammary tumours delayed for more than three months. This group tended to express little anxiety, to be less educated and to be unfamiliar with hospitals. A personality assessment showed a tendency to greater introversion in this group.

In a study of a consecutive series of 160 women admitted for breast tumour biopsy and interviewed the day prior to operation, Greer (1974) found that 33% of those subsequently proved to have malignant tumours delayed longer than three months but only 20% of those with benign tumours delayed for as long as this. In both groups the commonest principal reasons for delay appeared to be fear of cancer and fear of disfigurement. Bacon et al. (1952) found that 45% of their sample delayed for more than three months before consulting a doctor. This figure coincides exactly with that in the author's (Lyon, 1976) own series of 100 patients suffering from cancer of the breast, among whom 45% delayed for longer than three months. The mean delay for the total sample between noticing "a lump" and seeing a doctor was over 22 weeks. The reasons given for the delay were varied but correlated closely with the findings of the other authors mentioned.

Though frequently the patient apparently "denies" the illness, especially while pain is absent, the significance of her symptom is suspected but dismissed (Shands et al., 1951). A patient in this situation may seek aid by devious means such as seeing her doctor about something unrelated, "hoping" that he will divine the real cause of her concern. She eventually mentions it to her family or friend and then on their "direction" goes to her doctor immediately. One means of procrastination is to convince herself that she will tell her doctor "when I happen to see him". All these methods were prominent in the author's series. Among those who did *not* delay, however, the value of a cancer education programme was demonstrated; 17% had either practised self-examination or had gone immediately to their doctor because of their contact with such a programme (Lyon, 1976).

Conversely, denial can act as a valuable defence once treatment is undertaken. In the author's series (Lyon, 1976) of 100 patients with cancer of the breast, 21% were considered on several criteria to be showing a strong denial of illness while undergoing radiotherapy. Only one of this group spoke spontaneously of the possibility of cancer, whereas 40% of the total sample did so without prompting from the investigator. The one who did raise the subject said "I do feel sorry for these people, they all seem to have cancer; I'm so lucky that I don't". She had undergone a radical mastectomy and was currently attending for radiotherapy. Clearly to inform such a patient of her diagnosis would break down her defence and leave her very vulnerable. Any hint at the diagnosis would be rejected.

Whether or not patients with cancer should be told their diagnosis has been the subject of several papers. The findings are summarized and discussed by Hinton (1966). In general the population as a whole say that they would wish to know (Kelly and Freisen, 1950) but doctors are reluctant to tell them. Notably, radiotherapists responsible for treatment in the later stages of illness are the least likely to tell (Fitts and Ravdin, 1953). It is clear that there can be no universal answer to this question but that the decision must rest with the doctor and the particular patient. First, there are those showing an obvious strong defence by denial. These are best left alone. Many, given the opportunity, will convey to the physician how much they want to know (Hinton, 1967, 1973) and will arrive at their conclusion in their own way (Shands et al., 1951).

Not infrequently, a tacit conspiracy occurs where the doctor "spares the patient's misery" by not telling, and the patient "spares the staff's discomfort" by not asking, though she is aware of the diagnosis (Glaser and Strauss, 1965). Aitken-Swan and Easson (1959) found that in a series of 231 patients who had been told that they had cancer, 66% approved of being told, 7% disapproved and 19% denied ever having been told. If the patient does not really want to know, she cannot be told.

STAGE OF ANXIETY

A stage of overt anxiety is to be expected on the way to a realistic adaptation to illness. This anxiety is frequently delayed and is therefore not seen by the physician at the time of his interview, but occurs after the patient has left the doctor's office. This acute anxiety is usually short lived but may occasionally persist. Not infrequently, it recurs at "land marks" in the course of the illness, such as surgery, radiotherapy or the obvious presence of secondary deposits.

Psychological defences are likely to be mobilized

to cope with this anxiety. Such defences are often useful and constructive, but sometimes are unsuccessful in dealing with the anxiety, or the defence itself may lead to further problems. Dissociation may occur, when the patient protects herself by splitting into observer and actor; she herself becomes the observer and this may reach the stage of depersonalization. Identification with a patient she has known previously gives her certainty rather than the need to work out the future for herself. Unfortunately, this certainty may be both unpleasant and incorrect (Shands et al., 1951).

Regression frequently occurs as a response to anxiety. This may take the form of return towards infancy and a real dependency upon relatives, even to the stage of requiring bathing and dressing when the physical state does not require this. More often it will be seen as dependency, frequently upon the physician, who is now felt to hold the patient's life in his hands. This is usually directed to one person and is no respector of rank; it may be anyone from the medical student to the head of the clinic. If the former, some embarrassment may result, when only his advice and suggestions for treatment will be accepted.

Unfortunately, dependency is also a position of vulnerability for the patient because she may choose as the target for this dependency a person who leaves the clinic she attends. She may see a different member of the staff on each visit, thus precluding the possibility of any useful dependency. She will also be very sensitive to any change in attitude, which may in reality reflect no more than how busy the physician happens to be at the time. Some times the physician himself finds this dependency too much of a strain and withdraws from the contact and this may be interpreted by the patient as rejection. This in turn provokes anxiety which may appear openly, or may lead to such reactions as deserting the physician in retaliation (so abandoning treatment), or developing the belief that the physician has something against her.

Paranoid reactions may arise by this mechanism and are seen frequently as a means of "apportioning blame" in order to deal psychologically with the patient's awareness of illness. The surgeon performing a mastectomy is a common target for this. Some times it is the patient who blames herself, in which case it presents as a guilt reaction.

In the author's (Lyon, 1976) series of 100 patients undergoing radiotherapy for carcinoma of the breast, 62% had had a mastectomy. Of those who had undergone this surgery, 32% expressed hostility towards the surgeon. In the total sample, 6% held feelings against the radiotherapists and 8% felt that their illness was in retribution for some sin they had committed. This information was volunteered without the investigator seeking such information.

STAGE OF DEPRESSION

Some degree of depression is to be expected at each major event in the course of the illness, including discovery of "a lump", the initial visit to a doctor and the events of surgery or radiotherapy. Fortunately, this is usually of only a few days, duration but longer term reactions are by no means unusual. These will present as a persistent feeling of sadness (with or without weeping), a loss of interest and capacity for enjoyment, and variable insomnia. It is not advisable to treat such a low grade depression with antidepressant medication unless it remains unresolved for a substantial time, as this may prevent the patient from achieving a realistic adaptation.

It is often feared that this stage of depression may result in suicide and this is the reason frequently given for concealing the diagnosis from the patient. There is, however, little published evidence of suicide as a consequence of patients being informed that they have cancer. To many physicians, the fear that greater frankness may do immediately recognizable harm seems to outweigh the more insidious damage of secrecy, isolation and deception (Hinton, 1966). The presence of organic illness does however contribute to suicide (Stewart, 1960), and Sainsbury (1955) in a survey of suicides in London, found the incidence of cancer among suicides to be twenty times that expected in a normal population.

REACTIONS TO SURGERY IN GENERAL

Surgery is inevitably a stress both physiologically and psychiatrically. There are two principal forms of reaction to surgery which may present as psychiatric problems. Surgery may be followed by a "post-operative psychosis", or an acute or sub-acute psycho-organic syndrome may be encountered during the recovery phase.

The psycho-organic syndrome is variously described in the literature as "acute confusional state", "acute brain syndrome", "delirium" and is included by some under the heading of post-operative psychosis". It is certainly a psychosis but requires different treatment from the post-operative psychoses to be described later. The psycho-organic syndrome may occur at any time from immediately

after surgery. The cardinal symptom is clouding of consciousness with a lack of awareness and understanding of the environment. Judgement is impaired, attention and concentration are not maintained and the patient is easily distracted. The interpretation of sensory data is disturbed so that illusions are common and hallucinations (usually visual) may occur.

A failure of recent memory can lead to disorientation in time and place and the patient may confabulate to cover this loss. Emotional lability with irritability and swings from elation to depression occur. There tends to be an intolerance of noise. Increased suspiciousness may lead to delusional ideas though these are usually poorly organized, fleeting and quickly forgotten. The illness progresses to one of delirium, though in the middle aged and elderly it is more likely to resemble a Korsakov's psychosis with marked impairment of recent memory and confabulation.

The psycho-organic syndrome should be distinguished from the post-operative psychosis. There is usually a latent interval before the onset of the psychosis. The peak incidence is ten days after surgery but it may present up to nine weeks later (Stengel et al., 1958). The post-operative psychosis is not a specific entity but the patient may develop any one of the classical psychoses. This may be either pole of the manic-depressive psychosis or schizophrenia, and will present with the appropriate symptomatology. It may be coloured at times by an admixture of the "confusional state", especially of a degree of perplexity. The major differentiating features are the absence of any clouding of consciousness and the marked constancy of the symptoms; for example, should paranoid delusions occur, they will be organized and unchanging.

Stengel et al. (1958) described a series of 80 patients in whom a psychosis following surgery was of sufficient severity to warrant their removal to a psychiatric observation unit. Depression was much the commonest cause, occurring in 36 cases. There were nine instances of the opposite pole of mania and 12 of schizophrenia. He included in this series 21 "confusional states", eight of which were associated with dementia. The incidence of these psychoses was not any greater in cases of mastectomy than of other surgery, but he showed a higher incidence with increasing age.

Surgery in these cases appears to be the stress which acts as a precipitant of psychiatric illness to which the patient was already vulnerable. Thus, it occurs more commonly in those who have previously suffered from a similar psychotic illness or in whom there is a marked family incidence of such illness. History of puerperal psychosis in the past should also alert one to the possibility of a recurrence after surgery.

REACTIONS TO MASTECTOMY

Mastectomy inevitably disturbs the body image. Bressler et al. (1956) suggested that a "breast phantom" occurs in about half the patients following mastectomy. That this is rarely troublesome and very infrequently painful may be because the breast is not integrated into the primitive body image of the female child in the early years of growth. The mammary phantom may be discerned as a percept either of the whole breast or of the nipple. It is episodic, transient and less realistic than that of a limb, and is accentuated by menstruation and changes in the weather.

Failure to achieve a successful psychological adjustment to mastectomy is more likely to occur in those individuals in whom the integrity of the body image prior to illness was over-valued to maintain self-esteem. Renneker and Cutler (1952) found that successfully married women with children, adapted more easily and faster to the loss of the breast than those who were unmarried or whose marriage was unsuccessful. An inappropriate psychological response may occur following surgery at any of the stages of adaptation already described. Thus many surgeons are familiar with the patient who post-operatively denies having been told prior to surgery of the possibility of a mastectomy being performed and paranoid reactions against the surgeon sometimes appear.

A mourning reaction to the loss of the breast may occur and this may present as a depression with withdrawal, lowered self-esteem, anorexia and insomnia. Thoughts of suicide are not infrequent at this stage, often with a feeling of retaliation against the body that has betrayed them ("cutting off one's nose to spite one's face"). This is a primitive reaction which in most cases is fleeting.

"To unsex a woman is surely to maim or affect injuriously the integrity of her nervous system"; this was said in Hack Tuke's ' Dictionary of Psychological Medicine" in 1892. His remarks were made concerning the removal of the uterus and ovaries, but with the socio-cultural attitude held in the western world to the sexual significance of the breast, it must apply equally well. Katz et al (1970) in their study of 30 women awaiting an operation for breast cancer, felt

that the cosmetic issue of the breast loss seemed to be even more effective than the medical issue of the cancer in challenging their psychological defences.

In the author's series (Lyon, 1976), of the 62 patients who had undergone a mastectomy and were currently receiving radiotherapy, 80% expressed some doubt about their femininity; 70% showed a marked preoccupation with their body and its form; 12% said that they were unable to look in a mirror since the operation and were no longer willing to undress in front of their spouse; 8% said they were afraid of sexual intercourse since the operation. This should be distinguished from a loss of libido as such, which may occur as part of a depressive reaction or in response to radiotherapy.

A problem frequently encountered (24%) was the fear that the patient would be rejected by her sexual partner. This tended to be "confirmed" by his failure to make advances. The question had not been openly discussed between them. Encouraging such discussion or seeing both partners together usually showed that the man respected the woman's position and was awaiting some indication from her that the time was ripe. This she had not given for fear of rejection. Discussion resolved every case but one. In this instance, the husband became totally impotent. Enquiry showed that sexually he was very heavily "breast orientated" and his wife had indeed previously been well endowed in this respect. He was unable to adapt to the changed situation. A further 30% of the post-mastectomy patients said that they had passed through similar difficulties after the operation, but that because their partners were "so understanding" or "we were able to talk about it" the problem had already been overcome.

Another hurdle is the fear of rejection by society as a whole, especially by other women, as the patient may feel "no longer a woman". The greatest difficulty for many is their concern about personal appearance, and the adequacy (or otherwise) of a prosthesis. There is much anticipatory worry because of the fear that they will never again be able to wear a bathing costume or a low cut dress, and that their "deformity" and "mutilation" will be obvious to all. Indeed, the sight of another lady so attired may be the trigger for a flow of tears. They may respond by withdrawal from society or may develop hostile feelings against their own sex.

It is in this situation that discussion with a fellow patient who has successfully adapted to problems following mastectomy is so valuable. The patient is not at all likely to bring up such questions in the usual clinical situation. Not surprisingly these problems decrease with increasing age of the patient.

REACTIONS DURING RADIOTHERAPY

Lyon (1976) found that the psychological defences previously mentioned were very much in evidence during radiotherapy. For example, though 79% spontaneously expressed their considerable appreciation for the efforts of the radiotherapy staff, 6% projected blame for their illness onto them.

Perhaps the most striking reaction was the very high level of "faking good", and 21% of the sample appeared to be totally happy and entirely free of problems, both at interview and on several different forms of assessment of depression applied at various times during and after the course of radiotherapy. This group showed a mean lie score on the Eysenck Personality Inventory (Form A) of 6.00. Eysenck and Eysenck (1964) found a mean L score of 4.529 in a group of apprentices in whom the tests had been set up as part of a selection procedure, thus encouraging the "faking good" response. The mean score of a sample of the normal population was 2.263.

The position of the remainder of Lyon's sample is perhaps indicated by their mean lie score on the E.P.I. of 4.51 which is very close to that of the "faking good" apprentices, and similar to the findings of Greer and Morris (1975) who obtained a mean score of 4.42 in patients assessed the day before breast tumour biopsy. This psychological defence appeared to be effective in the majority, though somewhat brittle. There were several examples in which the defence broke down to be followed by a marked depressive reaction. Whether or not a patient had undergone mastectomy did not appear to be a factor in the development of this response.

In the same series an assessment of depression (Beck, 1961) indicated that 11% of the patients in the series suffered from a moderate or severe depression. This may be compared with a figure of 2% showing moderate depression in a sample of women from the general population of comparable age and social class to whom the same test was applied.

All the patients attending for radiotherapy also completed a visual analogue scale (Aitken, 1969) at each attendance. This revealed the variation in mood over the course of radiotherapy and afterwards. There was an initial low mood, possibly related to their uncertainty about what was to come, followed by a slight lift, but then a steady decline until shortly before the end of the course. This decline was more marked in those who had had a mastectomy. This measure also revealed a sudden severe depression lasting only one to five days which occurred in 51% of the patients. It may well have been missed in others who did not happen to attend for treatment

during the critical period which was found to occur anywhere between the fourth and twenty-fourth day of treatment.

The depression is severe. The only patient in the series to attempt suicide did so during such an episode, but 13% of the total sample expressed some thoughts of suicide during the course of radiotherapy. These ideas were most prominent near the beginning of the course. This figure had fallen to 5% when the patients were seen one month after completion of the course. This is a figure which does not differ significantly from the proportion of the control sample who expressed similar ideas.

The measures of personality and depression were applied to a different sample of women who had undergone both mastectomy and radiotherapy more than one year previously. The results did not differ significantly in any respect from those of the control sample. This tends to confirm the work of Craig et al. (1974) who found no evidence of increased psychosocial disability among breast cancer patients 5 years or more after their initial treatment.

LATE PSYCHIATRIC SYMPTOMS

Psychiatric symptoms in the absence of neurological signs may also be evidence of cerebral metastases. At first there may be no more than a subtle change in personality, perhaps some degree of disinhibition in a previously reticent person. In others it may present as irritability, nervousness, a loss of interest and apathy, which may be easily misdiagnosed as a neurotic reaction. It is the change from their previous pattern without apparent reason rather than the severity of the symptoms which provides the clue. In the course of a few weeks or months more obvious symptoms of an organic psychosis are likely to develop with disorientation in time and space, recent memory loss, impaired intellectual function and deterioration in social habits (Mitchell, 1967). Occasionally more specific localising psychiatric syndromes such as the "fatuous jocularity" of the frontal lobe syndrome become evident.

Rarely non-metastatic neuropsychiatric complications may occur. Brain and Henson (1958) include cases occurring in carcinoma of the breast in their discussion of the carcinomatous neuromyopathies. They presented usually with progressive intellectual impairment and memory failure leading ultimately to dementia. The mood was generally euphoric but the syndrome was occasionally preceded by a depression. It was often associated with cerebellar symptoms. Hypercalcaemia, should it occur, is not infrequently associated with psychiatric symptoms though their nature is variable. Apparent neurotic symptoms may appear unexpectedly or a psychosis may develop. Sometimes it presents as an "acute brain syndrome" (Lehrer and Levitt, 1960).

MANAGEMENT OF THE PATIENT

In dealing with the psychoses which may develop post-operatively or late in the disease, the opinion of a psychiatrist is needed and the patient will frequently require to be transferred to a psychiatric unit. In view of the co-existence of both physical and psychiatric problems the two specialties will need to work together. Where the patient is nursed will depend on the seriousness of the psychiatric illness and the degree of surgical or general medical care needed. Certainly a psychotic patient is difficult to nurse in a general ward but with the advice of a psychiatrist it is frequently possible. Conversely many psychiatric units do not have either the equipment or the skills to deal with the surgical aspect of the illness and may well need the support of the referring physician if the patient is transferred. Each case has to be decided on its merits by discussion and co-operation between the specialties.

Prevention is better than treatment in those cases where the processes of psychological adaptation to the illness have gone awry. It should be remembered that the psychoses are rare but a process of adaptation must be gone through by all with varying degrees of success. It is in this field that communication is of the greatest importance (Waxenberg, 1966). This communication is between the doctor and the patient, the staff of the unit and the patient, and between the patient and society, especially those close to her. Prevention begins before operation or any other treatment. Time spent in diminishing anxiety and building a good rapport between patient and doctor at this stage pays great dividends afterwards (Bard and Sutherland, 1955).

The physician must be aware also of his own attitudes and reactions. His view of cancer and the possibility of removing a sexually significant organ in a member of the opposite sex will be coloured by his personal experience, socio-cultural background and medical training. We too have our own reactions to the patient and must protect ourselves against the frustration and resentment produced in us by one who fails to get better despite our treatment, and may offer the ultimate affront by dying (Bronner-Huszar, 1971).

The tendency to brief communication with, and to

look away from, the dying patient on the medical round is well known. It must be remembered that the patient is likely to have a different socio-cultural background to that of the physician, and he must be careful not to project his own attitudes onto her, but to consider the values, reactions and roles imposed upon her by the patient's own background (Bard, 1966). He must also remember the roles, both useful and harmful, into which he may be cast by the patient, varying from the omnipotent healer to the evil creator of her discomfort.

Given the opportunity by a physician aware of the possible problems, the patient will usually give him the cue to open up further discussion. It is often introduced in a "by the way" remark late in the interview. This phrase nearly always heralds an important communication from the patient. Once the problem is in the open, it may be quite easily resolved. Should tears flow, then it is best to let them flow. The "stiff upper lip" can cover unresolved major difficulties.

Often the junior medical, nursing or radiotherapy staff are the ones that are selected in the search for help in these problems. The patient feels that senior doctors would not, or should not, be concerned in these "non-medical" matters, and contact with the nursing or radiotherapy staff may be both more frequent and more informal. This places a considerable responsibility on them. Excessive and unrealistic optimism on the part of the staff may do harm by preventing communication with the patient. It must be remembered that many will formulate their diagnosis correctly for themselves though they may not wish to be told directly. An unrealistic optimism may lead them to believe that they would never be told anything anyway, so any discussion would be useless.

Cosmetic, social and sexual reactions are very common problems but even if these subjects are brought up for discussion the patient may feel that reassurances or advice are shallow and unrealistic because "they haven't gone through this mutilation, how can they possibly know?". This is where the great values of discussion with another person who has reached successful adaptation may be so useful. She can see that a prosthesis may be very successful and can discuss social and perhaps sexual fears with "one who knows" (Lasser and Clarke, 1972).

Though such an approach is of the greatest value in the majority, those putting up a strong defence by denial may resent such an approach and the defence may be broken with harmful results. Care is needed in the selection of suitable people to undertake this work. All "volunteers" should not be taken at face value and the urge to teach others how to behave and to demonstrate their own "success" may be an attempt at mastery over many unresolved problems. Basic dissatisfaction will be only too apparent to the new patient and will result in more harm than good. In selecting which particular lady is to see a given patient it is important to bear in mind age differences and the socio-cultural background.

Though the psychological problems outlined can be disastrous for some and unpleasant for all, it is hopeful to know that most patients will have successfully overcome these difficulties within a year or so, but if we can make that path both easier and more successful, then we must do so.

REFERENCES

Aitken, R. C. B. (1969). A growing edge of management of feeling. *Proceedings of the Royal Society of Medicine 62*, 989.

Aitken-Swan, J. and Easson, E. C. (1959). Reactions of cancer patients on being told their diagnosis. *British Medical Journal 1*, 779.

Bacon, C. L., Renneker, R. and Cutler, M. (1952). A psychosomatic survey of cancer of the breast. *Psychosomatic Medicine 14*, 453.

Bard, M. (1966). Clues to the psychological management of patients with cancer. *Annals of the New York Academy of Science 125*, 995.

Bard, M. and Sutherland, A. M. (1955). Psychological impact of cancer and its treatment. IV Adaptation to radical mastectomy. *Cancer 8*, 656.

Beck, A. T. (1961). An inventory for measuring depression. *Archives of General Psychiatry 4*, 561.

Bronner-Huszar, J. (1971). The psychological aspects of cancer in man. *Psychosomatics 12*, 133.

Brain, R. and Henson, R. A. (1958). Neurological syndromes associated with carcinoma. *Lancet ii*, 971.

Bressler, B., Cohen, S. I. and Magnussen, F. (1956). The problems of phantom breast and phantom pain. *Journal of Nervous and Mental Diseases 123*, 181.

Cameron, A. and Hinton, J. (1968). Delay in seeking treatment for mammary tumours. *Cancer 21*, 1121.

Craig, T. J., Comstock, G. W. and Geiser, P. B. (1974). The quality of survival in breast cancer. *Cancer 33*, 1451.

Eysenck, H. J. and Eysenck, S. B. G. (1964). *Manual of the Eysenck Personality Inventory*, p. 10, University of London Press, London.

Fitts, W. T. and Ravdin, I. S. (1953). What Philadelphia Physicians tell patients with cancer. *Journal of the American Medical Association 153*, 901.

Glaser, B. G. and Strauss, A. L. (1965). *Awareness of Dying*, p. 64, Aldine Publishing Co., Chicago.

Greer, H. S. (1974). Delay in the treatment of breast cancer. *Proceedings of the Royal Society of Medicine 67*, 470.

Greer, H. S. and Morris, T. (1975). Psychological attributes of women who develop breast cancer. *Journal of Psychosomatic Research 19,* 147.

Henderson, J. G. (1966). Denial and regression as factors in the delay of patients with cancer presenting themselves to the Physician. *Annals of the New York Academy of Science 125,* 856.

Hinton, J. (1966). Facing death. *Journal of Psychosomatic Research 10,* 22.

Hinton, J. (1967). *Dying,* p. 132; Pelican Books, Harmondsworth, England.

Hinton, J. (1973). Patients' views in their care during terminal cancer. *Proceedings of the Royal Society of Medicine 66,* 610.

Holland, B. C. and Ward, R. S. (1966). *American Handbook of Psychiatry,* p. 359 Vol. 3, (Ed. S. Arieti). New York: Basic Books.

Katz, J. L., Ackman, P., Rothwax, Y., Sacher, E. J., Weiner, H., Hellman, L. and Gallagher, T. F. (1970). Psychoendocrine aspects of cancer of the breast. *Psychosomatic Medicine 32,* 1.

Kelly, W. D. and Freisen, S. R. (1950). Do cancer patients want to be told? *Surgery 27,* 822.

Lasser, T. and Clarke, W. K. (1972). *Reach to Recovery.* Simon and Schuster, New York.

Lehrer, G. M. and Levitt, M. F. (1960). Neuropsychiatric manifestations of hypercalcaemia. *Journal of the Mount Sinai Hospital 27,* 10.

Lyon, J. S. (1976). In preparation.

Mitchell, W. M. (1967). Etiological factors producing neuropsychiatric syndromes in patients with malignant disease. *International Journal of Neuropsychiatry 3,* 464.

Renneker, R. and Cutler, M. (1952). Psychological problems of adjustment to cancer of the breast. *Journal of the American Medical Association 148,* 833.

Sainsbury, P. (1955). *Suicide in London,* p. 82. Maudsley Monograph, No. 1. Chapman and Hall, London.

Shands, H. C., Finesinger, J. E., Cobb, S. and Abrams, R. D. (1951). Psychological mechanisms in patients with cancer. *Cancer 4,* 1159.

Stengel, E., Zeitlyn, B. B. and Rayner, E. H. (1958). Postoperative psychoses. *Journal of Mental Science 104,* 389.

Stewart, I. (1960). Suicide; the influence of organic disease. *Lancet ii,* 919.

Waxenberg, S. E. (1966). The importance of the communication of Feelings about cancer. *Annals of the New York Academy of Science 125,* 1000.

Index